Multiple Myeloma

METHODS IN MOLECULAR MEDICINE™

John M. Walker, SERIES EDITOR

METHODS IN MOLECULAR MEDICINE™

Multiple Myeloma

Methods and Protocols

Edited by

Ross D. Brown

*Institute of Haematology, Royal Prince Alfred Hospital,
Sydney, Australia*

P. Joy Ho

*Institute of Haematology, Royal Prince Alfred Hospital,
Sydney, Australia*

HUMANA PRESS ✴ TOTOWA, NEW JERSEY

Production Editor: Tracy Catanese
Cover design by Patricia F. Cleary

Cover illustration: Figure 4A,B from Chapter 19, "An In Vitro Osteoclast-Forming Assay to Measure Myeloma Cell-Derived Osteoclast-Activating Factors" by Andrew C. W. Zannettino, Amanda N. Farrugia, L. Bik To, and Gerald J. Atkins.

For additional copies, pricing for bulk purchases, and/or information about other Humana titles, contact Humana at the above address or at any of the following numbers: Tel.: 973-256-1699; Fax: 973-256-8341; E-mail: orders@humanapr.com or visit our website at www.humanapress.com

Printed in the United States of America. 10 9 8 7 6 5 4 3 2 1

e-ISBN: 1-59259-916-8

Library of Congress Cataloging in Publication Data

Multiple myeloma : methods and protocols / edited by Ross D. Brown, P. Joy Ho.
     p. ; cm. -- (Methods in molecular medicine ; 113)
 Includes bibliographical references and index.
 ISBN 1-58829-392-0 (alk. paper)
 1. Multiple myeloma--Molecular aspects--Laboratory manuals.
 [DNLM: 1. Multiple Myeloma--immunology--Laboratory Manuals. 2. Multiple Myeloma--genetics--Laboratory Manuals. WH 25 M961 2005] I. Brown, Ross D. II. Ho, P. Joy. III. Series.
 RC280.B6M855 2005
 616.99'418--dc22

                                                                                           2004019697

Preface

Basic research into the B-cell malignancies has often provided important insights into the pathogenesis of human cancer. Although a range of potentially curative therapeutic options has become available for patients with lymphoma, there is as yet no therapy that could be considered curative for patients with multiple myeloma. During the last decade, an increased focus on research into multiple myeloma has resulted in significant advances in our understanding of the abnormalities in cytogenetics, molecular rearrangements, intra- and intercellular signaling, gene expression, and cell survival pathways. Recent research has gained considerable momentum and there is currently a real prospect of applying these new discoveries to achieve a significant improvement in the response to therapy.

From the classic Plasma Cell Labeling Index methodology, which is used routinely in many laboratories around the world to determine prognosis, through to a final chapter on "Making Sense of Microarrays," *Multiple Myeloma: Methods and Protocols* details with step-by-step instructions a series of classic and proven methodologies which have been, and can continue to be, used in many laboratories for the investigation of this disease. As is usual for volumes in this series, a most helpful feature is the authors' Notes, which appear at the end of each chapter.

Ross Brown
P. Joy Ho

Contents

Contributors

KEWAL ASOSINGH • *Department of Hematology and Immunology, Free University Brussels, Brussels, Belgium*

MONICA ASTOLFI • *Divisione di Ematologia, Universita' di Torino, Torino, Italy*

GERALD J. ATKINS • *Department of Orthopaedics and Trauma, University of Adelaide, Adelaide, Australia*

MARIO BOCCADORO • *Divisione di Ematologia, Universita' di Torino, Torino, Italy*

ROSS D. BROWN • *Institute of Haematology, Royal Prince Alfred Hospital, Sydney, Australia*

LYNDA J. CAMPBELL • *Victorian Cancer Cytogenetics Service, St Vincents Hospital, Melbourne, Australia*

TIM CHAN • *Saskatoon Cancer Centre, University of Saskatchewan, Saskatoon, Canada*

MARA COMPAGNO • *Divisione di Ematologia, Universita' di Torino, Torino, Italy*

PEDRO COUCK • *Department of Clinical Chemistry, Academic Hospital of the Free University Brussels, Brussels, Belgium.*

PETER CROUCHER • *Division of Clinical Services, University of Sheffield Medical School, Sheffield, UK*

ALBERTO ORFAO DE MATOS • *Haematology Department, Hospital Universitario, Salamanca, Spain*

HENDRIK DE RAEVE • *Department of Pathology, University of Antwerp, Antwerp, Belgium*

JOSHUA EPSTEIN • *Myeloma Institute for Research and Therapy, University of Arkansas for Medical Science, Little Rock, AK*

AMANDA N. FARRUGIA • *Myeloma and Mesenchymal Research Laboratory, Institute of Medical and Veterinary Science, Adelaide, Australia*

RAFAEL FONSECA • *Associate Professor of Medicine, Mayo Clinic, Scottsdale, AZ*

OLIVER GALM • *Medizinische Klinik IV, Universitaetsklinikum Aachen, Aachen, Germany*

RAMÓN GARCIA-SANZ • *Haematology Service, University Hospital of Salamanca, Salamanca, Spain*

DAVID GONZÁLEZ • *Department of Haemato-Oncology, Institute of Cancer*

Research, Surrey, UK

FRANS GORUS • Department of Clinical Chemistry, Academic Hospital of the Free University Brussels, Brussels, Belgium

PHILIP R. GREIPP • Hematology, Mayo Clinic, Rochester, NY

SIGUO HAO • Saskatoon Cancer Centre, University of Saskatchewan, Saskatoon, Canada

ANDREW HALL • Northern Institute for Cancer Research, Medical School, Newcastle upon Tyne, UK

JAMES G. HERMAN • The Sidney Kimmel Comprehensive Cancer Centre at Johns Hopkins, Baltimore, MD

P. JOY HO • Institute of Haematology, Royal Prince Alfred Hospital, Sydney, Australia

JULIE IRVING • Northern Institute for Cancer Research, Medical School, Newcastle upon Tyne, UK

DOUGLAS JOSHUA • Institute of Haematology, Royal Prince Alfred Hospital, Sydney, Australia

JITRA KRIANGKUM • Cross Cancer Institute, University of Alberta, Edmonton, Canada

WALTER H. KOCH • Department of Pharmacogenetics, Roche Molecular Systems, Alameda, USA

SHAJI KUMAR • Hematology, Mayo Clinic, Rochester, NY

MARCO LADETTO • Divisione di Ematologia, Universita' di Torino, Torino, Italy

WEI-MIN LIU • Roche Molecular Systems, Alameda, USA

BARBARA MANTOAN • Divisione di Ematologia, Universita' di Torino, Torino, Italy

GEMA MATEO MANZANERA • Haematology Department, Hospital Universitario, Salamanca, Spain

ELIZABETH MATHESON • Northern Institute for Cancer Research, Medical School, Newcastle upon Tyne, UK

MALCOLM A. S. MOORE • Sloan Kettering Cancer Institute, New York, NY

LINDA M. PILARSKI • Cross Cancer Institute, University of Alberta, Edmonton, Canada

JESUS F. SAN MIGUEL IZQUIERDO • Haematology Department, Hospital Universatario, Salamanca, Spain

PULIVARTHI H. RAO • Texas Childrens Cancer Centre, Baylor College of Medicine, Houston, TX

SUNHEE K. RO • Roche Molecular Systems, Alameda, USA

SURINDER S. SAHOTA • Molecular Immunology Group, Tenovus Laboratory, Southampton University Hospitals, Southampton, UK

JEFFREY R. SAWYER • Myeloma Institute for Research and Therapy,

University of Arkansas for Medical Sciences, Little Rock, AK

FREDA K. STEVENSON • *Molecular Immunology Group, Tenovus Laboratory, Southampton University Hospitals, Southampton, UK*

ERIN R. STRACHAN • *Cross Cancer Institute, University of Alberta, Edmonton, Canada*

DANIEL M-Y. SZE • *Institute of Haematology, Royal Prince Alfred Hospital, Sydney, Australia*

BRIAN J. TAYLOR • *Cross Cancer Institute, University of Alberta, Edmonton, Canada*

L. BIK TO • *Myeloma and Mesenchymal Research Laboratory, Institute of Medical and Veterinary Science, Adelaide, Australia*

MARK TOWNSEND • *Molecular Immunology Group, Tenovus Laboratory, Southampton University Hospitals, Southampton, UK*

BEN VAN CAMP • *Department of Hematology and Immunology, Free University Brussels, Brussels, Belgium*

KARIN VANDERKERKEN • *Department of Hematology and Immunology, Free University Brussels, Brussels, Belgium*

SCOTT VANWIER • *Mayo Clinic, Scottsdale, AZ*

MARK VELANGI • *Northern Institute for Cancer Research, Medical School, Newcastle upon Tyne, UK*

ANGELO WILLEMS • *Department of Hematology and Immunology, Free University Brussels, Brussels, Belgium*

JUANITA WIZNIAK • *Cross Cancer Institute, University of Alberta, Edmonton, Canada*

KAI-DA WU • *Cell Biology Program, Sloan-Kettering Cancer Institute, New York, NY*

DAJING XIA • *Saskatoon Cancer Centre, University of Saskatchewan, Saskatoon, Canada*

JIM XIANG • *Saskatoon Cancer Centre, University of Saskatchewan, Saskatoon, Canada*

SHMUEL YACCOBY • *Myeloma Institute for Research and Therapy, University of Arkansas for Medical Science, Little Rock, AK*

EDNA YUEN • *Institute of Haematology, Royal Prince Alfreed Hospital, Sydney, Australia*

ANDREW C. W. ZANNETTINO • *Myeloma and Mesenchymal Research Laboratory, Institute of Medical and Veterinary Science, Adelaide, Australia*

Color Plates

Color plates 1–8 appear in an insert following p. 146.

1

Multiple Myeloma

Challenges and Opportunities

Douglas Joshua, Ross Brown, and P. Joy Ho

Multiple myeloma (MM) is a B-cell neoplasm in which malignant plasma cells accumulate in the bone marrow and produce lytic bone lesions and excessive amounts of a monoclonal protein (usually an immunoglobulin of the IgG or IgA type or free light chain). Approximately 14,000 new cases of MM are diagnosed each year in the United States, and the disease accounts for approx 1.9% of all cancer-related deaths *(1,2)*. Despite significant advances in therapy, the disease remains essentially incurable. The therapy of choice in younger patients is currently high-dose therapy with autologous stem cell transplantation; however, a range of novel therapeutic options have recently become available, creating new opportunities for clinical investigation. The major challenge facing clinicians is to determine which of these new agents or which combination of agents will prove to be the most effective and result in a cure for even a small proportion of patients.

Investigations into the pathogenetic mechanisms in myeloma have resulted in a diverse range of innovations in the treatment of myeloma. An unprecedented variety of new drugs for myeloma are under investigation in either animal models or clinical trials. For example, the antitumor activity of thalidomide has led to the production and trial of a range of thalidomide derivates, such as CC-5013 (Revimid®), that appear to have greater biological activity and fewer adverse effects than thalidomide *(3,4)*. The proteasome inhibitor PS-341 (Velcade®) induces growth arrest and apoptosis of MM cells via inactivation of the nuclear transcription factor nuclear factor-κB (NF-κB) and has been shown to have significant antitumor activity in patients with refractory disease *(3,5)*.

From: *Methods in Molecular Medicine, Vol. 113: Multiple Myeloma: Methods and Protocols*
Edited by: R. D. Brown and P. J. Ho © Humana Press Inc., Totowa, NJ

The recent discovery of the role of the receptor activator of NF-κB ligand (RANKL)/OPG system in bone formation and resorption has suggested that a range of potentially new agents that will inhibit either RANKL or macrophage inflammatory protein-1α (e.g., AMG-162, AMGN-007, and RANK-Fc) could be developed. These agents appear to inhibit not only bone resorption but also tumor growth *(3)*. Another approach has been to target ras mutations, which are relatively common in myeloma. Thus, there is an opportunity to target ras farnesylation with a farnesylation inhibitor *(6)*. Patients with myeloma have defects in the mitochondrial intrinsic pathway resulting from imbalances in the expression of bcl-2 and Mcl-1, the latter a target gene for the antiangiogenic agent Flavoperidol *(3)*. Bcl-2 may be a target for bcl-2 antisense therapy, which can increase the sensitivity of tumor cells to chemotherapy *(3,7)*. A subgroup of patients has been shown to exhibit t(4;14). Preclinical studies have validated FGFR3 as a therapeutic target in patients with t(4;14) myeloma, and plans for a clinical trial are under way *(8)*. Vascular endothelial growth factor receptor (VEGFR) triggers MM cell proliferation via a mitogen-activated protein kinase–dependent pathway and migration via a protein kinase C–dependent pathway; the tyrosine kinase inhibitor GW654652 inhibits all three VEGFRs with similar potency *(9)*.

The existence of these new therapeutic agents can be attributed to recent laboratory investigations that use a range of molecular and cellular methodologies to identify novel targets for therapy. An important aim of this volume is to establish a series of reliable and clearly defined laboratory protocols. The opportunity for real progress in the treatment of myeloma, a disease with no current curative therapy, has resulted in an increased number of basic scientists studying this disease during the last decade and, therefore, it is not surprising that the number of scientific publications per year related to MM has doubled.

The production of a monoclonal immunoglobulin by malignant plasma cells provides a unique molecular signature and an easily identifiable tumor-specific protein, a rarity among human cancers, but a valuable tool for the experimental scientist. This also may prove to be a valuable marker of residual disease if curative therapies become a reality. Cytogenetic abnormalities tend to be complex, and there is no known single molecular lesion responsible for the disease although the adverse prognostic impact of deletions of chromosome 13 is well established *(10,11)*. Whether this chromosome contains a yet to be discovered tumor suppressor gene is the focus of several investigations.

Many patients present with primary translocations resulting from errors in immunoglobulin heavy (IgH) chain switch recombinations. The five most common of these, which account for approx 40% of all patients, involve 11q13 (cyclin D1), 4p16.3 (FGFR3 and MMSET), 6p21 (cyclin D3), 16q23 (c-maf), and 20q11 (mafB). Gene expression microarrays have recently been used to screen for potentially new therapeutic targets in the tumor genome and to reclassify patients into clinically related subtypes according to Ig translocation present and cyclin D expression *(3)*. How to effectively interpret the vast amount of data generated by microarray analysis is a challenge for the basic scientist and the subject of the last chapter of this volume.

The postmicroarray era is providing opportunities to develop strategies to attack these newly identified tumor-specific targets. Classification according to subgroups of genes whose expression is linked to distinct transitions in late-stage B-cell differentiation *(12)* or to the translocation of oncogenes and cyclins has also been made *(13)*. Whether molecular classification of patients with MM can be used not only to predict the likely prognosis but also to identify the most appropriate therapy for subgroups of patients will be a major challenge for the future.

References

1. Greenlee, R. T., Hill-Harmon, M. B., Murray, T., and Thun, M. (2001) Cancer statistics, 2001. *CA Cancer J. Clin. 2001* **51,** 15–36.
2. Ries, L. A. G., Eisner, M. P., and Kosary, C. L. (2002) *SEER Cancer Statistics Review, 1973–1999.* National Cancer Institute, Bethesda, MD.
3. Barillé-Nion, S., Barlogie, B., Bataille, R., et al. (2003) Advances in biology and therapy of multiple myeloma. *Hematology (Am. Soc. Hematol. Educ. Program)* **2003,** 248–278.
4. Richardson, P., Schlossman, R, Weller, E., et al. (2002) Immunomodulatory drug CC-5013 overcomes drug resistance and is well tolerated in patients with relapsed multiple myeloma. *Blood* **100,** 3063–3067.
5. Richardson, P. G., Barlogie, B., Berenson, J., et al. (2003) A phase 2 study of bortezomib in relapsed, refractory myeloma. *N. Engl. J. Med.* **348,** 2609–2617.
6. Santucci, R., Mackley, P. A., Sebti, S., and Alsina, M. (2003) Farnesyltransferase inhibitors and their role in the treatment of multiple myeloma. *Cancer Control* **10,** 384–387.
7. Liu, Q. and Gazitt, Y. (2003) Potentiation of dexamethasone-, paclitaxel-, and Ad-p53-induced apoptosis by Bcl-2 antisense oligodeoxynucleotides in drug-resistant multiple myeloma cells. *Blood* **101,** 4105–4114.
8. Trudel, S., Ely, S., Farooqi, Y., Affer, M., Robbiani, D. F., and Bergsagel, P. (2004) Inhibition of fibroblast growth factor receptor 3 induces differentiation and apoptosis in t(4;14) myeloma. *Blood* **103,** 3521–3528.
9. Podar, K., Catley, L. P., Tai, Y. T., et al. (2004) The pan-inhibitor of VEGF receptors GW654652 blocks growth and migration of multiple myeloma cells in the bone marrow microenvironment. *Blood* **103,** 3474–3479.
10. Facon, T., Avet-Loiseau, H., Guillerm, G., et al. (2001) Chromosome 13 abnormalities identified by FISH analysis and serum beta2-microglobulin produce a powerful myeloma staging system for patients receiving high-dose therapy. *Blood* **97,** 1566–1571.

11. Desikan, R., Barlogie, B., Sawyer, J., et al. (2000) Results of high-dose therapy for 1000 patients with multiple myeloma: durable complete remissions and superior survival in the absence of chromosome 13 abnormalities. *Blood* **95,** 4008–4010.
12. Zhan, F., Tian, E., Bumm, K., Smith, R., Barlogie, B., and Shaughnessy, J., Jr. (2003) Gene expression profiling of human plasma cell differentiation and classification of multiple myeloma based on similarities to distinct stages of late-stage B-cell development. *Blood* **101,** 1128–1140.

2

Immunophenotyping of Plasma Cells in Multiple Myeloma

Gema Mateo Manzanera, Jesús F. San Miguel Izquierdo, and Alberto Orfao de Matos

Summary

Multiparametric immunophenotyping of multiple myeloma (MM) and other plasma cell (PC) dyscrasias represents an attractive approach not only for research purposes but also in clinical practice. Based on well-established antigenic patterns, discrimination between myelomatous and normal PCs can be easily achieved in various types of samples, and this can be particularly valuable for the differential diagnosis between MGUS and MM and for monitoring residual disease in the latter. In addition, immunophenotyping may be an alternative and more reproducible method than morphology for evaluating PC infiltration, as well as for specifically analyzing DNA content and the cell-cycle distribution of different subsets of PCs. Despite the widespread use, standardization of methods and protocols still remains a challenge. In this chapter, we describe in detail the protocols and precise instructions for specimen collection, sample preparation, together with the methods for staining PCs and flow cytometry, data acquisition, and data analysis, including the more recent developments in the field. We highlight the most frequent limitations, and provide troubleshooting and practical recommendations that could help to solve them. The goal of this chapter is to emphasize the relevance of methodological issues in order to obtain reproducible and high-quality results regarding the phenotypic analysis of PCs.

Key Words

Multiple myeloma; plasma cell; flow cytometry; immunophenotyping; antigen.

1. Introduction

During the last decade, immunophenotyping of multiple myeloma (MM) has been frequently debated. The complexity of assaying plasma cells (PCs) is owing, to a large extent, to their low representation in bone marrow aspirates, despite obvious morphological involvement in biopsy specimens. Additional

From: *Methods in Molecular Medicine, Vol. 113: Multiple Myeloma: Methods and Protocols*
Edited by: R. D. Brown and P. J. Ho © Humana Press Inc., Totowa, NJ

difficulties owing to the maturation-related loss of most of the B-lineage-associated markers, together with the intrinsic antigen heterogeneity of PCs *(1–3)*, have made it difficult to specifically characterize this cell population for many years. Moreover, a relatively large number of studies have been reported in which single or double antigen stainings were used, PCs were not specifically identified, and the total number of PCs evaluated was frequently relatively small; this would not allow appropriate assessment of weakly expressed antigens or antigens present in only a small proportion of all PCs. Altogether these and other factors may contribute to explaining some of the overt controversies found in the literature regarding the exact phenotype of myelomatous PCs and its clinical significance.

In recent years, efforts have been made to solve these methodological problems, to standardize the immunophenotyping protocols, and to gain further insight into the phenotype of normal and myelomatous PCs. The value of multi-parameter immunophenotyping by flow cytometry for distinguishing between normal/polyclonal and tumoral/clonal PCs is now well recognized, even when PCs are present in the sample at very low frequencies. Such distinction can be of clinical interest for the differential diagnosis between distinct PC dyscrasias *(4,5)*, for monitoring of residual disease after treatment *(6–8)* and for investigation of the presence of contaminating PCs in peripheral blood-derived products for an autologous transplant *(9,10)*. Consequently, immunophenotyping has progressively been incorporated into routine practice in many clinical laboratories, while also continuing to be a useful technique in basic research in MM. Accordingly, in parallel with the methodological advances, an increasingly large amount of knowledge has accumulated in recent years about the biology of MM, to which immunophenotyping has actively contributed by providing not only technical support but also intrinsically relevant information.

2. Materials

The materials described outline the type of specimens and samples and basic requirements for specimen collection, and the equipment and supplies as well as the reagents necessary to conduct immunophenotypic studies of PCs.

1. Specimens and samples: Specimens from patients with MM containing PCs that are susceptible to being studied by immunophenotypic approaches may include the following (*see* **Notes 1–4**):
    a. Bone marrow.
    b. Peripheral blood.
    c. Liquors or malignant effusions (e.g., ascitic or pleural effusions).
    d. Other solid tissues (e.g., plasmacytomas, tonsilar tissues, lymph nodes).
    e. Immortalized PCs.

2. Multiparameter flow cytometer with 488- and 653-nm double-excitation lasers and filters for the detection of at least green, orange, red, and deep-red fluorescence.
3. Fluorescence-activated cell sorter or magnetic cell-sorting equipment (optional).
4. Computer workstation equipped with calibration, quality control, and appropriate software for data acquisition, transfer, and analysis.
5. Additional computer support (PCs, CDs, ZIP drive).
6. Benchtop centrifuge at 540*g* adapted for 5-mL tubes and/or plates.
7. Refrigerator (at ≈4°C), for storage of reagent.
8. Polystyrene tubes (12 × 75 mm) or 96-well culture plates.
9. Set of precision-adjustable calibrated micropipets capable of dispensing in the range of 5–10 µL and in volumes of 100–1000 µL.
10. Appropriate pipet tips.
11. Vortex mixer.
12. Tube mixer/roller (optional).
13. Monoclonal antibodies (MAbs) directly conjugated to fluorochromes optimized for detection of cell surface and intracellular epitopes resistant to conditions of fixation and permeabilization. Staining reagents may be used as a multicolor cocktail.
14. Filtered (0.40-µm pore filter) phosphate-buffered saline (PBS) with 0.1–0.2% sodium azide and 0.1–2% protein solution (e.g., bovine serum albumin), pH 7.6, as cell wash buffer.
15. Red cell lysing solution (*see* **Note 5**).
16. Fixation and permeabilization solution for staining of intracellular antigens (*see* **Note 6**).
17. Reagents and cells for instrument setup (*see* **Note 7**).

3. Methods

Technical procedures used for the immunophenotypic analysis of human PCs typically may include up to five sequential steps:

1. Preparation of specimen and sample.
2. Staining of cells.
3. Acquisition of data.
4. Analysis of data.
5. Interpretation of the results.

3.1. Preparation of Specimen

The most important requirement of a specimen for multiparameter flow cytometry analysis is that it contain a single cell suspension that allows specific immunophenotypic characterization of individual cells and facilitates interaction of the antibody with the antigen. Since in the bone marrow and other solid tissue specimens cell aggregates exist, adequate mechanical disaggregation procedures should be used. Accordingly, these specimens should be passed several times through a 25-gage needle using a syringe either directly (bone marrow and fine-needle aspirates) or after the tissue has been placed in a Petri dish containing 1 to 2 mL of PBS and cut into small (1-mm^3) pieces (solid tissues); alternatively, semiautomated instruments, which are commercially available (BD Medimachine™, BDB Biosciences), can be used to disaggregate solid tissues mechanically. Just prior to starting staining procedures, a nucleated blood cell count should be performed and the cell concentration adjusted to a final count of 10^7 nucleated cells/mL. For that purpose, and if it is necessary, the sample should be diluted in filtered PBS and gently mixed.

3.2. Staining of Cells and Preparation of Samples

In this section, we discuss (1) the requisites to choose the most appropriate combinations of reagents and (2) techniques used to identify the antigens expressed, either at the cell surface or cytoplasmic/nuclear level, in PCs.

3.2.1. Panels of MAb Reagents

3.2.1.1. COMBINATIONS OF MABS

For the immunophenotypic analysis of PCs, two different groups of MAbs should be combined for simultaneous assessment of their expression. First, MAbs aimed at the specific identification of PCs or their subsets should be chosen from a relatively restricted number of reagents. Second, these should be further combined with a set of one or more reagents selected for characterization of the PCs and/or their subsets of interest. Despite the increasingly large number of antigens known to be expressed by normal and pathological PCs, CD38 and CD138 are the most efficient ones for their specific identification. Both antigens are considered to be highly sensitive and specific for the identification of PCs. However, note that PCs that express low levels of CD138 can be frequently found, and this antigen can also be expressed on nonhematopoietic cells; in turn, CD38 is an antigen widely expressed on both hematopoietic and nonhematopoietic cells that shows uniquely high amounts on normal PCs but that can be expressed at lower levels in myelomatous PCs. Consequently, some researchers (5,11–13) have proposed the combined assessment of both markers for a more efficient identification of PCs. In addition to CD38 and CD138, other surface and cytoplasmic antigens, such as CD13, CD19, CD20, CD28, CD33, CD40, CD52, CD56, CD45, CD86, and CD117, as well as surface and cytoplasmic immunoglobulin (Ig) κ and λ light chains, have been shown to be of variable utility for the specific identification within the PC compartment of normal/polyclonal vs pathological/clonal PCs in patients with monoclonal gammopathies. If enumeration of PCs or their subsets is pursued, the use of CD45 or a DNA dye can be of great help in creating a common denominator of all leukocytes or nucleated cells present in the sample, respectively.

Accordingly, overall consensus exists on the use of the CD38/CD56/CD19/CD45 or CD38/CD56/CD19/CD45/CD138 four- or five-color combinations of MAb reagents for the specific identification and enumeration of normal and pathological PCs from a sample. In addition to these markers, an increasingly large number of surface and intracytoplasmic molecules have been found to be of relevance in MM. According to their functional role, these may be classified as (1) coreceptors for signal transduction that modulate PC response to various stimuli, (2) crucial molecules in the cell-cell and cell-matrix interactions, (3) molecules involved in the differentiation and maturation of PCs, as well as (4) proteins associated with apoptosis and cell survival. **Table 1** summarizes the most relevant molecules that have been described on myelomatous PCs. Many high-quality and validated MAb reagents that specifically bind to unique epitopes of these molecules are currently available *(14)*.

3.2.1.2. FLUOROCHROMES

Primary MAbs can be labeled with different fluorescent molecules or fluorochrome tandems from which fluorescein isothiocyanate (FITC), phycoerythrin (PE), allophycocyanin (APC), PE/cyanin-5 (PE/Cy5), peridin/chlorophyll protein (PerCP)/Cy5, PE/Cy7, APC/Cy7, and PE/Texas red (TR) are the most frequently used. In recent years, new fluorochromes have been incorporated into fluorochrome-conjugated MAbs, including pacific blue and the Alexa® 647 and 488 dyes; such an increase in the number of available fluorochrome conjugates has been pushed by the development of new flow cytometry instruments that allow the simultaneous detection of more than 10 different fluorescent signals. However, note that once conjugated to an MAb, each fluorochrome behaves differently regarding fluorescence intensity, requirements for fluorescence compensation, or fluorescence-resonance energy transfer properties, among others. As a result, fluorochrome conjugates should be carefully selected for each MAb reagent to be included in a multicolor combination. As an example for the four-color combination of MAbs just listed, the following combinations of fluorochrome-conjugated reagents would be recommended: CD38 FITC/CD56 PE/CD19 PerCPCy5 or PE/TR/CD45 APC or PE/Cy5 depending on the characteristics of the flow cytometer. Additionally, differences in the reactivity obtained for different MAb clones and in the quality of the reagents available from different manufacturers might also be observed.

3.2.1.3. CONTROLS

Parallel measurement of a negative control specifically stained for PCs is required, because PCs show variable levels of intrinsic autofluorescence that differ from those of other nucleated cells. Negative controls are necessary to establish a cutoff for positivity based on the levels of natural

Table 1
Summary of Most Relevant Molecules Described in PCs

Molecules involved in differentiation/maturation process of PCs
PCs represent the last stage of B-cell development. Maturation of B-lymphocytes toward PCs is a multistep process in which a coordinated acquisition/loss of surface and intracellular antigens occurs. During malignant transformation of PCs, the expression of these antigens may be altered.

CD19	pan-B-cell marker that functions as a general rheostat for defining signaling thresholds critical for expansion of B-cells. Specific loss in malignant/clonal PCs (~98% of myeloma cases) correlates with altered PAX-5, a gene that encodes for the transcriptional positive regulatory factor BSAP (B-cell-specific activating protein), necessary for CD19 expression.
CD20	B-cell-specific antigen that is expressed from intermediate stages of B-cell maturation in BM and is downregulated in normal PCs. In ~20% of MM patients and up to 50% of "PC leukemia" cases, partial or total expression of CD20 is seen, suggesting the potential utility of CD20-directed serotherapy (Rituximab®).
CD38	A transmembrane glycoprotein with enzymatic activity that is widely expressed on both hematopoietic and nonhematopoietic cells. It has a discontinuous and variable pattern of expression in B-cells with PCs showing uniquely high amounts of CD38. CD38 is downregulated in PCs from ~80% of all myeloma cases. It is one of the most useful markers for the specific identification of PCs.

CD45 (leukocyte common antigen)

Protein tyrosine phosphatase required for activation of lymphocytes and development. Its expression decreases during PC differentiation. In most MM cases, PCs lack CD45 expression. Brighter CD45 expression has been correlated with a higher proliferative capacity and a high degree of immaturity of PCs.

CD52 (CDw52)	Characterized as a human leukocyte differentiation antigen. It is present on the surface of malignant PCs from MGUS and MM patients. It is a potential target for specific immunotherapies (e.g., Alemtuzubab®, Campath-1H) for MM and other hematological disorders.

Cytokine/chemokine receptors
Cytokines are soluble proteins produced and secreted by different hematopoietic cells including PCs (IL-6, IGF-1, TNF-α, VEGF). IL-6 is a key growth and survival factor for PCs (induces PC proliferation and inhibits apoptosis) as well as a major morbidity

Table 1 *(continued)*

---

factor (bone destruction, hypercalcemia, renal failure) in MM. Chemokines are a superfamily of cytokines that play a critical role in selective cell trafficking and homing acting through specific receptors on the cell surface.

- **IL-6 receptor**

    CD126 subunit (IL-6Rα, gp 80)

    > α-chain of the IL-6R that specifically binds IL-6. High levels of soluble IL-6R have been associated with poor prognosis in MM.

    CD130 subunit (IL-6Rβ, gp 130)

    > Common β-chain of the IL-6R that is responsible for signal transduction. IL-6 triggers proliferation via the Ras/Raf/MEK/MAPK cascade and promotes PC survival through phosphorylation of STAT3 and upregulation of antiapoptotic molecules (Mcl-1, Bcl-xL, and bcl-2). IL-6 interaction protects against dexamethasone through PI3K/AKT signaling.

- **SCF receptor**

    CD117 (c-kit ligand)

    > Class III family tyrosine kinase strongly expressed by mast cells, stem cells and myeloid precursors. It is also present in PCs from ≈1/3 of myeloma patients. SCF induces via CD117 an increased in PC proliferation. It is a potential target for novel drugs (Imatinib mesylate, STI571, Gleevec®) for treatment of myeloma.

- **Chemokine SDF-1 receptor**

    CXCR4   A chemokine receptor for SDF-1 that induces chemotaxis of PC toward BM. In addition, it modulates the adhesion activity of VLA-4 (α4β1 integrin).

- **RANTES and MIP-α ligand**

    CCR1   BM in MM produces high levels of RANTES and/or MIP-α. Both chemoattractants bind to the CCR1 receptor on PCs, inducing migration and homing.

Cell adhesion

Adhesion molecules bind to their ligands on BMSCs, or on extracellular matrix proteins and proteoglycans, allowing individual cells to form and stabilize close contacts relevant for the maintenance of a higher order of tissue specialization and facilitate transfer of information. Adhesive interactions play a crucial role in the pathogenesis of the growth and survival of MM.

(continued)

Table 1 *(continued)*

- **Integrin family**

β1-integrins   Ligation of VLA-4 (CD49d/CD29; α4/β1 integrin) via vascular cellular adhesion molecule-1 present on BMSCs upregulates IL-6 secretion by BMSCs, induces proliferation, and blocks apoptosis of myeloma PCs. Altogether, it decreases secretion of osteoprotegerin and increases expression of RANKL, promoting osteolysis.

VLA-5 (CD49e) binds to fibronectin. Expression of CD49e identifies "mature" PCs, whereas negativity for CD49e correlates with more "immature" PCs with a higher proliferation rate and resistance to chemotherapy.

β2-integrins   LFA-1 (CD11a-CD18) interacts with ICAM-1 on BMSCs; expression on myeloma PCs has been correlated with a higher tumor cell growth.

LFA-3 (CD58) mediates adhesion to T-cells via CD2, stimulating them to produce those cytokines necessary for MM growth. CD58 is not expressed by normal PCs but is commonly positive on malignant PCs.

- **Ig superfamily**

CD56 (NCAM)   Typically, CD56 is weakly expressed on normal/polyclonal PCs and strongly positive on the surface of myelomatous/clonal PCs (≈60% of myeloma cases) and stromal cells. PC leukemia usually lacks on CD56, suggesting disease progression. It is a useful marker for follow-up of minimal residual disease.

- **Cell-surface proteoglycans**

CD138 (BB4; syndecan-1)

CD138 is a heparan sulfate proteoglycan that promotes cell-surface adhesion to type I collagen, fibronectin, and thrombospondin. In BM, CD138 is expressed exclusively by PCs. This molecule is rapidly lost in apoptotic cells and shed from the surface of PCs into the serum in advanced phases of the disease (e.g., PC leukemia). It is commonly used for the identification and purification of myeloma PCs from clinical samples.

Other markers of interest

- **Costimulatory molecules**

CD28   CD28, a T-cell-restricted antigen, is also present in both normal and myelomatous PCs from >20% of the cases. The activation

Table 1 *(continued)*

	and function of CD28 in myelomatous PCs are not well known, but its overexpression correlates with disease progression and relapse, suggesting an important contribution of CD28 signaling to myeloma cell survival.
CD40	Normal and malignant PCs retain CD40 antigen at varying levels of expression. CD40 signaling inhibits apoptosis via nuclear factor-kB-mediated pathways, suggesting the possible use of proteasome inhibitors (PS341, Velcade®) and CD40 antagonists for the treatment of myeloma.
CD80 (B7-1) CD86 (B7-2)	CD80 is expressed by antigen-presenting cells (macrophages, activated B-cells, and dendritic cells) whereas CD86 is present on immature unstimulated antigen-presenting cells. On PCs, CD86 is variably expressed and CD80 is almost constantly absent. Studies have reported that a high expression of CD86 on malignant PCs may confer a poor prognosis in myeloma patients.

- **Myelomonocytic-associated antigens**

CD13 CD33	Both antigens are expressed by normal and malignant PCs. Their biological function and clinical significance in a PC that belongs to a different cell lineage remain unclear. CD13 and CD33 are useful markers for follow-up investigations of minimal residual disease in about 15% of all MM patients.

[a]BM = bone marrow; MGUS = monoclonal gammopathy of undetermined significance; IL-6 = interleukin-6; IGF-1 = insulin-like growth factor-1; TNF-α = tumor necrosis factor-α; VEGF = vascular endothelial growth factor; MEK = MAPK/ERK (extracellular signal-regulated)/ kinase; MAPK = mitogen-activated protein kinase; PI3K = phosphatidylinositol 3-kinase; AKT = also known as protein kinase B; SCF = stem cell factor; SDF-1 = stromal cell–derived factor-1; MIP-1α = macrophage inflammatory protein-α; BMSCs = bone marrow stromal cells; NCAM = neural cell adhesion molecule; RANKL = receptor activator of nuclear factor-κB ligand.

autofluorescence and/or nonspecific staining, and they are typically a sample aliquot treated in a way identical to that of the test sample. At present, it is well established that isotype-matched fluorochrome-conjugated mouse Igs are not the most appropriate control for specific fluorescence, especially when a large panel of MAbs of different isotypes is used. Accordingly, most appropriate negative controls include the specific measurement of basal autofluorescence levels of PCs **(Fig. 1A)** together with the confirmation that the expected reactivity is observed for the markers analyzed in the normal cells also present in the sample, including those cellular compartments

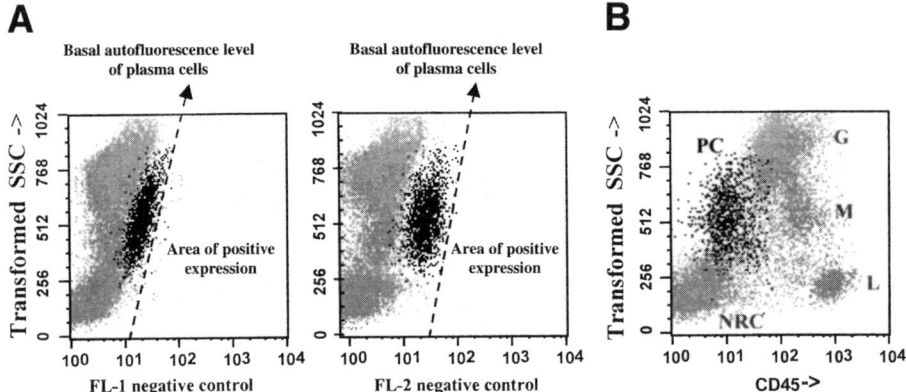

Fig. 1. (A) Level of natural autofluorescence of PCs (in black) and/or nonspecific green (FL-1; left dot plot) and orange (FL-2; middle dot plot) fluorescence. Negative controls are necessary to establish a cutoff for positivity. (B) SSC vs CD45 dot plot showing position of PCs (PC) referred to other normal cell populations present in sample. CD45 expression on PCs could be considered as negative because it is comparable with CD45-negative nucleated red cells (NRC). CD45 expression on positive cells—lymphocytes (L), monocytes (M), and granulocytes (G)—can be used as an internal positive control for this marker.

expressing high amounts of FcIg receptors. The use of a relatively large panel of MAbs also provides adequate positive controls. As an example, CD45 should be strongly expressed on lymphocytes, whereas neutrophils show low positivity for CD45, and nucleated red cells lack reactivity for this antigen (Fig. 1B).

3.2.2. Antigen Staining

3.2.2.1. Previous Considerations

Immunophenotyping staining assays on blood-containing samples (e.g., peripheral blood or bone marrow) are based on three steps: (1) lysing of non-nucleated red cells, (2) staining, and (3) washing with a fixation of nucleated cells. Erythrocyte contamination of leukocyte preparations is particularly vexing for flow cytometry procedures; consequently, samples must be depleted from erythrocytes prior to analysis. As stated in **Note 5**, there are several types of red cell lysing solutions that can be used either prior to or, more frequently, immediately after the staining of whole blood or bone marrow samples with the appropriate panel of MAbs. Usually, it is preferable first to stain and then to lyse and wash because lysing solutions may start to damage cells or even facilitate an increase in intracellular specific or nonspecific staining, especially if they contain fixatives. Depletion of erythrocytes through density gradient centrifugation (e.g., Ficoll-Hypaque) procedures for the purification of mononuclear cells to be used for further staining and analysis of PCs is currently not recommended owing to the high degree of manipulation that the sample is submitted to and the occurrence of an uncontrolled variable degree of cell loss.

3.2.2.2. DIRECT IMMUNOFLUORESCENCE TECHNIQUES

In this section, the exact steps used for the staining of surface antigens alone or in combination with intracytoplasmic markers on PCs are described. Such procedures can be simplified in nonnucleated red cell–free samples (e.g., cell lines, isolated/purified PCs) as pointed out in **Note 8**.

3.2.2.2.1. Protocol I: Staining for Surface Antigens

1. Label the tubes according to the MAb combinations (see the combinations listed in **Subheading 3.2.1.1.**).
2. Add the appropriate amounts of each of the selected MAbs (typically between 0.1 and 1.5 µg of antibody in a volume of 5–10 µL) to a final incubation volume of ≤250 µL.
3. In each of the tubes, place 100 µL of the PBS-diluted bone marrow sample containing 10^6 nucleated cells; gently mix the tubes for 10 s.
4. Incubate for 15 min at room temperature in the dark.
5. Add 2 mL/tube of lysing solution and gently mix.
6. Incubate for 10 min at room temperature in the dark.
7. Centrifuge the nonnucleated red cell-lysed sample for 5 min at 500g.
8. Discard the supernatant with a Pasteur pipet, and resuspend the cell pellet.
9. Add 2 mL/tube of filtered PBS.
10. Centrifuge for 5 min at 500g.
11. Discard the supernatant with a Pasteur pipet, resuspend the cell pellet, and add 0.5 mL/tube of filtered PBS containing 1% paraformaldehyde.
12. Read in a flow cytometer or store at 4°C for a maximum of 24 h. Preferentially, samples should be acquired just after being processed, although they can be stored at 4°C overnight.

3.2.2.2.2. Protocol II: Staining for Surface Ig κ and λ Light Chains (or Ig Heavy Chains) and Other Membrane Antigens

For the surface detection of Ig κ and λ light chains ($_s$κ and $_s$λ) or Ig heavy chains, it is recommended that the soluble Ig molecules potentially present in the sample in high amounts (e.g., peripheral blood and bone marrow) be eliminated. Soluble Igs specifically bind to the anti-Ig MAb reagents, and this decreases the intensity of staining for the Ig present at the surface of PCs toward undetectable levels. Accordingly, the following protocol should be followed:

1. Add 2 mL of filtered PBS to a tube.
2. Place 100 µL of the PBS-diluted bone marrow sample containing 10^6 nucleated cells in that tube, and vortex the sample for a few seconds.
3. Centrifuge for 5 min at 500g.
4. Discard the supernatant with a Pasteur pipet and resuspend the cell pellet; add 2 mL/tube of filtered PBS and gently mix for a few seconds.
5. Centrifuge for 5 min at 500g.
6. Discard the supernatant with a Pasteur pipet and resuspend the cell pellet.
7. Label the tubes according to the MAb combinations containing anti-Ig reagents in combination with other PC markers.
8. Proceed with **steps 2–12** of protocol I (*see* **Subheading 3.2.2.2.1.**).

3.2.2.2.3. Protocol III: Staining for Intracellular and Surface Antigens

When an antigenic target is sequestered or is present inside a cell, in the cytoplasmic or another intracellular compartment, its appropriate staining requires permeabilization of the cellular membranes to allow the antibody to enter the cell structures where the target protein is localized. To avoid extensive cell damage and cell loss, fixation procedures should be applied prior to permeabilization of the cellular membranes. The technique described next combines staining for intracellular antigens with detection of antigens expressed at the cell surface, which is useful for the identification of the target PCs (e.g., double staining with CD38 and CD138 on the cell surface to identify the PC and cytoplasmatic κ and λ Ig light chains to assess clonality).

1. Label the tubes according to the MAb combinations to be applied.
2. Add the appropriate amounts of each of the MAbs directed against the surface antigens.
3. To each tube add 100 µL of sample containing approx 10^6 nucleated cells; gently mix the tubes for a few seconds.
4. Incubate for 15 min at room temperature in the dark.
5. Add 2 mL/tube of filtered PBS.
6. Centrifuge for 5 min at 500g.
7. Discard the supernatant with a Pasteur pipet, and resuspend the cell pellet in a volume of <50 µL.
8. Add 100 µL/tube of a fixative reagent as detailed in **Note 6**; gently mix.
9. Incubate for 15 min at room temperature in the dark.
10. Add 2 mL/tube of filtered PBS.
11. Centrifuge for 5 min at 500g.
12. Discard the supernatant with a Pasteur pipet, and resuspend the cell pellet in a volume of <50 µL.
13. Add 100 µL/tube of a permeabilizing solution (*see* **Note 6**) and the appropriate amounts of those MAbs directed against the intracellular antigens to be detected; gently mix.
14. Incubate for 15 min at room temperature in the dark.

15. Add 2 mL/tube of filtered PBS.
16. Centrifuge for 5 min at 500*g*.
17. Discard the supernatant with a Pasteur pipet and resuspend the cell pellet.
18. Add 0.5 mL/tube of filtered PBS.
19. Read in a flow cytometer or store at 4°C for a maximum of 24 h. Preferentially, samples should be acquired just after being stained, although they can be stored overnight at 4°C.

3.3. Acquisition of Data on PC Phenotypes

Prior to acquisition of the data on the distribution of PCs in the sample and their phenotypes in a flow cytometer, instrument settings should be placed in optimal conditions for measurement.

3.3.1. Instrument Setup

Appropriate instrument settings should be preferentially established according to the protocol proposed by the European Working Group in Clinical Cell Analysis (EWGCCA) *(15)*; alternatively, the instrument setup protocol specifically recommended by the manufacturer may be used, either automatically, or manually if instrument setup software is not available. Typically, a threshold is set in forward scatter (FSC) at a relatively low channel value. A four-decade logarithmic amplification with a minimum 256-channel resolution is required for appropriate detection of immunofluorescence signals in conventional benchtop flow cytometers. Linear amplification of the forward and 90° light scatter amplifiers with the voltage of detectors set to provide the best discrimination between debris/platelets and different populations of nucleated cells is preferentially used. Although in most currently available benchtop flow cytometers, fluorescence compensation is done electronically after the voltages of the photomultiplier tubes have been set and prior to data acquisition, it can also be performed during or after data acquisition by software. In such cases, appropriate uncompensated files containing a set of single-antigen-stained samples with all fluorochromes/fluorochrome tandems used should be acquired with identical instrument settings to those used to measure the test sample *(16)*. Once established, instrument settings may be optimized by running unstained or stained PCs as described in the EWGCCA protocol *(15)*.

3.3.2. Acquisition of Data

All commercially available flow cytometer instruments are equipped with a proprietary software for data acquisition. Two-dimensional dot plots should be generated in which light scatter parameters (FSC and side scatter [SSC]) are correlated between them and with each fluorescence emission. Additional bivariate plots of all possible combinations of fluorescence emission should be created. After appropriately labeling the files to be stored, the data acquisition protocol should be established. Because of the limited capabilities of most software programs regarding the maximum number of events that they may handle for one file and the relatively low frequency of PCs in many samples, in these latter samples, it is recommended that data acquisition be performed in two consecutive steps for each combination of MAbs.

In the first step, fluorescence emissions and light scatter signals from 20 to 30×10^3 nucleated cells corresponding to the whole sample cellularity are acquired and stored in a list mode file without any selection of regions or gates apart from the threshold set in FSC. Acquisition of data on the normal cellular components of the sample together with those of the myelomatous PCs is necessary because it provides ideal internal negative and positive controls and will allow subsequent enumeration of the percentage of myelomatous PCs present in the sample (**Fig. 2**). After storing the first data file, broad electronic regions are set in an FSC vs SSC dot plot (R1 in **Fig. 2**) to exclude cell debris and in a CD38 vs CD138 dot plot (R2 in **Fig. 2**); in R1 all cells present in the sample are included; R1 plus R2 is enriched in PCs and includes all PCs. An alternative region to R1 (R3 in **Fig. 2**) may be drawn on FSC vs SSC to better define the population of PCs, especially when PCs show abnormally low CD38 and CD138 expression.

If information on <10,000 PCs of interest was acquired in the first step, as occurs for studies of minimal residual disease (MRD), a second acquisition step should be performed by activating an electronic live gate (R4 = R2 plus R3), with information specifically stored for the PCs present in a total of up to 10^6 nucleated cells (*see* **Note 9**).

3.4. Analysis of Data

Analysis of flow cytometry data stored in list mode files (FSC format) is performed using dedicated software programs. During analysis of data, the following steps are typically performed for the study of each of the populations of cells of interest: (1) identification, (2) enumeration, and (3) phenotypic characterization of the populations of PCs of interest; information on the intensity and homogeneity/heterogeneity of both antigen expression and light scatter features of each population of PCs in comparison with the pattern of expression observed for the same antigens in the other cells present in the sample should be recorded. If a combination of CD19, CD38, CD56, and CD45 has been employed to stain the sample, the following protocol can be used for data analysis:

1. Use the FSC/SSC dot plot to exclude dead cells and debris.
2. In an SSC/CD38 bivariate dot plot, gate on CD38 strong-positive cells.

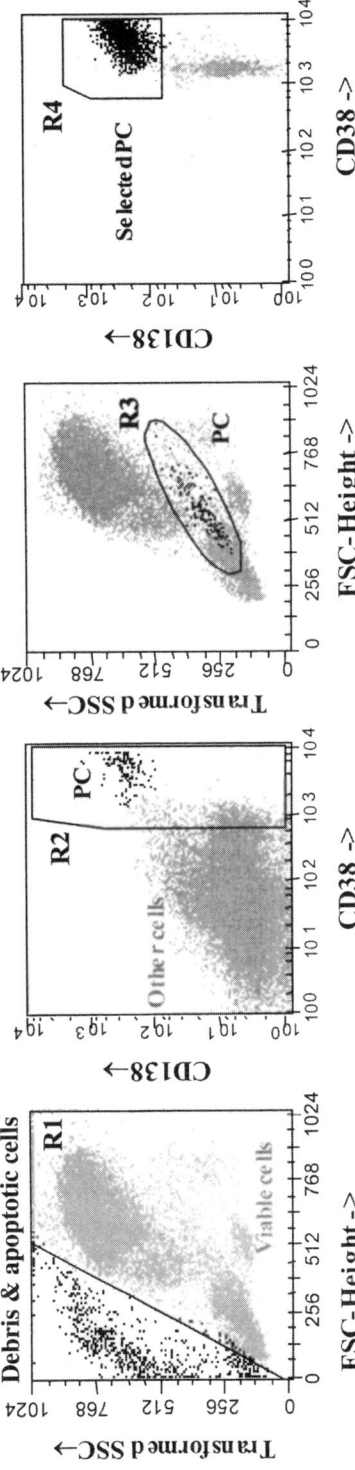

Fig. 2. Representative bivariate dot plots showing appropriate gate regions for correct acquisition of PCs. Based on the light scatter properties, it is possible to exclude debris and apoptotic cells (R1) while including PCs in a well-defined area of size (FSC) and internal complexity (SSC) (R3). The coexpression of CD38 and CD138 is used to specifically identify the PCs and distinguish them from other cells in the same sample (R2); such an analytical strategy can be further used to specifically acquire information on a higher number of PCs in a second-step acquisition through an electronic live gate as shown in the dot plot on the right (R4).

3. Redefine the gated CD38 strong-positive PCs in an FSC/SSC bivariate dot plot as a homogeneous population of cells in SCC with a relatively heterogeneous FSC distribution.
4. Report the percentage of PCs as defined in **step 3**.
5. Report on the mean and coefficient of variation (CV) of PCs for CD38, FL2 (orange), FL3 (red), and FL4 (deep-red) associated-fluorescence emissions.
6. Report on the immunophenotypic characteristics of the CD38 strong-positive PCs:
   a. Define the presence of normal PCs as low SSC/low FSC/CD38^{high} and CD56$^-$ and most expressing CD19 and CD45.
   b. Define the phenotypic characteristics of myelomatous PCs and report on its percentage from the total CD38^{high}CD138$^+$ PCs and both the mean and CV of the fluorescence emissions associated with the CD38, CD19, CD56, and CD45 markers.
7. Report on the percentage of events being the PC population of interest from the total number of events acquired, after excluding those corresponding to debris/platelets.

3.5. Interpretation of Results

Typically in MM, most of the myelomatous PCs accumulate in the bone marrow. In the marrow of patients with MM, normal PCs are either undectable or outnumbered by the myelomatous PC compartment. Compared with normal PCs, myelomatous PCs frequently show decreased expression of CD38, strong expression of CD56, and negativity for both CD19 and CD45 **(Fig. 3)**. In addition, other markers that are negative (CD117, CD20) or only dimly expressed in a small proportion of all normal PCs (CD28 and CD33) might also be strongly expressed by myelomatous PCs in up to 25% of all cases. In other monoclonal gammopathies such as monoclonal gammopathies of undetermined significance (MGUS), clonal PCs predominantly infiltrate the bone marrow as well, and they display a similar phenotype to that of MM; however, these clonal PCs from MGUS coexist in the bone marrow with the normal PCs at frequencies constantly lower than 97% of all PCs *(4)*. In contrast to MGUS and MM, in primary PC leukemias and primary plasmacytomas, pathological PCs infiltrate other tissues with variable levels of bone marrow involvement. Interestingly, in the two latter conditions, PCs more frequently display a CD56$^{(-)}$ and CD45$^{(+)}$ phenotype *(13,17)*. Actually, in other more immature disease conditions in which clonal PCs are also detected (e.g., Waldenström's macroglobulinemia *[18]*), clonal PCs show an aberrant, but clearly different, immunophenotype: CD56$^{(-)}$, CD19$^{(+)}$, CD20$^{(+)}$, CD22$^{(-/+)}$, CD45$^{(+)}$, and sIg$^+$ (typically with κ light chain restriction).

Once clearly identified, further characterization of antigen expression on clonal/myelomatous PCs should be performed. For each antigen analyzed, the following may be of utility: (1) the presence or absence of antigenic expression,

Selected-CD38^{high} plasma cells

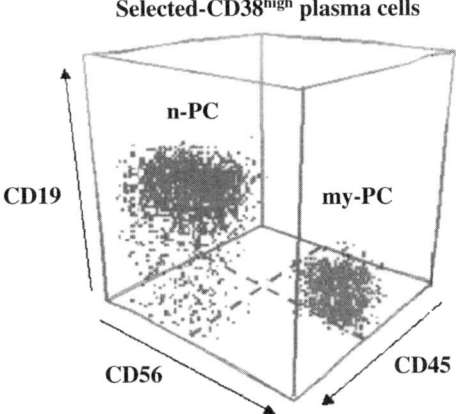

Fig. 3. Representative trivariate dot plot showing antigenic differences between myelomatous PCs (my-PC) and normal PCs (n-PC) among all CD38^{high} cells selected from a bone marrow sample. The combination of the four markers shown—CD19, CD45, CD56, and CD38—for selective gating of PCs represents the best combination of markers for a clear distinction between my-PC and n-PC in most patients with monoclonal gammopathies.

(2) the median amount of antigen expressed per cell within a given population of PCs as expressed by the median fluorescence intensity or other equivalent standardized units (molecules equivalent of soluble fluorochrome [MESF]; antibody binding capacity [ABC]), and (3) the pattern of antigen expression (homogeneous vs heterogeneous) as expressed by the CV for the reactivity observed for a particular antigen specifically on the population of PCs under analysis.

4. Notes

1. Bone marrow is the specimen most frequently used for immunophenotypic studies in myeloma because it usually contains the highest proportion of clonal PCs. However, there are specific clinical situations in which the investigation of other specimens, such as peripheral blood infiltrated with malignant PCs in advanced phases of the disease (in the so-called plasma cell leukemia) as well as solid tissues (e.g., plasmacytomas) or malignant effusions involved in extramedullarly disease, are required. From all these different types of biological specimens, cells of interest can be directly studied in a sample aliquot or submitted to subsequent procedures to be further used with the patient's informed consent in basic research or in routine clinical practice. Among others these may include the following:
   a. Isolation/purification of PCs: Highly enriched PC fractions are typically obtained using magnetic activated cell sorting (MACS) procedures after specifically labeling PCs with PC-specific antibodies (e.g., CD138) coupled to

magnetic particles of different sizes; or single-cell-based fluorescence activated cell sorting (FACS), which currently allows simultaneous isolation of up to four different populations of PCs that might coexist in a sample. An increasingly high number of alternative cell-sorting procedures are currently available and have been reviewed in detail elsewhere *(19)*.

b. Immortalization: The generation of cell lines derived from human myelomatous PCs through different procedures, including Epstein-Barr virus infection, can be done. These procedures have been detailed elsewhere *(20)*.

2. Specimen collection procedures: Bone marrow and peripheral blood specimens are obtained by conventional aspiration or venipuncture procedures, respectively; once obtained, they should be placed in a sterile tube containing a sufficient amount of anticoagulant. Ideally, 1 to 2 mL is required for immunophenotyping, but it depends on the assay to be performed. Pleural effusions or ascitic fluid are obtained by conventional thoracic and abdominal puncture procedures. Cellular specimens derived from solid tissues may be collected by either fine-needle aspiration or surgical procedures; once obtained, these specimens should be immediately placed in a sterile isotonic saline solution.

3. Anticoagulant used in collection: EDTA is the preferred anticoagulant for immunophenotypic studies for all types of specimens because it preserves cell morphology and phenotype the best. However, in cases in which the specimen will also be used for additional functional studies (e.g., in vitro cell culture experiments), sodium heparin can be alternatively employed.

4. Storage conditions and specimen integrity: Freshly obtained peripheral blood, bone marrow, and other body fluid specimens should be preferentially stored at stable room temperature (18–22°C) for no longer than 24 h. Longer storage periods should be avoided in order to prevent significant changes in the surface expression of specific antigens and/or selective loss of cells (e.g., under inadequate conditions PCs may lose CD138 expression and rapidly enter apoptosis) *(21,22)*. However, if required, storage for longer periods should be performed at lower temperatures ($\approx$2–8°C). In the case of samples aged longer than recommended or any specimens showing evidence of freezing, hemolysis, or clotting, cell viability should be assessed prior to phenotypic studies. The criteria for rejection of sample based on suboptimal conditions that may preclude successful analysis may vary, depending on the specific goals of the immunophenotypic studies. Stabilizing agents and solutions such as TransFix™ and Cytocheck (Cytochecks Laboratory) might allow prolonged storage of samples, but at present they have not been specifically and extensively tested for the preservation of PCs.

5. Red cell lysing solutions that contain a fixative or one fixative free can be used. The most frequently used solutions including those commercially available include 1X ammonium chloride, Optilyse and Versalyse (both from Immunotech, Marseille, France), FACSLysing (Becton/Dickinson, San José, CA), Quicklysis (Cytognos, Salamanca, Spain), Whole Blood Lysing Solution (Caltag, San Francisco, CA), and Uti-Lyse™ (DAKOCytomation, Glostrup, Denmark).

6. The following commercially available reagent kits containing both permeabilization and fixation reagents can be applied as reference reagents: Fix & Perm (Caltag), Intraprep (Immunotech), Intrastain (DAKOCytomation).
7. For instrument setup follow the protocol proposed by EWGCCA guidelines *(15)*.
8. In the case of samples corresponding to single cell suspensions that do not contain nonnucleated red cells, the lysing steps can be detected from protocols I (**steps 5–8**) and II (**steps 5–8** of protocol I in **step 8** of protocol II).
9. In any case, for their phenotypic characterization, a minimum of 10^3 PCs should be acquired using a single- or double-step acquisition. For studies of MRD, at least 100 events corresponding to pathological PCs should be collected to allow their unequivocal identification and accurate enumeration (CV of <10%).

Acknowledgment

This work was supported in part by a grant from the Instituto de Salud Carlos III for the "Spanish Myeloma Network" (G03-136).

References

1. Harada, H., Kawano, M. M., Huang, N., et al. (1993) Phenotypic difference of normal plasma cells from mature myeloma cells. *Blood* **81,** 2658–2663.
2. Terstappen, L. W. (1990) Identification and characterization of plasma cells in normal human bone marrow by high-resolution flow cytometry. *Blood* **76,** 1739–1747.
3. San Miguel, J. F. (1991) Immunophenotypic heterogeneity of multiple myeloma: influence on the biology and clinical course of the disease. Castellano-Leones (Spain) Cooperative Group for the Study of Monoclonal Gammopathies. *Br. J. Haematol.* **77,** 185–190.
4. Ocqueteau, M., Orfao, A., Almeida, J., et al. (1998) Immunophenotypic characterization of plasma cells from monoclonal gammopathy of undetermined significance patients: implications for the differential diagnosis between MGUS and multiple myeloma. *Am. J. Pathol.* **152,** 1655–1665.
5. Almeida, J., Orfao, A., Mateo, G., et al. (1999) Immunophenotypic and DNA content characteristics of plasma cells in multiple myeloma and monoclonal gammopathy of undetermined significance. *Pathol. Biol. (Paris)* **47,** 119–127.
6. Rawstron, A. C., Davies, F. E., DasGupta, R., et al. (2002) Flow cytometric disease monitoring in multiple myeloma: the relationship between normal and neoplastic plasma cells predicts outcome after transplantation. *Blood* **100,** 3095–3100.
7. San Miguel, J. F., Almcida, J., Mateo, G., et al. (2002) Immunophenotypic evaluation of the plasma cell compartment in multiple myeloma: a tool for comparing the efficacy of different treatment strategies and predicting outcome. *Blood* **99,** 1853–1856.
8. Almeida, J., Orfao, A., Ocqueteau, M., et al. (1999) High-sensitive immunophenotyping and DNA ploidy studies for the investigation of minimal residual disease in multiple myeloma. *Br. J. Haematol.* **107,** 121–131.

9. Pope, B., Brown, R., Gibson, J., and Joshua, D. (1997) Plasma cells in peripheral blood stem cell harvests from patients with multiple myeloma are predominantly polyclonal. *Bone Marrow Transplant.* **20**, 205–210.

10. Mateo, G., Corral, M., Almeida, J., et al. (2003) Immunophenotypic analysis of peripheral blood stem cell harvests from patients with multiple myeloma. *Haematologica* **88**, 1013–1021.

11. Rawstron, A. C., Barrans, S. L., Blythe, D., et al. (2001) In multiple myeloma, only a single stage of neoplastic plasma cell differentiation can be identified by VLA-5 and CD45 expression. *Br. J. Haematol.* **113**, 794–802.

12. Jego, G., Robillard, N., Puthier, D., et al. (1999) Reactive plasmacytoses are expansions of plasmablasts retaining the capacity to differentiate into plasma cells. *Blood* **94**, 701–712.

13. Garcia-Sanz, R., Orfao, A., Gonzalez, M., et al. (1999) Primary plasma cell leukemia: clinical, immunophenotypic, DNA ploidy, and cytogenetic characteristics. *Blood* **93**, 1032–1037.

14. Mason, D., Andre, P., Bensussan, A., et al. (2002) CD antigens 2002. *Blood* **99**, 3877–3880.

15. Papa, S. (2002) European Working Group on Clinical Cell Analysis (EWGCCA): 6 years on. *J. Biol. Regul. Homeost. Agents* **16**, 253–256.

16. Kraan, J., Gratama, J. W., Keeney, M., and D'Hautcourt, J. L. (2003) Setting up and calibration of a flow cytometer for multicolor immunophenotyping. *J. Biol. Regul. Homeost. Agents* **17**, 223–233.

17. Dahl, I. M., Rasmussen, T., Kauric, G., and Husebekk, A. (2002) Differential expression of CD56 and CD44 in the evolution of extramedullary myeloma. *Br. J. Haematol.* **116**, 273–277.

18. San Miguel, J. F., Vidriales, M. B., Ocio, E., et al. (2003) Immunophenotypic analysis of Waldenstrom's macroglobulinemia. *Semin. Oncol.* **30**, 187–195.

19. Radbruch, A. (2000) *Flow Cytometry and Cell Sorting*, Springer Verlag, New York.

20. Drexler, H. G. and Matsuo, Y. (2000) Malignant hematopoietic cell lines: in vitro models for the study of multiple myeloma and plasma cell leukemia. *Leuka. Res.* **24**, 681–703.

21. Jourdan, M., Ferlin, M., Legouffe, E., et al. (1998) The myeloma cell antigen syndecan-1 is lost by apoptotic myeloma cells. *Br. J. Haematol.* **100**, 637–646.

22. Bharti, A. C., Shishodia, S., Reuben, J. M., et al. (2003) Nuclear factor-κB and STAT3 are constitutively active in CD138+ cells derived from multiple myeloma patients, and their suppression leads to apoptosis. *Blood* **103**, 3175–3184.

3

Plasma Cell Labeling Index

Philip R. Greipp and Shaji Kumar

Summary

Multiple myeloma is characterized by proliferation of monoclonal plasma cells (PCs), mostly in the bone marrow. The proliferative rate of the malignant plasma cell is an important determinant of the disease biology and can be measured as the percentage of PCs in the S-phase of the cell cycle. This percentage, or PC labeling index, can be measured using a slide-based immunofluorescence method using an antibody against 5-bromo-2′-deoxyuridine, which is actively incorporated by DNA of the dividing PCs. This technique, which can be performed using bone marrow or peripheral blood specimens, also utilizes concurrent cytoplasmic staining against immunoglobulin as well as κ and λ light chains. Employment of cytoplasmic immunoglobulin staining allows more specific identification of PCs as well as confirmation of the monoclonal nature of the PC population. The staining procedure, which can be done manually or using an automated stainer, as well as the process of reading and interpreting these slides is described in detail. The bone marrow peripheral blood labeling index is an important clinical test, providing valuable diagnostic and prognostic information.

Key Words

Multiple myeloma; plasma cell; cell proliferation; bromodeoxyuridine; cell cycle; immunofluorescence microscopy; cell kinetics; labeling index.

1. Introduction

Multiple myeloma (MM) is characterized by proliferation of monoclonal plasma cells (PCs) in the bone marrow. Circulating PCs and B-lymphocytes belonging to the malignant clone can also be detected in the peripheral blood in a proportion of patients, depending on the stage of the disease (*1*). In addition to their characteristic morphology, PCs are characterized by the presence of cytoplasmic immunoglobulin, which can be detected by using antibody to κ or λ Ig light chains. As with most of the malignancies, the proliferative rate, or the percentage of malignant cells, in S-phase is an important prognostic factor

From: *Methods in Molecular Medicine, Vol. 113: Multiple Myeloma: Methods and Protocols*
Edited by: R. D. Brown and P. J. Ho © Humana Press Inc., Totowa, NJ

in myeloma. Various methods can be used to identify or "label" cells that are actively undergoing mitosis, thus allowing determination of the percentage of dividing cells, or labeling index (LI). Initial methods of determining labeling index in myeloma utilized the incorporation of radioactive thymidine by replicating DNA in order to label cells *(2,3)*. The percentage of labeled cells was then determined by autoradiography. PCs in the S-phase of the cell cycle actively incorporate 5-bromo-2'-deoxyuridine (BrdU). The development of antibodies against bromodeoxyuridine (BrdU) using hybridoma technology allowed the development of a slide-based immunofluorescence method for identifying dividing PCs that will be labeled with the BrdU *(2)*. Further refinement of this method using anti-BrdU antibodies with intrinsic DNase activity resulted in a more sensitive and specific method of determining labeling index, which is currently in use and is detailed in this chapter *(4)*. The DNase activity allows detection of incorporated BrdU without the necessity of using acid or alkali DNA denaturation, a process that often alters the Ig reactivity and PC morphology. In addition to avoiding the use of radioactivity, the current immunofluorescence method allows morphological confirmation of PC identity of the labeled cell, thus improving specificity over the autoradiographic method. The method provides a reliable way of identifying Ig-positive PCs that are in S-phase, enabling accurate determination of the LI. Additionally, by using concurrent staining of the cytoplasmic immunoglobulin for the κ or λ light chain, the percentage of κ and λ PCs can be determined. A κ/λ ratio of >4 or <0.5 confirms the monoclonal nature of the plasmacytosis.

The uses of the bone marrow plasma cell labeling index (PCLI) test in the diagnosis and management of MM are manyfold *(1,5–7)*. First, the test provides valuable information regarding the disease stage at diagnosis. It allows discrimination of patients with stable disease not requiring treatment including monoclonal gammopathy of undetermined significance (MGUS) and smoldering myeloma from patients with active myeloma requiring treatment for their disease *(3,8)*. Second, it provides valuable prognostic information in these patients. Patients with smoldering myeloma who have a high LI are at a high risk of progressing to active myeloma in the short term. In patients with active MM, a high LI at diagnosis portends a shorter overall survival and, conversely, a low LI is a good prognostic sign *(9,10)*. This allows the combination of LI with other prognostic factors such as β_2-microgobulin to identify high-risk patients. Third, it reflects disease activity following therapy for the disease. Patients in the plateau phase of the disease have a bone marrow LI of <0.2% compared with patients with relapsed disease, for which the LI is usually >1%. PCLI also has utility in other PC disorders such as primary systemic amyloidosis, for which LI is usually very low. A high LI in this disorder also has prognostic value in terms of survival *(1,5,11–14)*. Additional important information can be obtained from this test. For example, detection of small numbers of monoclonal PCs is important in patients with myeloma and other PC disorders in whom no monoclonal protein is identified in the serum or urine. Furthermore, the slide-based method allows identification of plasmablasts. Identification of the subset of patients with plasmablastic morphology (>2% plasmablasts) is important because these patients have a very poor prognosis. Finally, it allows a reliable estimation of the degree of bone marrow infiltration with PCs.

In addition to determining the LI of PCs from the bone marrow of patients with myeloma, the same technique can be extended to identify PCs circulating in the peripheral blood and their LI. The immunofluorescence method when used on peripheral blood provides several pieces of crucial information. It enables detection of circulating PCs as well as confirmation of their clonal nature and the LI of these PCs. The presence of circulating clonal PCs as well as a high LI of these cells has been correlated with a poorer prognosis in patients with MGUS, smoldering myeloma, active multiple myeloma, and primary amyloidosis.

2. Materials

2.1. Reagents

1. 1X Phosphate-buffered saline (PBS) without azide: Adjust pH to 7.6 ± 0.2; store at room temperature for up to 3 mo.
2. PBS-Tween: PBS with 0.05% Tween-80; store at room temperature for up to 3 mo.
3. S-0 Medium: 500 mL of RPMI-1640 with 5 mL of L-glutamine and 5 mL of penicillin/streptomycin; store at 4°C for 1 mo.
4. S-10 Medium: 90 mL of S-0 medium, 10 mL of newborn calf serum; store at 4°C for 2 wk.
5. S-1 Tween: 1 mL of S-10 + 9 mL of PBS/Tween. Make fresh each time.
6. Ficoll-Paque™ Plus (Amersham Pharmacia Biotech): Store at room temperature for up to 1 yr.
7. Absolute ethanol: *Caution: flammable.* Keep away from heat, sparks, and open flame. It may cause an explosive mixture with air.
8. Immersion oil (Zeiss 000000-1111-806).
9. *N*-Propyl gallate (mounting fluid): 0.95 g of *N*-propyl gallate in 4 mL of 1% PBS without azide and 34 mL of glycerol. Mix at low heat, and adjust the pH to 8.0 ± 0.2 with 6 *N* NAOH; store at room temperature for up to 2 mo.
10. BU-1 antibody: This is a monoclonal antibody directed against BrdUrd obtained from the culture fluid of the BU-1 hybridoma. It is available with DNase commercially from Amersham. Each vial contains 5 mL of concentrated antibody

(1X) that has been lyophilized. The lyophilized preparation should be dissolved in S-0 medium. For each new lot of antibody, the optimal dilution for staining must be determined by staining slides made from the same sample. The ideal dilution will give bright-staining BU-1-positive nuclei with little background staining. Working dilutions usually range from 1:1 to 1:3 of the 1X solution made from the lyophilized product (*see* **Note 1**). Store lyophilized reagent at –20°C and the rehydrated reagent at 4°C; the expiration is 2 wk.

11. Newborn calf serum; store 500 mL at –70°C. Thaw and aliquot into 10-mL tubes. Store the aliquots at –20°C. Frozen aliquots are stable indefinitely.

12. Goat antihuman, fluorescein isothiocyanate (FITC) conjugated (Biosource): Each vial contains 1 mL of antibody. Make a stock 1:5 dilution with S-10 medium. Store 1-mL aliquots of this stock dilution at –20°C for up to 1 yr. Thawed antibody can be kept for 1 mo.

13. Goat antimouse, IgG rhodamine conjugate (Chemicon): Make a stock solution per the manufacturer's recommendations. Use a 1:25 dilution of the stock for the test. Refrigerate at 4°C for up to 2 mo.

14. Goat antihuman κ, FITC conjugate (Biosource): Each new lot of antibody should be titered for optimal staining using known κ-positive bone marrow sides to give the brightest FITC staining with the least background as well as the least amount of crossreactivity with λ-positive PCs. If crossreactivity is too bright, repeat using a lesser dilution (*see* **Note 2**). Store frozen (–20°C) at the selected dilution in 2-mL Nunc vials (2 mL/vial).

15. Goat antihuman λ, FITC conjugate (Biosource): Each new lot of antibody should be titered for optimal staining using known λ-positive bone marrow sides to give the brightest FITC staining with the least background as well as the least amount of crossreactivity with κ-positive PCs. If crossreactivity is too bright, repeat using a lesser dilution (*see* **Note 3**). Store frozen (–20°C) at the selected dilution in 2-mL Nunc vials (2 mL/vial).

16. Preservative-free heparin (Sigma, St. Louis, MO): Powder form comes with 100,000 U/vial. Dilute the powder form with 10 mL of distilled water/vial to a final dilution of 10,000 U/mL. Store at –20°C for up to 1 yr.

17. 1 M Thymidine (Sigma): Dilute in 1% PBS without azide, pH 7.4 ± 0.1; store 1X at 4°C.

18. 6 N NaOH: Dissolve 24 g of NaOH in 100 mL of distilled water. *Caution: Caustic substance.* Precautions are necessary while handling. Store at room temperature for up to 6 mo.

19. Concentrated HCL: *Caution: corrosive.* Avoid contact with skin. Wear gloves and a protective eye shield.

2.2. Instruments

1. Olympus (Provis A × 70) or equivalent fluorescent microscope (100 W) equipped with filters (green) for detection of FITC (red), for detection of rhodamine, and mixed for detection of dual staining. The microscope should have capabilities for regular light microscope work.

2. AcT 10—(Coulter counter or equivalent).

3. Methods

3.1. Preparation of Pulsing (Collection) Tube

1. Weigh out approx 1 mg of BrdU (mol wt = 307.11) and 0.6 mg of 5-fluoro 2′-deoxyuridine (FdU) (mol wt = 246.2) in two separate glass tubes (12 × 75 mm).
2. Divide actual milligrams of BrdU by 3.07, and add that many milliliters of 1X PBS to give a 10 mM solution. Place the tubes at 37°C in a water bath for approx 5 min to dissolve the BrdU.
3. Divide actual milligrams of FdU by 2.46, and add that many milliliters of 1X PBS to give a 10 mM solution. Make a 1:10 dilution of this FdU solution.
4. In a conical flask, mix together 7.8 mL of 1X PBS, 0.1 mL each of the BrdU solution and the 1:10 FdU solution, and 2 mL of preservative-free heparin.
5. Add 0.125 mL of this final solution to 20 × 125 mm culture tubes with screw caps, and place the tubes (uncapped but covered) in a –20°C freezer for approx 4 h.
6. Transfer the tubes with the frozen solution to a lyophilizer on wire racks and let dry overnight. Remove and cap the tubes the next day. The tubes can be stored in the dark for 1 yr when kept desiccated.

3.2. Collection, Transport, and Processing of Sample

1. Draw 1 to 2 mL of bone marrow aspirate, place it in the pulsing tube, and mix gently.
2. Transport the tube to the laboratory at 37°C (the sample can be maintained at this temperature using a thermos bottle containing a thermal bag), and incubate for 1 h at 37°C (from the time of sample collection).
3. At the end of the 1-h incubation, use 1X thymidine solution to stop the reaction in the pulsing tube (if processing is delayed until the following day). Use 0.3 mL for bone marrow and 0.5 mL for peripheral blood.
4. Add 6 mL of PBS to the bone marrow and mix well. Place 4 mL of Ficoll in a 15-mL conical centrifuge tube. Carefully layer the diluted marrow (7 to 8 mL) over the Ficoll without any mixing. Cap the tube tightly and centrifuge for 20–30 min at 1500 rpm (approx 400g).
5. Aspirate the supernatant to within 0.5 in. of the mononuclear cell layer and discard. Transfer the mononuclear cell layer with a disposable transfer pipet to a new 15-mL conical centrifuge tube, filtering the sample using a piece of 40-µ mesh as it is transferred. If the mononuclear layer appears grossly contaminated with red cells, repeating the Ficoll separation procedure may be useful. Dispose of the Ficoll tube and filter.
6. Fill the tube with PBS to the 14-mL mark, cap, and invert to mix. Centrifuge for 5 min at 1500 rpm (400g) and aspirate the supernatant.
7. Add 1 mL of S-10 to the cell button and mix gently with a disposable transfer pipet. Perform a cell count on the final sample, and add 0.7–1.0 × 10^6 cells to 1 mL of S-10 in a 12 × 75 Sarstedt tube.
8. Make six cytospin slides per patient, using approx 100 µL of the final dilution for each slide. Centrifuge on a table top instrument for 4 min at 200 rpm or an

appropriate speed for cytospin. Remove the slides, being careful not to disrupt the cell spot, and place the slides in a rack to dry.

9. Fix the slides for 5 min with 200-proof alcohol in a Coplin jar and dry in a slide rack.

3.3. Staining (see Notes 4–6)

1. Select three slides for each patient; mark one each for κ light chain, λ light chain, and polyclonal. Use supercured slides when it is known in advance that manual staining will be necessary. Extra slides can be wrapped in foil and stored in a –20°C freezer (or long term at –70°C).
2. Soak in PBS-Tween for at least 10 min. Dry the slides and place them on a moist paper towel.
3. Add 100 μL of BU-1 antibody to each slide. Incubate for 30–40 min at room temperature. Rinse individual slides with a squirt bottle of PBS-Tween. Place in a rinse jar of PBS-Tween for 10 min.
4. Remove the slides and dry in a slide rack.
5. Label three tubes as follows: G/M (goat antimouse rhodamine conjugated), G/H (goat antihuman FITC conjugated: κ), and G/H (goat antihuman FITC conjugated: λ). Prepare the second set of antibodies as follows.
   a. G/M dilution (tube 1): Multiply the total number of slides (polyclonal, κ, and λ) by 50 to obtain the volume of S-10 medium required (μL). Divide this by 25 (dilution factor) to obtain the volume of G/M (μL) required. Mix well together.
   b. κ dilution (tube 2): Multiply the number of κ slides by 50 to obtain the G/M (μL) dilution or microliters of κ antibody required.
   c. λ dilution (tube 3): Multiply the number of κ slides by 50 to obtain the G/M (μL) dilution or microliters of κ antibody required.
   d. G/H dilution: Use this dilution on the polyclonal slides. Multiply the number of polyclonal slides by 50 to obtain the volume of S-10 medium required (μL) (add this to the remainder of the G/M dilution). Divide this by 7.5 (dilution factor) to obtain the volume of G/H (μL) required. Mix well together.
6. Place the dried slides on a moist paper towel again. Add 100 μL of freshly prepared antibody dilutions to the appropriate slides. Incubate for 30–40 min.
7. Rinse individual slides with PBS-Tween using a squirt bottle, place all the slides in PBS-Tween, and soak for 10 min. Remove and dry on a slide rack.

3.4. Immunofluorescence Microscopy (see Note 7)

1. Organize slide trays with each patient's three slides (poly, κ, and λ) together.
2. Place a small drop of *n*-propyl gallate on each cell spot and cover slip. Press down gently with a tissue.
3. Add a drop of immersion oil onto each cover slip, and read the slides under a fluorescent microscope.
4. Count a total of 500 mononuclear cells on each slide. The cytoplasm of PCs will stain green (FITC) if positive. PCs are identified by the cytoplasmic immunoglob-

Table 1
Interpretation of LI Results

LI results (%)	Interpretation
0.0–0.2	Very low
>0.2–0.99	Intermediate
1.0–3.0	High
>3.0	Very high

ulin staining (FITC-green) and their characteristic morphology. The PCs on each slide are quantitated as a percentage of mononuclear cells (no. of PCs/mononuclear cells × 100).

5. Determine the κ-to-λ ratio (κ/λ) as a ratio of PC percentages from the κ and λ slides. At least 20 PCs must be counted to determine clonality. $\kappa/\lambda \geq 4$ is a clonal excess of κ; $\kappa/\lambda \leq 0.5$ is a clonal excess of λ.

6. To determine the LI, count a total of 500 PCs (on the clonal slide, if applicable). Count the positive BU-1-stained nucleus (this will be red; rhodamine positive) (no. of red nucleus labeled cells/500 PCs × 100). They will be in the range of 0.0–3.0% or greater. At least 100 PCs must be counted to report an LI. If 100 cells are not seen on the clonal slide, count the polyclonal slide.

3.5. Test Interpretation (see Notes 8–12)

The presence of monoclonal PCs is determined based on the ratio of κ and λ PCs as described in **Subheading 3.4., step 5**. The LI is categorized as in **Table 1**.

Bone marrow with <10% PCs and a PCLI of 0.0–0.8% is consistent with MGUS, smoldering MM, or MM in plateau phase and good-prognosis MM. Bone marrow plasmacytosis of >10% and LI ≥1% suggests active myeloma. Patients with an LI of <0.8% and 10–30% PCs may have smoldering myeloma, and those with a similar LI and >30% PCs usually have good-prognosis myeloma. The results of PCLI should be used in conjunction with the results of other tests and clinical features in making clinical decisions.

4. Notes

1. Regarding BU-1 antibody dilutions, rehydrate a lyophilized vial with 5 mL of S-0. This is the original volume before lyophilization (1X). Prepare the following dilutions from the 5-mL original volume (1X):
   a. 1:1 = 1 mL (1X) run as a straight dilution.
   b. 1:2.6 = 1 mL (1X) plus 1.3 mL of S-0.
   c. 1:2 = 1 mL (1X) plus 1 mL of S-0.
   d. 1:3 = 1 mL (1X) plus 2 mL of S-0.

Further dilutions can be made as necessary. Stain manually using the same patient slides to determine the degree of labeling. Use 100 µL/slide. Read the slides using a fluorescent microscope. With the optimal dilution, slides should have bright-staining BU-1-positive nuclei with little background staining.

2. The standard dilution for goat antihuman κ, FITC conjugated is 1:25. Each new lot of the antibody should be tested for the optimal dilutions. To check for optimal cytoplasmic staining, do additional dilutions of 1:10 and 1:50. After preparing these dilutions, stain a set of slides from the same sample from a known κ patient as described in **Subheading 3.3.** Use S-10 instead of G/M dilution, and use 100 µL of final dilution/slide. In addition, run one slide on a known λ patient at the 1:25 dilution, to examine for crossreactivity. Read the slides with a fluorescence microscope as described. At optimal dilution, the slides should stain for both weakly and strongly staining Ig-positive PCs, with little background staining.

3. The standard dilution for goat antihuman λ, FITC conjugated is 1:50. Each new lot of the antibody should be tested for the optimal dilutions. To check for optimal cytoplasmic staining, do additional dilutions of 1:75 and 1:100. After preparing these dilutions, stain a set of slides from the same sample from a known λ patient as described in **Subheading 3.3.** Use S-10 instead of G/M dilution, and use 100 µL of final dilution per slide. In addition, run one slide on a known κ patient at the 1:50 dilution, to examine for crossreactivity. Read the slides with a fluorescence microscope as described. At optimal dilution, the slides should stain for both weakly and strongly staining Ig-positive PCs, with little background staining.

4. When processed in large numbers in the clinical setting, an automated stainer such as the Tech Mate 500 from Ventana Systems can be used. Staining procedures should follow the manufacturer's instructions and are not detailed here. Optimal antibody dilutions should be determined using the automatic stainer.

5. Scan each slide for homodeoxyuridine (BrdU) uptake and proper rhodamine staining. It is important to study the immunofluorescence slide prior to counting the PCLI to be sure that there are BrdU-positive cells. Every properly prepared marrow will contain some BrdU-positive cells. Positive cells will include morphologically identifiable erythroid and myeloid elements. Positively stained cells act as internal controls and should be positively identified on each preparation before starting the PCLI count. If BrdU-positive cells are not identified anywhere on the preparation, one cannot ensure the adequacy of the BrdU labeling of the PCs.

6. Additionally, controls can be used to ensure adequacy of the methods. Pulse cells from a cell line such as Daudi with BrdU. Prepare appropriate cell dilution and slides using the same methods. These control slides can be prepared in sufficient numbers and stored at –70°C for up to 1 yr. One control slide can be included with the daily run to ensure consistency.

7. At our institution, the slides are read by a technologist skilled in the methods of determining PCLI and verified by a trained hematologist. The slides are examined to ensure the adequacy of BrdU labeling; accurate identification of PCs; accurate determination of the percentage and monoclonality of the PCs and the PCLI; and

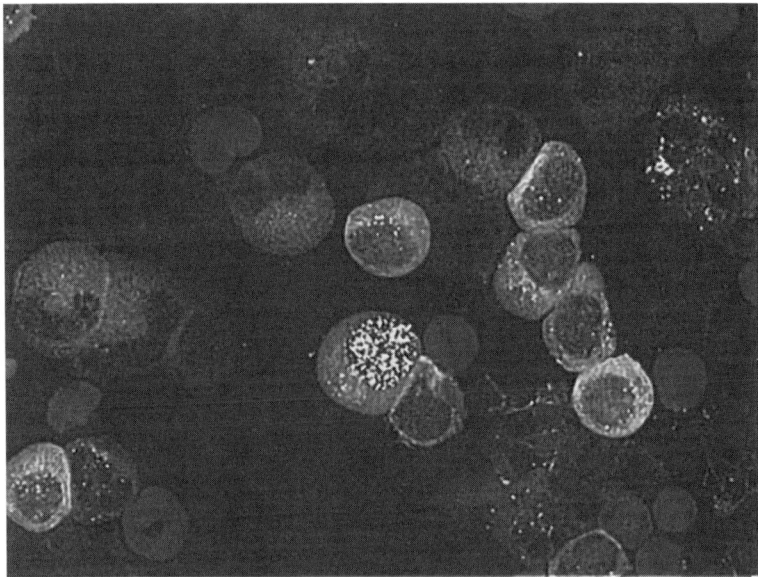

Fig. 1. Note the brightly labeled nucleus and the eccentric placement of the nucleus in the labeled PC. Also seen are nonlabeled PCs with similar morphology.

identification of the plasmablastic morphology, if present. The concordance for high and low values on separate assays on the same sample is >90% in our laboratory.

8. It is important to identify accurately the PCs and distinguish them from other cells that may be positive for cytoplasmic Ig. Other Ig-positive cells include lymphocytes, other lymphoid cells, monocytoid cells, and macrophages. Occasionally, megakaryocytes also stain positive for Ig. PCs classically have bright cytoplasmic Ig stain, an eccentrically placed nucleus, and often a well-defined cytoplasmic hof **(Fig. 1)**. Lymphocytes and lymphoid cells have only a thin rim of Ig stain and are rarely confused with PCs, except in patients with lymphocytoid myeloma or Waldenström macroglobulinemia. Monocytoid cells and macrophages are distinguished from PCs by their indented nuclei, and they have more brightly granular cytoplasm than the accompanying PCs. Monocytoid cells often can have a high LI of 20–30%. They are rarely observed, but if labeled monocytoid cells are inappropriately included in the PCLI, they can spuriously elevate the result. It is good practice to study carefully the morphology of the monoclonal PC population in each immunofluorescence preparation before starting the PCLI count, to avoid including any Ig-staining cells that cannot be certainly identified as PCs.

9. Scattered rhodamine staining can often be seen in the immunofluorescence slide and may overlay the cell, giving the appearance of a labeled nucleus. In a truly labeled nucleus, the bright orange dots of rhodamine-stained nuclear material are confined within the nuclear boundary.

10. The pH of the solutions can significantly affect the results. The pH of the medium used for BrdU antibodies should be 7.5 ± 0.2 for optimal binding and that of the mounting medium (*n*-propyl gallate) should be 8.5 ± 0.2 for optimal fluorescence.
11. The fluorescent light source should be replaced regularly for optimal fluorescence. Bulbs should generally be replaced after every 400–500 h of use, but this may vary.
12. The results of κ λ analysis should be compared with that of the immuno-electrophoresis to confirm the type of light chain.

References

1. Witzig, T. E., Gonchoroff, N. J., Katzmann, J. A., Therneau, T. M., Kyle, R. A., and Greipp, P. R. (1988) Peripheral blood B cell labeling indices are a measure of disease activity in patients with monoclonal gammopathies. *J. Clin. Oncol.* **6,** 1041–1046.
2. Greipp, P. R., Witzig, T. E., and Gonchoroff, N. J. (1985) Immunofluorescent plasma cell labeling indices (LI) using a monoclonal antibody (BU-1). *Am. J. Hematol.* **20,** 289–292.
3. Greipp, P. R. and Kyle, R. A. (1983) Clinical, morphological, and cell kinetic differences among multiple myeloma, monoclonal gammopathy of undetermined significance, and smoldering multiple myeloma. *Blood* **62,** 166–171.
4. Gonchoroff, N. J., Katzmann, J. A., Currie, R. M., et al. (1986) S-phase detection with an antibody to bromodeoxyuridine: role of DNase pretreatment. *J. Immunol. Methods* **93,** 97–101.
5. Witzig, T. E., Dhodapkar, M. V., Kyle, R. A., and Greipp, P. R. (1993) Quantitation of circulating peripheral blood plasma cells and their relationship to disease activity in patients with multiple myeloma. *Cancer* **72,** 108–113.
6. Greipp, P. R., Witzig, T. E., Gonchoroff, N. J., et al. (1987) Immunofluorescence labeling indices in myeloma and related monoclonal gammopathies. *Mayo Clin. Proc.* **62,** 969–977.
7. Witzig, T. E., Gonchoroff, N. J., Ahmann, G. A., Katzmann, J. A., and Greipp, P. R. (1991) T cell depletion using anti-CD2 coated magnetic beads simplifies the detection of peripheral blood plasma cells. *J. Immunol. Methods* **144,** 253–256.
8. Durie, B. G., Salmon, S. E., and Moon, T. E. (1980) Pretreatment tumor mass, cell kinetics, and prognosis in multiple myeloma. *Blood* **55,** 364–372.
9. Greipp, P. R., Katzmann, J. A., O'Fallon, W. M., and Kyle, R. A. (1988) Value of beta 2-microglobulin level and plasma cell labeling indices as prognostic factors in patients with newly diagnosed myeloma. *Blood* **72,** 219–223.
10. Greipp, P. R., Lust, J. A., O'Fallon, W. M., Katzmann, J. A., Witzig, T. E., and Kyle, R. A. (1993) Plasma cell labeling index and beta 2-microglobulin predict survival independent of thymidine kinase and C-reactive protein in multiple myeloma. *Blood* **81,** 3382–3387.
11. Pettersson, D., Mellstedt, H., and Holm, G. (1980) Monoclonal B lymphocytes in multiple myeloma. *Scand. J. Immunol.* **12,** 375–382.

12. Witzig, T. E., Kimlinger, T. K., Ahmann, G. J., Katzmann, J. A., and Greipp, P. R. (1996) Detection of myeloma cells in the peripheral blood by flow cytometry. *Cytometry* **26,** 113–120.
13. Billadeau, D., Greipp, P., Ahmann, G., Witzig, T., and Van Ness, B. (1995) Detection of B-cells clonally related to the tumor population in multiple myeloma and MGUS. *Curr. Top. Microbiol. Immunol.* **194,** 9–16.
14. Berenson, J., Wong, R., Kim, K., Brown, N., and Lichtenstein, A. (1987) Evidence for peripheral blood B lymphocyte but not T lymphocyte involvement in multiple myeloma. *Blood* **70,** 1550–1553.

4

Conventional Cytogenetics in Myeloma

Lynda J. Campbell

Summary

Chromosome analysis has become an important diagnostic tool in the assessment of patients with multiple myeloma. Conventional cytogenetic analysis of myeloma cells is complicated by the difficulty in inducing myeloma cells to divide. A method for the culture and harvest of bone marrow samples from patients with myeloma is presented together with a protocol for producing G-banded metaphases for microscopic analysis. It is recommended that two or more cultures be established from each sample. There is extensive literature describing the use of various cocktails of mitogens to assist in obtaining dividing myeloma cells with little consensus as to the optimal method. A protocol is given for stimulating cells to divide using interleukin-4, the method in routine use in the Victorian Cancer Cytogenetics Service.

Key Words

Cytogenetics; multiple myeloma; chromosome abnormalities; tissue culture; interleukin-4.

1. Introduction

Since the first cytogenetic abnormality was detected in chronic myeloid leukemia in 1960, studies of chromosomes have been used to understand the genetic basis of tumorigenesis. In early studies of multiple myeloma (MM), bone marrow cells were cultured under the same conditions as used for leukemias, and abnormal karyotypes were obtained in a minority of cases, mostly in patients with advanced, refractory disease. However, these studies were able to identify some of the common abnormalities seen in MM; for example, hyperdiploidy with chromosome counts of 53–55 and t(11;14) (q13;q32) were described in an early article (1). A prospective study of 82 patients in which bone marrow cells were harvested directly or after short-term culture in mitogen-free medium demonstrated an abnormal clone in 27%, but it was evident that this method of harvest enabled the karyotypes of only the

From: *Methods in Molecular Medicine, Vol. 113: Multiple Myeloma: Methods and Protocols*
Edited by: R. D. Brown and P. J. Ho © Humana Press Inc., Totowa, NJ

most aggressive and rapidly dividing myeloma cells to be identified *(2)*. Furthermore, many of these patients were subsequently found to have therapy-related myelodysplastic syndromes or acute leukemia, accounting for their chromosomal abnormalities.

Subsequent investigators attempted to improve the culture conditions to allow the karyotype of myeloma cells with a lower proliferative capacity to be studied. A number of different cytokines and culture times have been tried, with cultures extending from 1 to 7 d and stimulated with various combinations of granulocyte macrophage colony-stimulating factor (GM-CSF), interleukin-2 (IL-2), IL-3, IL-4, IL-6, and/or tumor necrosis factor-α *(3–7)*. Despite the multitude of methods, there is still little consensus regarding the optimal technique. The failure to identify an abnormal karyotype in more than 50% of myeloma cases has led to the development of strategies to circumvent this problem, particularly the use of fluorescent *in situ* hybridization (FISH), which is discussed elsewhere in this volume.

Despite the problems associated with obtaining an abnormal karyotype in MM, many investigators have established the clinical significance of partial or complete loss of the long arm of chromosome 13 [del(13q) or monosomy 13] *(8–11)*. There has been considerable debate as to whether del(13q) detected by FISH alone is an independent prognostic indicator, but all series confirm the prognostic impact of del(13q) as detected by conventional cytogenetics. Other abnormalities have also been correlated with prognosis. For instance, hypodiploidy, although often seen in association with loss of chromosome 13, has been shown to be an independent poor prognostic indicator *(12,13)*. The 11;14 translocation that is characteristic of mantle cell lymphoma and has been observed in approx 16% of multiple myelomas *(14)* has been noted recently to correlate with small mature plasma cell morphology *(15)*. Chromosome analysis has become an important diagnostic tool in the initial assessment of patients with myeloma.

Conventional cytogenetic analysis relies on inducing cells in culture to divide. The cells are then harvested so that metaphase spreads of chromosomes are available for analysis via microscopy. After a period of time in culture at 37°C, the first step of harvesting is the addition of Colcemid™, a synthetic colchicine analog, which arrests cell division at metaphase, when the chromosomes are at their most condensed and, therefore, most easily visualized. It acts by preventing the formation of spindle fibers, which would normally allow movement of the chromatids to opposite poles of the cell before cell division. The cells are then treated with a hypotonic salt solution (KCl), which causes lysis of the unwanted red blood cells and swelling of the nucleated cells, so that the chromosomes separate and untwine from each other. Finally, the cells are permanently fixed using Carnoy's solution, a mixture of methanol and glacial acetic acid. After changes of fixative, the cell suspension is ready to be dropped onto clean glass slides. The slides are air-dried, aged, and G (Giemsa)-banded; a microscopic analysis is performed; and chromosome karyotypes are assembled. The resulting karyotype is described according to ISCN 1995 nomenclature *(16)*.

The reluctance of myeloma cells to divide in culture has resulted in the microscopic analysis of nonmyeloma cell metaphases in the majority of instances, thus leading to a normal karyotype being obtained. Identifying a cytogenetic abnormality in the myeloma cells is dependent on a number of factors.

The percentage of plasma cells (PCs) in the bone marrow aspirate is critical. In my and my colleagues' experience, the presence of 30% or more PCs will increase the likelihood of finding a cytogenetic abnormality significantly. Of the last 200 cases of myeloma analyzed in our laboratory, a cytogenetic abnormality was observed in 91 (45.5%), excluding those patients with loss of the Y chromosome as a sole abnormality. The median percentage of PCs in cases with an abnormal karyotype was 48% compared with a median of 25% for the cases from which a normal karyotype was obtained.

As already detailed, many different combinations of mitogens and growth factors have been used in an attempt to increase the number of myeloma cells dividing in culture, but there appears to be no clear advantage for any particular cocktail of mitogens. There is, however, evidence that the more cultures established from a sample, the higher the likelihood of finding a cytogenetic abnormality in that sample *(5)*. In my laboratory, we set up a minimum of two cultures: a 24-h unstimulated culture and a 72-h culture stimulated with IL-4 *(7)*. If there is sufficient sample, we establish a third culture, an unstimulated 72-h culture. Whereas many researchers advocate a 5-d culture, we have found that the cell growth falls off after 3 d, perhaps owing to exhaustion of the medium's nutritional supply. Many advocate the addition of IL-6, but this has not been shown to improve the abnormality rate compared with unstimulated cultures *(4–7)*.

After cells are harvested, slides are made and a G-banding technique is applied to produce the distinctive pattern of dark and light bands that enables individual chromosomes to be identified. Chromosomal proteins appear to contribute to the production of the G-banding pattern, the trypsin preferentially attacking the chromosomal histones in the adenine-thymine (AT)-rich band regions, leading to an enhanced accessibility of the AT-rich regions for dye molecules compared with the guanine-cytosine-rich regions. A considerable number of protocols capable of inducing G-banding have been developed *(17)*.

The methods presented herein are those in routine use in the Victorian Cancer Cytogenetics Service for culturing and harvesting bone marrow samples from patients with MM to produce chromosome spreads for cytogenetic analysis.

2. Materials

The materials listed have been divided into separate sections according to the stage at which they are required in the preparation of cytogenetic suspension from bone marrow samples.

2.1. Bone Marrow Culture

1. Bone marrow aspirate: Collect 0.5–1.0 mL in a sterile syringe or tube containing approx 100 U of preservative-free heparin.
2. RPMI-1640 medium with L-glutamine and HEPES: Store the powdered form at 4°C. Prepare the medium by dissolving the powder in distilled H_2O with 2 g of sodium bicarbonate, adjust the pH to 7.2–7.3 using 1 N HCl or 1 N NaOH, and sterilize by filtration. Aseptically decant the medium into sterile bottles and store at 4°C for 1 to 2 wk. The medium should not be used if it becomes opaque, changes color, or acquires floating particles.
3. Fetal calf (bovine) serum (FCS): Store at –20°C in aliquots (i.e., 20-mL aliquots for addition to 200-mL bottles of medium to produce a 10% solution). This should be thawed and added to medium immediately before use.
4. L-Glutamine-penicillin-streptomycin (PSG): a mixture containing 200 mM L-glutamine, 10,000 U of penicillin, and 10 mg of streptomycin/mL. Store at –20°C, and add 1 mL to a 200-mL bottle of medium immediately prior to use.
5. IL-4: 1 μg/mL solution stored at –20°C in 50-μL aliquots.
6. Sterile vented 50-mL tissue culture flasks.
7. Sterile pipets.

2.2. Harvest

1. Colcemid®: 10 μg/mL solution.
2. Hypotonic solution (0.075 mol/L of KCl): a 5.59 g/L solution of KCl (mol wt = 74.55).
3. Carnoy's solution: 3:1 (v/v) methanol/glacial acetic acid, made fresh just before use.
4. Plastic, nonsterile screw-top centrifuge tubes (15 mL).
5. Microscope glass slides: 76 × 26 mm superfrost slides with ground edges.

2.3. Banding

1. Trypsin: desiccated tryptic enzyme rehydrated in 10 mL of sterile distilled H_2O and aliquots stored at –20°C. Make a fresh working solution daily by adding 0.25 mL of trypsin solution to 35 mL of trypsin diluent (*see* **item 2**) and 35 mL of distilled H_2O in a Coplin jar.
2. Trypsin diluent: Dissolve NaCl (8.0 g), KCl (0.4 g), Na_2HPO_4 (0.06 g), KH_2PO_4 (0.06 g), and $NaHCO_3$ (0.5 g) in 1 L of distilled H_2O and store at 4°C prior to use.
3. Ca^{2+}/Mg^{2+}-free solution: Dissolve NaCl (8.0 g), KCl (0.2 g), Na_2HPO_4 (1.15 g), and KH_2PO_4 (0.2 g) in 1 L of distilled H_2O and store at 4°C prior to use.

4. Leishman's solution (eosin methylene blue compound) (*see* **Note 1**): Store in powdered form at room temperature. Add Leishman's stain powder (2.8 g) to 1 L of analytical-grade methanol and mix with a magnetic stirrer for 3 h. Incubate the resulting solution at 37°C for at least 1 wk. To prepare a working solution, filter 100 mL through Whatman No. 1 filter paper. Store the rest in the dark at room temperature until required. Then dilute the filtered Leishman's stain 1 in 10 in Giemsa buffer (*see* **item 5**) immediately prior to use.
5. Giemsa buffer: Dissolve one Gurr® buffer tablet (pH 6.8) in 1 L of distilled H_2O and store at 4°C prior to use.
6. DPX mounting solution: Store at room temperature.
7. Glass cover slips (24 × 50 mm).

3. Methods

The following methods outline (1) the establishment of three separate cultures of bone marrow cells from patients with MM and the harvesting of cells from each culture after varying periods of incubation, and (2) slide making and the production of banded metaphase spreads for microscopic analysis.

3.1. Culture and Harvest Methods

3.1.1. Culture 1: Overnight Unstimulated Culture

1. Place 10 mL of RPMI-1640 medium supplemented with PSG and 10% FCS into a sterile vented 50-mL tissue culture flask.
2. Using a sterile pipet, inoculate the medium with an appropriate amount of bone marrow (*see* **Note 2**).
3. Lie the flask flat and incubate at 37°C in 5% CO_2 for approx 24 h.
4. Add 0.2 mL of 10 μg/mL Colcemid to the culture and incubate at 37°C for a further 30 min.
5. Transfer the culture to a harvesting tube and centrifuge for 10 min at approx 1000 rpm (200g) in a sealed bucket centrifuge.
6. Discard the supernatant.
7. Resuspend the cell pellet in 8 mL of KCl and place in a 37°C water bath for 20 min.
8. Centrifuge for 8–10 min at 1000 rpm (200g).
9. Discard the supernatant.
10. Resuspend in 5 mL of fresh fixative (3 : 1 methanol : glacial acetic acid) by adding the fix drop by drop initially with thorough mixing to avoid cell clumping (*see* **Note 3**).
11. Refrigerate the cell suspension at 4°C for 15 min.
12. Repeat **steps 8–10** at least once. Replace the fixative until the suspension appears clear without any trace of a brown tinge. Finally, spin the suspension and dilute if necessary with fixative to produce a slightly cloudy appearance. Store the cell suspension at –20°C until slide making (*see* **Subheading 3.2.**).

3.1.2. Culture 2: 72-h IL-4-Stimulated Culture

1. Place 10 mL of RPMI-1640 medium supplemented with PSG and 20% FCS into a sterile vented 50-mL tissue culture flask labeled as a 3-d stimulated culture. Record the date of harvest on worksheets.
2. To this culture, add 50 µL of 1 µg/mL IL-4 (*see* **Note 4**).
3. Using a sterile pipet, inoculate the medium with an appropriate amount of bone marrow (*see* **Note 2**).
4. Lie the flask flat and incubate at 37°C in 5% CO_2 for approx 72 h.
5. Add 0.2 mL (200 µL) of 10 µg/mL Colcemid to the culture and incubate at 37°C for a further 60 min.
6. Undertake all further steps in harvesting as per **steps 5–12** in the overnight culture method described in **Subheading 3.1.1.**

3.1.3. Culture 3: 72-h Unstimulated Culture

1. Place 10 mL of RPMI-1640 medium supplemented with PSG and 20% FCS into a sterile vented 50-mL tissue culture flask labeled as a 3-d unstimulated culture. Record the date of harvest on worksheets.
2. Using a sterile pipet, inoculate the medium with an appropriate amount of bone marrow (*see* **Note 2**).
3. Lie the flask flat and incubate at 37°C in 5% CO_2 for approx 72 h.
4. Add 0.2 mL (200 µL) of 10 µg/mL Colcemid to the culture and incubate at 37°C for a further 60 min.
5. Undertake all further steps in harvesting as per **steps 5–12** in the overnight culture method described in **Subheading 3.1.1.**

3.2. Slide Making and G-Banding

Slide preparation is important for optimal G-banding. Ideally, slides are made when the temperature is 22°C and the humidity is 40–45% (*see* **Note 5**).

1. Place the cell suspension on the bench and allow it to warm to room temperature. This usually takes approx 15 min (*see* **Note 5**).
2. Clean the slides by filling a Coplin jar with 100% ethanol, dipping the slides into ethanol, wiping clean with a lint-free tissue, and allowing to air-dry.
3. Using a clean Pasteur pipet, drop three to five drops of suspension evenly along each slide. Allow the slides to air-dry (*see* **Note 6**).
4. Assess the quality of the slides by phase contrast microscopy. The chromosomes should appear medium gray in contrast and be well spread (*see* **Note 7**).
5. Age the slides prior to banding to reduce fuzziness and to produce clear, crisp G-bands (*see* **Fig. 1**). A number of methods are available. The following steps are designed to produce successful G-banding on the day slides are made (*see* **Note 8**).

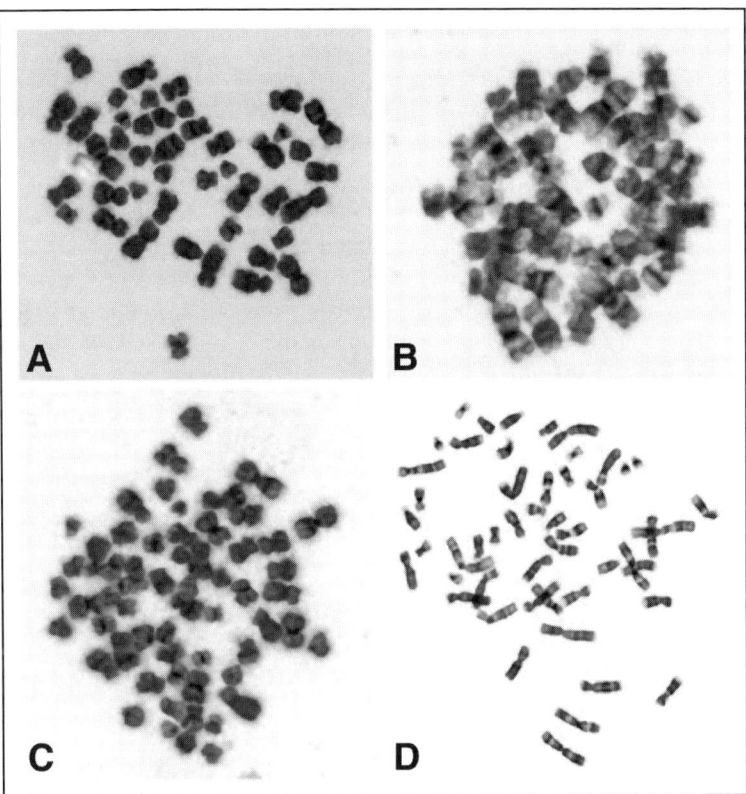

Fig. 1. Four examples of myeloma cell metaphases are shown. (**A**) A cell with 44 chromosomes and a t(11;14)(q13;q32). Although analyzable, the chromosomes are fuzzy around the edges and the banding is not crisp. It is likely that the slide was allowed to dry too slowly and not aged sufficiently. (**B**) A metaphase with 45 chromosomes that also contains a t(11;14)(q13;q32). The banding is crisper but the metaphase is not well spread, making analysis difficult. (**C**) A metaphase with 61 chromosomes but only one copy of chromosome 13. The chromosomes in this metaphase are underbanded. It is possible that the slide dried too quickly. Increasing the trypsin time may improve the banding, but slides that dry too fast may become trypsin resistant. (**D**) A metaphase with 51 chromosomes, mainly numerical abnormalities including monosomy 13. It is well banded and reasonably well spread although a number of chromosomes are crossed over one another.

6. Allow the freshly made slides to air-dry at room temperature for 30 min (*see* **Note 9**).
7. Prior to commencing banding, set up one Coplin jar with a working solution of diluted trypsin and two Coplin jars with Ca^{2+}/Mg^{2+}-free solution and let stand at room temperature.

8. Place the slides on a hot plate at 100°C for 8–10 min (*see* **Note 10**).
9. Without allowing the slides to cool, dip into the diluted trypsin and agitate for approx 8–10 s (*see* **Note 11**).
10. Rinse in two changes of Ca^{2+}/Mg^{2+}-free solution.
11. Shake off excess moisture and place the slides on a staining rack. Pipet Leishman's solution onto the slides and let stand for 8–10 min or longer if necessary (*see* **Note 12**).
12. Rinse off the stain under running tap water.
13. Allow the slides to air-dry.
14. Cover-slip the slides by placing three small drops of DPX Mounting Medium at intervals along the cover slip. Gently place the air-dried slides face down onto the cover slips, invert, and place the slides on a 37°C hot plate for a sufficient time to allow the DPX to set. The G-banded slides are now ready for microscopic analysis (*see* **Note 13**). Because only a minority of metaphases from each culture may contain chromosome abnormalities, at least 20 metaphases from each culture should be fully analyzed. This may involve the scanning of more than one G-banded slide from each culture (*see* **Note 14**).

4. Notes

1. The G-banding method given here uses Leishman's solution because we have found this method to be the most reliable and least given to fading over time. However, other methods commonly used in cytogenetics laboratories involve the use of Giemsa stain or Wright's stain.
2. The amount of bone marrow aspirate inoculated into each culture is dependent on the cellularity of the aspirate and the degree of blood dilution. If a cell count is performed on the aspirate, approx 1×10^7 nucleated cells should be added to each 10-mL culture. Alternatively, the viscosity of the marrow specimen may be assessed. If the marrow appears to be quite thick and viscous, add 5–7 drops to each culture using a sterile pipet; if only slightly viscous, add 8–11 drops; and if quite thin and blood diluted, add 12–14 drops. Care should be taken not to exceed this quantity because an excess of red cells added to the culture may affect cell growth.
3. All harvesting to the point of first adding fixative should be performed while wearing disposable gloves and in a class II biohazard cabinet. All centrifuging to the first fix stage should be in a centrifuge with sealed, autoclavable buckets.
4. IL-4, once thawed, can be kept at 4°C for 3 mo.
5. High humidity causes slides to dry too slowly and, thus, chromosomes to overspread (*see* **Fig. 1A**). If humidity is above 45–50%, the slides may be warmed briefly on a hot plate prior to dropping suspension onto the slides. Alternatively, low humidity causes slides to dry too fast and, thus, chromosomes become clumped and underspread (*see* **Fig. 1B**). Below 40% humidity, slides may be rested on a freezer block for a few seconds prior to dropping suspension onto the

slides. An alternate method of slide making when the humidity is low is to use cell suspension that has just been removed from the freezer, rather than allowing the suspension to warm to room temperature.

6. Small amounts of suspension should not be left uncapped on the bench at room temperature for long periods of time. As soon as the slides have been made, recap and store the suspension in a freezer.

7. The following steps may be tried to enhance spreading:
   a. Breathe warm, moist air onto clean slides and drop the sample onto the misted surface.
   b. Place clean slides in a freezer until the surface is misted and then drop the sample as just described.
   c. Hold the slides on an angle when dropping the suspension.
   d. Dip the slides in a 60% acetic acid solution and drop the sample onto the wet slides.

   To reduce overspreading, the slides may be heated on a 60°C hot plate prior to dropping suspension onto the slides.

8. Slides may be "aged" by a variety of methods, including placing the slides in a 60°C oven or in a desiccator for 1 to 2 d or as long as required.

9. Slides can continue to be aged in this manner for a number of hours after being made (30 min is not a critical time period). However, it only works well if performed the same day on which the slides are made.

10. Although most slides require between 8 and 10 min on a 100°C hot plate to age sufficiently, up to 20 min may be required in some cases when banding is being attempted on the same day as the slides are prepared.

11. The time needed for each slide to be immersed in trypsin may vary depending on the quality of chromosome morphology; less time may be required for chromosome preparations of poor quality. One slide should be tested at a time to estimate the optimum time for producing satisfactory G-bands for each specimen. Depending on the appearance of the banded spreads, the time in trypsin solution can be varied for additional slides (*see* **Fig. 1C**).

12. Hot plate-aged slides tend to be paler staining than slides aged by alternative methods and, thus, may require a longer application of Leishman's solution.

13. If the banding is not distinct, microscopic analysis of myeloma cases presents a challenge to even the most experienced cytogeneticists. The number of abnormal metaphases found is not proportional to the percentage of PCs in a marrow sample, so if an abnormal metaphase is seen, large numbers of metaphases may need to be analyzed to find another with the same abnormalities.

14. Only clonal abnormalities can be included in the karyotype (*16*). Thus, structural abnormalities or gains of whole chromosomes must be observed in at least two metaphases and loss of a whole chromosome must be observed in at least three metaphases to establish the clonality of an abnormality. The low mitotic index of myeloma cells makes conventional cytogenetics an inappropriate test of response to therapy or assessment of minimal residual disease.

References

1. Liang, W., Hopper, J. E., and Rowley, J. D. (1979) Karyotypic abnormalities and clinical aspects of patients with multiple myeloma and related paraproteinemic disorders. *Cancer* **44,** 630–644.

2. Dewald, G. W., Kyle, R. A., Hicks, G. A., and Greipp, P. R. (1985) The clinical significance of cytogenetic studies in 100 patients with multiple myeloma, plasma cell leukemia or amyloidosis. *Blood* **66,** 380–390.

3. Lai, J. L., Zandecki, M., Mary, J. Y., et al. (1995) Improved cytogenetics in multiple myeloma: a study of 151 patients including 117 patients at diagnosis. *Blood* **85,** 2490–2497.

4. Smadja, N. V., Louvet, C., Isnard, F., et al. (1995) Cytogenetic study in multiple myeloma at diagnosis: comparison of two techniques. *Br. J. Haematol.* **90,** 619–624.

5. Brigadeau, C., Trimoreau, F., Gachard, N., et al. (1997) Cytogenetic study of 30 patients with multiple myeloma: comparison of 3 and 6 day bone marrow cultures stimulated or not with cytokines by using a miniaturized karyotypic method. *Br. J. Haematol.* **96,** 594–600.

6. Nilsson, T., Lenhoff, S., Turesson, I., et al. (2002) Cytogenetic features of multiple myeloma: impact of gender, age, disease phase, culture time, and cytokine stimulation. *Eur. J. Haematol.* **68,** 345–353.

7. Hernandez, J. M., Gutièrrez, N. C., Almeida, J., et al. (1998) IL-4 improves the detection of cytogenetic abnormalities in multiple myeloma and increases the proportion of clonally abnormal metaphases. *Br. J. Haematol.* **103,** 163–167.

8. Tricot, G., Barlogie, B., Jagannath, S., et al. (1995) Poor prognosis in multiple myeloma is associated only with partial or complete deletions of chromosome 13 or abnormalities involving 11q and not with other karyotype abnormalities. *Blood* **86,** 4250–4256.

9. Seong, C., Delasalle, K., Hayes, K., et al. (1998) Prognostic value of cytogenetics in multiple myeloma. *Br. J. Haematol.* **101,** 189–194.

10. Desikan, R., Barlogie, B., Sawyer, J., et al. (2000) Results of high-dose therapy for 1000 patients with multiple myeloma: durable complete remissions and superior survival in the absence of chromosome 13 abnormalities. *Blood* **95,** 4008–4010.

11. Zojer, N., Konigsberg, R., Ackermann, J., et al. (2000) Deletion of 13q14 remains an independent adverse prognostic variable in multiple myeloma despite its frequent detection by interphase fluorescence in situ hybridisation. *Blood* **95,** 1925–1930.

12. Smadja, N. V., Bastard, C., Brigaudeau, C., Lerouz, D., and Fruchart, C., on behalf of the Groupe Francais de Cytogenetique Hematologique. (2001) Hypodiploidy is a major prognostic factor in multiple myeloma. *Blood* **98,** 2229–2238.

13. Fassas, A. B. T., Spencer, T., Sawyer, J., et al. (2002) Both hypodiploidy and deletion of chromosome 13 independently confer poor prognosis in multiple myeloma. *Br. J. Haematol.* **118,** 1041–1047.

14. Fonseca, R., Blood, E. A., Oken, M. M., et al. (2002) Myeloma and the t(11;14) (q13;q32): evidence for a biologically defined unique subset of patients. *Blood* **99,** 3735–3741.

15. Robillard, N., Avet-Loiseau, H., Garand, R., et al. (2003) CD20 is associated with a small mature plasma cell morphology and t(11;14) in multiple myeloma. *Blood* **102,** 1070–1071.
16. Mitelman, F. (ed.). (1995) *ISCN (1995): An International System for Human Cytogenetic Nomenclature,* S. Karger, Basel, Switzerland.
17. Barch, M. J., Knutsen, T., and Spurbeck, J. (eds.). (1997) *The AGT Cytogenetics Laboratory Manual,* 3rd ed. Lippincott-Raven, Philadelphia.

5

Multicolor Spectral Karyotyping in Multiple Myeloma

Jeffrey R. Sawyer

Summary

Multiple myeloma is a plasma cell disorder characterized at the cytogenetic level by aneuploid karyotypes with numerous complex structural aberrations. Unfortunately, conventional chromosome-banding techniques are unable to resolve many of these aberrations. Multicolor Spectral Karyotyping (SKY) is a molecular cytogenetic technique that utilizes chromosome-painting probes for characterizing complex structural chromosome aberrations. This innovative technology allows the simultaneous display of each of the 24 different chromosomes in a different color. Chromosomal sites of rearrangement or translocation between different chromosomes are visualized by a change in the color at the point of the aberration. The SKY technique makes possible the identification of chromosomal bands of unknown origin, including translocations, insertions, complex rearrangements, and marker chromosomes, which, in many cases, go unresolved by traditional banding methods.

Key Words

Multiple myeloma; spectral karyotyping; chromosomes; fluorescent *in situ* hybridization.

1. Introduction

Multiple myeloma (MM) is a plasma cell (PC) disorder characterized at the cytogenetic level by karyotypes with both hypodiploid and hyperdiploid cell lines as well as numerous complex structural aberrations. Unfortunately, conventional chromosome-banding techniques are unable to resolve many of these complex aberrations. The molecular cytogenetic technique of fluorescent *in situ* hybridization (FISH) allows the detection of whole chromosomes or specific loci by the use of selected chromosome-specific DNA probes. In extremely complex metaphase karyotypes, however, FISH is not the optimal approach. Multicolor Spectral Karyotyping (SKY) is a newer molecular cyto-

From: *Methods in Molecular Medicine, Vol. 113: Multiple Myeloma: Methods and Protocols*
Edited by: R. D. Brown and P. J. Ho © Humana Press Inc., Totowa, NJ

genetic technique that allows the simultaneous display of each chromosome in a different color *(1)*. SKY provides an important technical advantage over FISH because it provides for the simultaneous hybridization of 24 differentially labeled chromosome-painting probes to metaphase chromosomes. Chromosomal sites of rearrangement or translocation between different chromosomes are visualized by a change in the color at the point of the aberration (**Fig. 1**). This technique makes it possible to identify chromosomal bands of unknown origin, including translocations, insertions, complex rearrangements, and marker chromosomes found in the myeloma karyotypes *(2–6)*.

The system developed by Applied Spectral Imaging (ASI) (Vista, CA) for spectral karyotyping combines Fourier spectroscopy (interferometry), charge-coupled device (CCD) imaging, and optical microscopy to measure simultaneously all points in the chromosome emission spectrum in the visible and near-infrared spectral range *(1)*. Measurement of a discrete spectrum at every pixel in the image makes it possible to discriminate multiple and spectrally overlapping fluorochromes in a single data acquisition *(7)*. With this system, every pixel of an image with the same spectral information is subsequently assigned the same pseudocolor, allowing the spectral classification of all chromosomes *(7)*. The spectral karyotyping technique represents an important technical advancement over conventional FISH chromosome-painting technique. Unlike standard FISH procedures, which base fluorochrome discrimination on the measurement of only a single or a few probes, SKY is based on the combinatorial labeling of painting probes to include all chromosomes in a single hybridization procedure. The probes for SKY are derived from chromosome libraries produced by amplifying flow-sorted chromosomes utilizing a degenerate oligonucleotide–primed polymerase chain reaction *(8)*. The probes are labeled through the incorporation of either haptenized (biotin and digoxigenin) or directly labeled nucleotides. The generated chromosome-specific probes are pooled, precipitated with an excess of Cot-1 DNA to suppress repetitive sequences, and hybridized to metaphase chromosomes.

All cytogenetic techniques have certain advantages and limitations *(5)*. One of the main limitations of conventional FISH is that it requires some prior knowledge of the origin of the abnormal chromosome in order to select the appropriate probe. This is not the case with SKY, because the combination of probes allows the coloring of the entire karyotype. The dyes have overlapping spectra (some outside the visual range) that cannot be distinguished by the human eye, nor can they be easily imaged through a filter without the loss of signal intensity. The SKY technique is limited in some respects by its inability to detect intrachromosomal events such as pericentric or paracentric inversions, very small deletions, and duplications, which do not lead to color changes within the chromosome. In addition, the limits of sensitivity of the SKY system

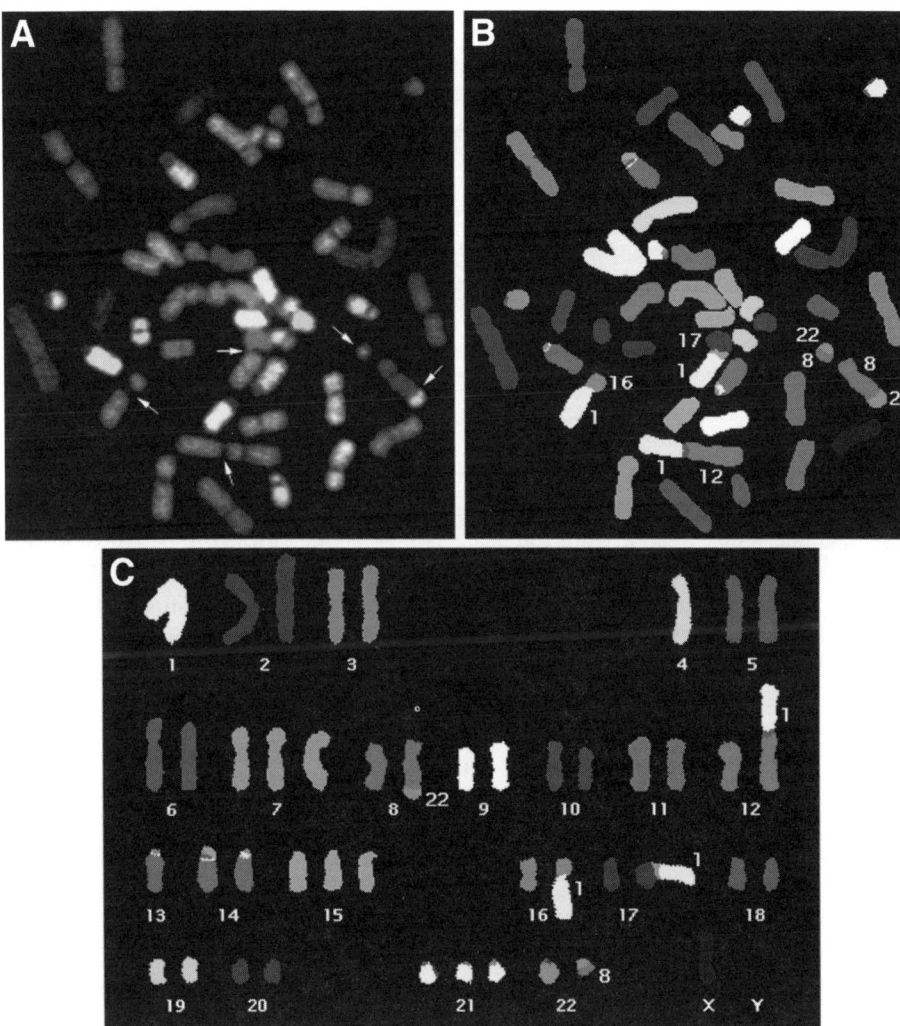

Fig. 1. Spectral karyotyping of bone marrow sample of a patient with MM. The simultaneous hybridization of 24 combinatorially labeled chromosome painting probes is demonstrated. (**A**) Metaphase shown in display colors as seen through microscope; (**B**) same metaphase cell shown in classification colors after spectral classification of chromosomes in pseudocolors; (**C**) spectral karyotype of same metaphase shown in classification colors. Note that multiple translocations are identified by changes in color patterns.

with painting probes have been estimated to be between 500 and 1500 kbp; therefore, the inability to detect very small chromosomal events is hampered (*1*). Other small insertions or small translocations are also difficult to identify with SKY and should be confirmed by additional FISH techniques.

2. Materials

1. SKY probes: These are supplied as kits (totaling five vials) from ASI. Alternatively, the probes can be can be prepared according to Telenius et al. *(8)* or Hilgenfeld et al. *(9)*. The five vials in the ASI kit are as follows:
   a. Vial 1: human spectral karyotyping reagent.
   b. Vial 2: blocking reagent.
   c. Vial 3: Cy5 staining reagent.
   d. Vial 4: Cy5.5 staining reagent.
   e. Vial 5: antifade/4′,6-diamidino-2-phenylindole (DAPI) reagent.
2. Pepsin (cat. no. P6887; Sigma, St. Louis, MO): Prepare 10% pepsin stock solution (100 mg/mL) in sterile distilled water. Aliquot into microcentrifuge tubes. Store at –20°C.
3. Saline sodium citrate (SSC) (cat. no. S6639; Sigma): To prepare 4X SSC/0.1% Tween-20, add 1 mL of Tween-20 to 200 mL of 20X SSC and then add 790 mL of distilled H_2O. Adjust the pH to 7.0. Store at room temperature.
4. Formamide (molecular biology grade) (cat. no. F7503; Sigma): To prepare formamide/SSC wash solution, add 75 mL of formamide to 15 mL of 20X SSC and 60 mL of distilled H_2O. Adjust the pH to 7.0 with HCl.
5. 2.0 *N* HCl (cat. no. 251-26; Sigma): To prepare 0.01 *M* HCl solution, add 0.5 mL of 1 *M* HCl to 49.5 mL of distilled H_2O.
6. $MgCl_2$ (cat. no. M82667; Sigma): To prepare 1 *M* $MgCl_2$, add 20.33 g of $MgCl_2$ to 100 mL of distilled H_2O (filter the solution). Store at room temperature. To prepare 1X phosphate-buffered saline (PBS)/$MgCl_2$, add 50 mL of 1 *M* $MgCl_2$ to 950 mL of PBS. Store at room temperature; protect from light.
7. Tween-20 (cat. no. P-9416; Sigma).
8. Formaldehyde: Prepare 1% formaldehyde solution. Add 2.7 mL of 37% formaldehyde to 100 mL of 1X PBS/$MgCL_2$.
9. PBS (cat. no. 1000-3; Sigma).
10. Ethanol (cat. no. A962; Fisher, Fairview, NJ) (90% anhydrous ethyl alcohol; 100% reagent alcohol). Prepare 100 mL each of 70, 80, and 100% ethanol. Prepare two series of three ethanols (50 mL each), one to be kept at room temperature and the other at –20°C. Place the –20°C series in a freezer for at least 2 to 3 h prior to use.
11. Distilled H_2O.
12. Rubber cement.
13. Cover slips (plastic and glass).

3. Methods

The SKY methods described next are modified from the protocol of ASI. Clinical cytogenetic techniques for the culture of myeloma bone marrow cells involve a range of times, including direct harvest, 24 h, 48 h, and synchronized harvest *(10)*. Prior to beginning the procedure, the metaphase slide preparations should be prepared from the best cell pellet available. The metaphase spreads should be dropped onto slides 2 to 3 d prior to d 1 of the procedure (*see* **Note 1**). The hybridization procedure for SKY takes 3 d to complete and an indefinite period of time for image acquisition and analysis. Day 1 consists of pretreatment of the chromosome preparations (*see* **Subheading 3.2.**), denaturation of chromosomes (*see* **Subheading 3.3.**), denaturation of probe (*see* **Subheading 3.4.**), and initiation of hybridization. Day 2 is a continuation of the hybridization procedure with the slides maintained in a 37°C incubator (for at least 48 h). Day 3 consists of preparation of the slides for signal detection (*see* **Subheading 3.6.**) and imaging procedures (*see* **Subheading 3.7.**).

3.1. Day 1 Preparation

1. Using a good-quality phase contrast microscope, scan the slides for an area of higher mitotic index and good spreads (*see* **Note 2**). Select an area of each slide to be hybridized and mark the best area (22 × 22 mm) on the back (underside) of the slide with a diamond pencil.
2. Prepare denaturation solution by combining 28 mL of formamide, 4 mL of 20X SSC, and 8 mL of distilled H_2O. Adjust the pH to 7.0 with HCl. Preheat the denaturation solution to 72°C (this will denature four slides).
3. Prepare three Coplin jars of 1X PBS. Prepare one Coplin jar of $PBS/MgCl_2$.

3.2. Pepsin Pretreatment

1. Preheat 50 mL of 0.01 *M* HCl to 37°C in a glass Coplin jar. Add 7 µL pepsin to 50 mL of 0.01 *M* HCl solution at 37°C in a Coplin jar and mix well. Immerse the slides in pepsin solution for 4 min, 30 s at 37°C. This time may very depending on the amount of cytoplasmic background (*see* **Note 3**).
2. Transfer the slides to 1X PBS wash solution at room temperature for 5 min.
3. Transfer the slides to a second 1X PBS wash for 5 min.
4. Wash the slides in 1X $PBS/MgCl_2$ at room temperature for 5 min.
5. Transfer the slides to a Coplin jar containing 1% formaldehyde, and incubate for 10 min at room temperature.
6. Transfer the slides to a third 1X PBS wash for 5 min.
7. Transfer the slides to an ethanol series of 70, 80, and 100% for 2 min each. Air-dry the slides.

3.3. Chromosome Denaturation

1. Warm 40 mL of denaturation solution to 70–72°C in a glass Coplin jar in a water bath. Do not place the Coplin jar directly in an 80°C water bath because this may crack the glass. Preheat the solution and Coplin jar together in the water bath by slowly raising the temperature to 70–72°C. Place the slides one at a time in the denatured solution for 1 to 2 min. Be careful not to overdenature.
2. Immediately transfer the slides to a –20°C ethanol series of 70, 80, and 100% ethanol for 2 min each. Air-dry the slides.

3.4. Probe Denaturation and Hybridization

1. Briefly microcentrifuge vial 1 (ASR1001H). Mix the contents of the vial (including any red precipitation) by pipetting up and down. Using 10 µL for each slide, place the probe in a microcentriofuge tube and denature by floating the tube in an 80°C water bath for 7 min.
2. Transfer the probe to a 37°C water bath for 1 h.
3. Add 10 µL of the denatured probe (vial 1) to the selected areas of the denatured slides.
4. Place an 18 × 18 mm glass cover slip over the selected probe area, being careful not to introduce any bubbles under the cover slip. Carefully seal the edges with rubber cement. Transfer the slides to a humidified plastic box and place in an incubator at 37°C for 48 h.

3.5. Preparation for d 3 Detection (48 h later)

1. Pour 50 mL of 50% formamide/SSC wash into three plastic Coplin jars and preheat to 45°C.
2. Preheat two Coplin jars of washing solution II (1X SSC) to 45°C.
3. Pour seven jars of 4X SSC/0.1% Tween.
4. Add 10 µL of Cy5 staining reagent (vial 3 from CAD kit) to 1 mL of 4X SSC. This antibody-containing reagent solution is unstable; discard at the end of each day.
5. Add 5 µL of Cy5.5 staining reagent (vial 4 from CAD kit) to 1 mL of 4X SSC. This antibody-containing reagent solution is unstable; discard at the end of each day.

3.6. Detection Procedure

   Slides should remain wet and protected from direct light during this procedure.

1. Remove the slides from the incubator and humidified chamber. Carefully remove the rubber cement.
2. Transfer the slides to a Coplin jar in a shaking water bath containing formamide wash solution I (50% formamide in 2X SSC) for 5 min at 45°C with mild agitation.
3. Transfer the slides to a second formamide wash for 5 min at 45°C with mild agitation.
4. Transfer the slides to a third formamide wash for 5 min at 45°C with mild agitation.
5. Transfer the slides to a Coplin jar containing washing solution II (1X SSC) for 5 min at 45°C.
6. Transfer the slides to a second washing solution II for 5 min at 45°C.
7. Transfer the slides to a washing solution III (4X SSC/0.1% Tween-20) for 2 min at room temperature. Drain excess solution from the slides without drying.

8. Apply 80 µL of blocking reagent (vial 2) per slide. Place a plastic cover slip over the area and incubate at 37°C for 30 min.
9. Remove the cover slip, drain the fluid from the slides, but do not allow to dry. Apply 80 µL of diluted Cy5 staining reagent (vial 3) and place a plastic cover slip over the area. Incubate the slides at 37°C for an additional 45 min.
10. Wash the slides three times in solution III (4X SSC/0.1% Tween-20) at 45°C for 3 min each with mild agitation. Remove the slides from the third wash, drain excess liquid, but keep wet.
11. Apply 80 µL of diluted Cy5.5 staining reagent (vial 4) to each slide, place a plastic cover slip over the area, and incubate for 45 min at 37°C.
12. Wash the slides three times in solution III (4X SSC/0.1% Tween-20) at 45°C for 3 min each with mild agitation.
13. Wash the slides briefly in tap water and air-dry the slides.
14. Apply 20 µL of the antifade/DAPI reagent (vial 5) to the hybridization area and place a 24 × 60 mm glass cover slip on the surface. Be careful not to introduce air bubbles under the cover slip. The slides are now ready to be viewed under a microscope.

3.7. Image Acquisition

Image acquisition and analysis are based on a combination of Fourier spectroscopy, CCD imaging, and optical microscopy. Following completion of the hybridization procedure, the specimen is exposed to a 150-W xenon light source and the combination of dyes (chromosome-painting probes) is excited simultaneously (*see* **Note 4**); the emission spectra of the differently labeled probes are measured with a single exposure through a custom-designed optical triple band-pass filter (Chroma Technologies, Brattleboro, VT). The emitted light then passes through the interferometer to the CCD camera of the Spectracube™ system (SD200; ASI). Fourier transformation algorithms are used to convert the interferogram (this is deduced from a sequence of intensity measurements acquired at varying optical path differences of the light emitted from the different painting probes and also depends on the wavelength of the emitted fluorescence) produced for each pixel of the CCD image into spectra curves of each image point. Once the spectral image is acquired the SKYVIEW™ software compares the acquired spectral image with the spectra measured for the normal metaphase chromosomes, which are stored as reference spectra in a spectral library (*1*). Conversion of emission spectra into the visualization of display colors is achieved by assigning blue, green, and red to specific spectral ranges. Automated classification of test metaphase is based on a pixel-by-pixel comparison of the measured spectra in the test sample and the stored reference spectra. Image points showing the same spectra are highlighted with the same classification color, thus revealing chromosome identification. The red, green, blue display renders a similar color to that of chromosomes that are labeled with spectrally overlapping fluorochromes. Based on the measurement of the discrete emission spectra at all pixels of the image, the hybridization colors **(Fig. 1A)** are then converted into classification colors **(Fig. 1B)** by applying an algorithm that results in the assignment of a discrete color to all pixels with an identical spectrum. DAPI banding images are acquired as part of the image acquisition process and analyzed using a DAPI-specific optical filter. The DAPI images (not shown) are used in conjunction with spectral classification for the identification of chromosome aberrations and construction of the final spectral karyotype **(Fig. 1C)** (*see* **Note 5**).

4. Notes

1. As with any conventional metaphase cytogenetic technique, the quality of the final karyotypes is most directly related to the quality of the metaphase slide preparations. In this regard, great care in the harvesting technique is critical to obtaining excellent slide preparations. Perhaps the most important step in the harvest procedure for obtaining good spreads with good morphology is the first fixation. Most laboratories use a 3:1 methanol:acetic acid fixative; however, variations on the basic methanol:acetic acid fix such as a 5:2 ratio may work equally well or better. Following hypotonic treatment, the pellet should be carefully resuspended and the first fix added drop by drop while gently shaking the cell suspension. Fixative should be changed at least three times. To make slide preparations, resuspend and dilute the pellet in fixative and drop on a test slide. If spreading is not optimal, a final concentration of 5:3 methanol:acetic acid fix ratio may improve the results. Wet and cold, as well as dry, room temperature slides should be tested, because one method may be more successful than the other with a given pellet or time of year. For example, wet and cold slides may work best in winter and dry room temperature slides in summer. Generally, slides should be dry within 1 min; if slides dry too fast or too slow, residual cytoplasm will be evident. Typically, direct harvest preparations should not be used; select the best pellet from the 24- or 48-h cell cultures. Slides should be dropped at least 2 d before hybridization and kept at room temperature. Cell pellets can be stored in fixative at –20°C for several years.

2. Low mitotic index is a common problem in MM because PCs do not typically divide. A large number of variations of Colcemid® times and concentrations have been advocated for harvesting bone marrow. If the length of Colcemid time is extended, the concentration should be lowered. Excessive time or Colcemid concentration will result in short, highly condensed chromosomes, which will be suboptimal for SKY. Cell pellets can be spun down and the concentration of cell suspension increased to enhance the number of metaphases in the hybridization region. Slides should be viewed on a high-quality phase microscope to determine the best area for hybridization.

3. Pepsin pretreatment will vary depending on the amount of cytoplasmic background. High background may require lengthening pepsin times. Be careful not to overtreat, because this may lead to lower signal intensity from the SKY probes *(8)*.

4. It is important to view chromosomes in the display colors in order to assess the quality of the hybridization prior to additional computation (**Fig. 1A**). A poor-quality hybridization is characterized by a lack of distinct color separation of the pure dyes and indicates that subsequent analysis may be less than optimal. This indicates that the hybridization may need to be repeated if possible. It is preferable to repeat the hybridization rather than try to do the analysis from suboptimal cells.

5. The assumption that the color assignments of SKY will ease the interpretation of complex karyotypes and therefore eliminate the need for highly experienced cytogenetic technologists is incorrect. It is important that the individuals performing the SKY analysis on very complex karyotypes such as MM have previous bone marrow harvesting and G-banding experience with the same types of specimens. Owing to the use of combinatorial labeling of probes, in some cases the SKY system will assign multiple chromosome numbers to the same region; therefore, it is necessary to analyze as many different cells as possible to resolve the discrepancies. Conventional G-band karyotypes made from the same cell pellet or harvest should also be used in the analysis. Very small translocations or other rearrangements need to be confirmed by the use of locus-specific FISH probes.

Acknowledgments

I thank Regina Lichti Binz for excellent technical assistance. This work was supported in part by grant CA55819 from the National Cancer Institute, Bethesda, MD.

References

1. Schröck, E., du Manoir, T., Veldman, T., et al. (1996) Multicolor spectral karyotyping of human chromosomes. *Science* **273,** 494–497.
2. Rao, P. H., Cigudos, J., Ning, Y., et al. (1998) Karyotypic complexity of multiple myeloma defined by multicolour spectral karyotyping (SKY). *Blood* **92,** 1743–1748.
3. Sawyer, J. R., Lukacs, J. L., Munshi, N., et al. (1998) Identification of new nonrandom translocations in multiple myeloma with multicolor spectral karyoytping. *Blood* **92,** 4269–4278.
4. Sawyer, J. R., Lukacs, J. L., Thomas, E. L., et al. (2001) Multicolor spectral karyotyping identifies new translocations and a recurring pathway for chromosome instability in multiple myeloma. *Br. J. Haematol.* **112,** 167–174.
5. Ho, P. J., Campell, L. J., Gibson, J., Brown, R., and Joshua, D. (2002) The biology and cytogenetics of multiple myeloma. *Rev. Clin. Exp. Hematol.* **6,** 276–300.

6. Bayani, J. M. and Squire, J. A. (2002) Applications of SKY in cancer cytogenetics. *Cancer Invest.* **20,** 373–386.
7. Garini, Y., Macville, M., du Manoir, S., et al. (1996) Spectral karyotyping. *Bioimaging* **4,** 65–72.
8. Telenius, H., Pelear, A. H., Tunnacliffe, A., et al. (1992) Cytogentic analysis by chromosome painting using DOP-PCR amplified flow-sorted chromosomes. *Genes Chromosomes Cancer* **4,** 257–263.
9. Hilgenfeld, E., Mantagna, C., Padilla-Nash, H., Stapleton, L., Heselmeyer-Haddad, K., and Reid, T. (2002) Spectral karyotyping in cancer cytogenetics. *Methods Mol. Med.* **68,** 29–44.
10. Sawyer, J. R., Waldron, J. A., Jagannath, S., and Barlogie, B. (1995) Cytogenetic findings in 200 patients with multiple myeloma. *Cancer Genet. Cytogenet.* **82,** 41–49.

6

Detection of Chromosome 13 Deletions by Fluorescent *In Situ* Hybridization

Scott VanWier and Rafael Fonseca

Summary

Multiple myeloma (MM), like other hematological malignancies, has both normal and clonal neoplastic cells coresiding in the bone marrow. To perform interphase fluorescent *in situ* hybridization (FISH) analysis accurately, for the detection of clonal chromosome abnormalities, it is crucial to restrict the analysis to the tumoral cells. The correct detection of these abnormalities may have diagnostic, prognostic, and therapeutic implications. Our laboratory has developed a clone-specific cytoplasmic immunoglobulin (cIg) staining method coupled with FISH (cIg-FISH) for the study of plasma cell (PC) neoplasms. An unlimited combination of DNA probes can be used with this technique to examine the genetic changes that frequently occur in patients with these diseases, one of which is abnormalities of chromosome 13. Using the two techniques simultaneously (i.e., cIg-FISH), we have demonstrated that approx 50% of patients with MM have abnormalities of chromosome 13, mostly monosomy, and when present involving the majority of the cells. In this chapter, we present the technical methodology for detecting chromosome abnormalities and how to restrict the analysis to the clonal PCs.

Key Words

Multiple myeloma; light chain; fluorescent *in situ* hybridization; plasma cell; clone.

1. Introduction

Complex and varied chromosome abnormalities are present in the clonal plasma cells (PCs) of patients with multiple myeloma (MM) and related conditions. Classic cytogenetics reports only 30% of MM patients having chromosome abnormalities by karyotype analysis *(1–3)*. The low proliferative rate of the PC coupled with the uncertainty of whether the karyotype came from the malignant clone results in an inadequate means of studying patients with MM. Fluorescent *in situ* hybridization (FISH) has bridged the gap between classic

From: *Methods in Molecular Medicine, Vol. 113: Multiple Myeloma: Methods and Protocols*
Edited by: R. D. Brown and P. J. Ho © Humana Press Inc., Totowa, NJ

cytogenetics and molecular genetics and has been instrumental in finding that all patients with MM have detectable chromosome abnormalities *(4–6)*.

Chromosome 13 abnormalities have been detected in slightly over 50% of patients with MM, and monosomy is the predominant abnormality seen (85% of those with abnormalities) *(7–10)*. Patients with MM with chromosome 13 abnormalities have an overall shorter survival and lower likelihood of response to therapy *(11)*. Identifying the malignant cells from the normal cells is critical for diagnosis and treatment decisions (for further details regarding the clinical implications of chromosome 13 abnormalities, refer to the papers of Facon *[9]*, Fonseca *[11]* and Desikan *[12]*).

Given the variable involvement of the bone marrow by the clonal PCs, it is imperative to restrict the scoring to only the PCs. This can be achieved either by selecting the cells (e.g., by flow cytometry or, more commonly, by magnetic bead separation) or by performing combined FISH with morphological and immunohistochemical/immunofluorescence detection of the cells (i.e., cIg-FISH or FICTION). Staining PCs with immunofluorescent-labeled antibodies can detect cytoplasmic light chains and accurately identify the same light chain as the monoclonal protein, thus limiting study to the malignant clone (clone-specific analysis) *(13)* (**Fig. 1**). A previous article by us illustrates the processing of a sample and making of cytospin slides *(14)*.

Although this chapter primarily deals with the techniques necessary for the study of chromosome 13, the same principles apply to the study of any other chromosome abnormality for which there are validated FISH probes. In addition, this chapter does not deal with the clinical implication of methods of detection of chromosome 13 deletion, i.e., karyotype analysis vs FISH detection. Although much debate has ensued regarding the best method of detection, each of the methods has advantages and disadvantages. Nevertheless, FISH is a much more sensitive technique that allows detection of nearly all patients with chromosome 13 deletion/monosomy (>98% vs 30% of patients with monosomy/deletion, FISH vs karyotype, respectively).

2. Materials

All reagents are potentially hazardous. Use appropriate safety procedures when handling these materials. Avoid contact with skin and mucous membranes.

2.1. Pretreatment of Slides

1. AMCA Anti-Human Lambda Chain (cat. no. CI-3070; Vector). Store at 4°C.
2. AMCA Anti-Human Kappa Chain (cat. no. CI-3060; Vector). Store at 4°C.
3. AMCA Anti-Goat IgG (H+L) (cat. no. CI-5000; Vector). Store at 4°C.
4. 100% Ethanol: molecular-grade pure grain alcohol. Store at room temperature.

cIg Staining

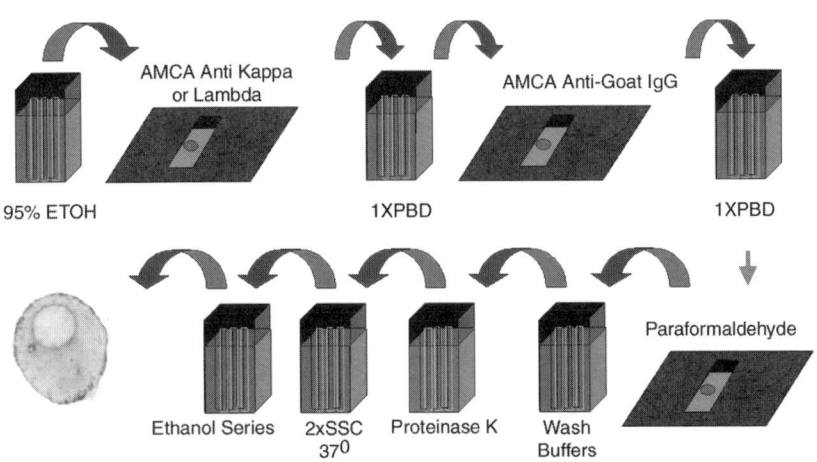

Fig. 1. Cytoplasmic immunoglobulin (cIg) staining procedure. PBD = phosphate-buffered detergent.

5. 95% Ethanol: Add 25 mL of distilled water to 475 mL of 100% ethanol. Store at room temperature.
6. 85% Ethanol: Add 75 mL of distilled water to 425 mL of 100% ethanol. Store at room temperature.
7. 70% Ethanol: Add 150 mL of distilled water to 350 mL of 100% ethanol. Store at room temperature.
8. Culture medium: 90% RPMI-1640, 10% fetal calf serum (FCS) (Gibco-BRL, Gaithersburg, MD).
9. 2% Paraformaldehyde: Heat 80 mL of distilled water to 70°C, stir in 2.0 g of paraformaldehyde, add 6 *M* NaOH until the paraformaldehyde goes into solution, add 10 mL of 10X phosphate-buffered saline (PBS), adjust the pH to 7.2 with 6 *N* HCl, and distilled water to 100 mL. Do not use until cooled to room temperature. Make fresh monthly.
10. 10X PBS: 10X concentrate (Sigma, St. Louis, MO).
11. Proteinase K: 100-mg lots. Store at –20°C. See the product label sheet for expiration (Sigma).
12. Proteinase K stock solution (2.5%): Add 0.025 g of proteinase K to 1 mL of distilled water. Aliquot into 32-µL lots. Store at –20°C.
13. Proteinase K working solution (0.002%): Add 32 µL of stock solution to 40 mL of 2X saline sodium citrate (SSC).
14. 20X SSC buffer: 3.0 *M* NaCl, 0.3 *M* sodium citrate, pH 7.0. Store at room temperature (Roche, Indianapolis, IN).
15. 2X SSC buffer: Mix 50 mL of 20X SSC with 450 mL of distilled water. Store at room temperature. Use within 6 mo.

16. Mild detergents: Use either APK (Oncor), Np40 (Vysis), or Tween-20 (Roche). Follow the manufacturer's suggested dilutions.
17. Staining dishes and Coplin jars.
18. Super Pap™ pen (cat. no. 00-8899; Zymed).
19. Test tubes: 5-mL polystyrene round-bottomed tubes or equivalent.
20. 37°C Water bath.
21. Platform rotator.

2.2. Hybridization

1. 13q14 DNA probes: LSI 13 (13q14) SpectrumGreen and LSI D13S319 (13q14.3) SpectrumOrange (cat. no. 32-192018 and 32-190045, respectively; (Vysis).
2. Hybridization buffer: supplied with commercial probes.
3. Sterile water.
4. Programmable hot plate.
5. Glass cover slips: Fisherbrand microscope cover glass (cat. no. 12-545-80; Fisher, Fairview, NJ).
6. No-wrinkle rubber cement (Elmers).
7. Humidified chamber.
8. 37°C incubator.

2.3. Washing

1. 0.4X SSC buffer: Mix 10 mL of 20X SSC with 490 mL of distilled water. Store at room temperature. Use within 6 mo.
2. Coplin jars.
3. 70°C Water bath.
4. Mild detergent (e.g., NP-40, Tween).
5. Vectashield mounting medium for fluorescence (*important:* buy Vectashield without 4′,6-diamidino-2-phenylindole [DAPI]) (cat. no. H-1000; Vector). Store at 4°C.
6. Glass cover slips: Fisherbrand microscope cover glass (cat. no. 12-542-B; Fisher).

2.4. Analysis

1. Epifluorescence microscope with proper objectives and filter sets (*see* **Note 1**).
2. 100-W Mercury lamp source.

3. Methods
3.1. Pretreatment of Slides

1. Artificially age freshly made cytospin slides before any treatment is done on the specimen. Slides can be dried in an oven set at 80°C for 20–30 min or left on the bench for several days. Place slides in a Coplin jar of 95% ethanol for 5 min and air-dry. For slides stored in a freezer, immediately placed in 95% ethanol for 5 min at the time of retrieval and air-dry (*see* **Note 2**).
2. Measure 40 mL of 2X SSC in a Coplin jar and place in a 37°C water bath.

3. Using a Super Pap pen, draw a circle around the cytospin spot approximately the circumference of a dime.

4. In a 5-mL test tube, place 90 µL of RPMI-1640/FCS, and add 10 µL of goat anti-human κ or λ chain (depending on the monoclonal protein of the patient) conjugated with 7-amino-4-methylcoumarin-3-acetic acid (AMCA). Vortex the tube quickly, apply 100 µL of the 10% solution to the cytospin spot, and place the slide in the dark at room temperature for 20–30 min (*see* **Note 3**).

5. Tap the slide on the side of a waste container to remove the solution on the surface and place the slide in a staining dish. Flood the slide with 1X APK or other mild detergent. Using a platform rotator, gently shake the dish for 2 min. Pour off the detergent and repeat the wash. Remove the slide from the staining dish, and air-dry at 37°C for 5 min in the dark.

6. To enhance the intensity of the AMCA staining, mix 90 µL of RPMI/FCS and 10 µL of anti-goat immunoglobulin conjugated with AMCA. Apply 100 µL of the 10% solution to the cytospin spot, and place in the dark at room temperature for 20–30 min (*see* **Note 3**).

7. Repeat **step 5**.

8. Flood the cytospin spot with 2% paraformaldehyde for 5 min at room temperature in the dark (*see* **Note 4**).

9. Repeat **step 5** substituting 2X SSC for the second wash.

10. Incubate the slide for 15 min at room temperature in a Coplin jar containing proteinase K working solution (0.002%) (*see* **Note 5**).

11. Remove the slide from the coplin jar and place in a staining dish. Flood the slide with 2X SSC and gently rotate for 2 min. Pour off the 2X SSC and repeat the wash.

12. Place the slide in the prewarmed Coplin jar containing 2X SSC and incubate the slide 30–60 min.

13. Remove the slide and place in a Coplin jar containing 70% ethanol for 1 min. Repeat with 85 and 100% ethanol. Blot the bottom of the slide and wipe the underside of the slide dry with a paper towel.

14. Adjust a hot plate to 37°C and place the slide on the surface to evaporate any remaining ethanol (*see* **Note 6**).

3.2. Hybridization

1. Remove both vials of probe and hybridization buffer from the freezer and allow them to reach room temperature in the dark (*see* **Note 7**).

2. Spin down each vial in a minicentrifuge for 3 s. Pipet up and down the contents of each vial and spin down again.

3. In a microcentrifuge tube, add 7 µL of hybridization buffer, 1 µL of LSI 13 probe, 1 µL of LSI D13S319 probe, and 1 µL of water. Spin down the probe mixture, and pipet up and down the contents until mixed well (*see* **Note 8**).

4. Apply 3 µL of probe mixture to the slide and then cover with a circle glass cover slip. Make sure the probe mix spreads evenly over the hybridization area. If bubbles are seen, gently press on the cover slip until the bubbles disperse. Seal the outer edges of the cover slip with rubber cement.

5. Codenature the slide by programming the hot plate to ramp to 75°C and hold for 5 min. After 5 min have the hot plate ramp down to 37°C (*see* **Note 9**).
6. Place the slide in a prewarmed humidified box and place in a 37°C incubator. Let the slide hybridize for 12–16 h (*see* **Note 10**).

3.3. Washing

1. Thirty minutes prior to use, prepare a Coplin jar with 0.4X SSC and place in a 70°C water bath.
2. Carefully remove the rubber cement from the slide, and gently tease the cover slip off the hybridization area (*see* **Note 11**).
3. Place the slide in the Coplin jar containing 70°C 0.4X SSC for 3 min (*see* **Note 12**).
4. Remove the slide and place in a coplin jar containing room temperature 1X APK solution. Agitate the slide for 1–3 s, and then let stand in the solution for 2 min.
5. Remove the slide and air-dry in the dark.
6. Apply 5–10 µL of Vectashield mounting medium to the hybridization area and cover with a 22 × 22-mm glass cover slip. Gently blot any excess Vectashield with a paper towel (*see* **Note 13**).

3.4. Analysis

1. Switch on the power supply for the fluorescent microscope, and let the bulb warm up for 5 min.
2. Place a drop of immersion oil on the cover slip, and find the plane of focus using a single-pass DAPI filter. The monotypic PCs should be seen as stained blue from the AMCA and distinctive PC morphology should be observed (*see* **Note 14**).
3. Use an appropriate filter set to visualize the probes. The signals should be seen in the nucleus of the cell and have the look of either compact oval shapes or stringy, diffuse oval shapes (*see* **Note 15**).
4. Adjust the depth of focus, look for a "three-dimensional effect," and become familiar with the size and shape of the target signals.
5. Analyze hybridization only in cells displaying a combination of PC morphology and AMCA staining.
6. Analyze only nonoverlapping cells (single-pass DAPI is optimal for distinguishing overlapping cells).
7. Focus up and down to find all the signals present in the nucleus. A normal pattern consists of two pairs of closely associated signals. An abnormal pattern will consist of loss of one signal or both from one pair (**Fig. 2**).
8. Score 100 PCs and record the results.

Fig. 2. (*see facing page*) PCs with both (**A**) normal and (**B**) abnormal pattern seen in MM. Because the bone marrow contains both clonal and normal myeloid cells, FISH scoring can be done only on the clonal PCs as determined by their light chain.

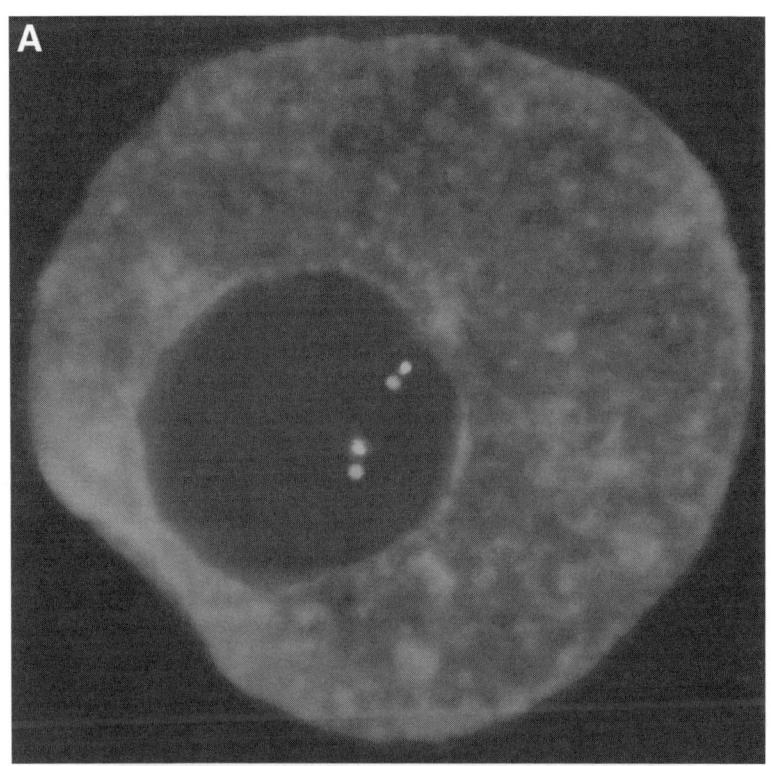

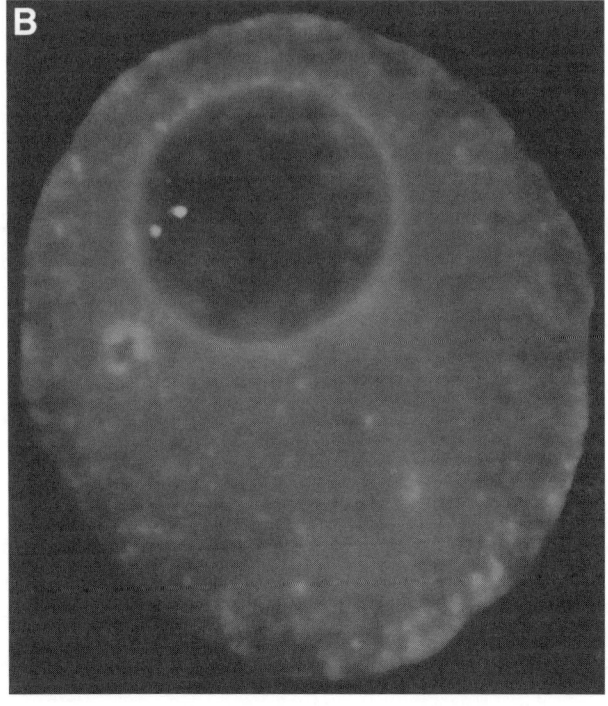

3.5. Interpretation of Results

When analyzing the specimen, one should have approx 90% of all cells showing signal for this particular probe set. The nonstaining cells serve as an internal control for this assay in that if signals are seen in these cells, the probe is performing properly and these cells most likely will display a normal pattern. Take note if they do not. In our laboratory, we have used the 10% cutoff to call a specimen abnormal. This is rarely an issue because the abnormal PCs are favored with clonal expansion and will display the abnormality in the majority of the PCs scored. In instances when one is near the cutoff or just over, such as 15%, have a second observer confirm the findings, or if that is not an option repeat the hybridization on the same patient and duplicate the first finding. Polyploid or 4N cells are a frequent occurrence when studying PCs from patients with MM, and they will be seen along with diploid or 2N cells in the same specimen. The polyploid cells tend to have a much larger nucleus owing to the extra DNA in the cell and will display four paired signals. It is not uncommon for an abnormal specimen to display an abnormal pattern in the smaller PCs whereas the larger PCs score as normal. These larger cells are likely abnormal polyploid versions of the diploid lineage but are usually scored as normal. Because of the coexistence of polyploidy cells with cells having only the 2N version of the chromosome complement, chromosome 13 is rarely if ever missed by FISH analysis.

4. Notes

1. Having optimum objectives and filter sets is critical for any FISH experiment. Plan Apochromat objectives represent the best filters available and the most expensive but are well worth the money if photoimaging is to be done. The filters used will need to be able to detect three fluorochromes and their particular spectral characteristics: AMCA with excitation/emission of 350 nm/450 nm, SpectrumGreen with 497 nm/524 nm, and SpectrumOrange with 559 nm/588 nm. Occasionally, one can use a filter designed for a certain spectrum to visualize a similar spectrum. In our laboratory, we use a DAPI filter to view the AMCA staining. For reasons such as this, it is a good idea to visit with a representative from a company that specializes in fluorescent microscopy for your particular needs.

2. Intracellular ice crystals may have formed during the storage in or immediately after extraction from the freezer. The crystals may burst and cause damage to the cell and decrease the success of the assay. To avoid complication, we immediately place slides pulled from the freezer into an ethanol solution.

3. Leaving the stain dry on the slide will cause autofluorescence when viewing with the microscope. This makes visualizing the probe signals difficult and may cause the assay to fail altogether.

4. Do not exceed 5 min. This step serves to preserve tissue morphology and to minimize loss of nucleic acids. Prolonged treatment causes excessive crosslinking of proteins, and the tissue becomes inaccessible for the probe. A permeabilization step with proteinase K may then be required.

5. Proteinase K acts by unmasking nucleic acids from associated proteins, leaving the tissue accessible for the probe. Overdigestion can cause loss of cells from the slides and create a "spilling out" of the probe signals from the nucleus, making analysis of the cell difficult, if not impossible. For this reason, we usually try to perform the FISH assay without the enzyme treatment on the initial specimen.

6. A cover should be placed over the hot plate to keep the slide protected from light.

7. Failure to bring the probe and hybridization buffer to room temperature will result in an increase in viscosity, leading to inaccurate measurement. This is a key mistake made by first-time users and will most likely result in failure of the assay.

8. Excess probe mix can be stored in a –20°C freezer and reused.

9. If a programmable hot plate is unavailable, a standard hot plate, an oven, or an incubator set to 75°C can be used and the slide removed after the allotted time. The important aspect is that the bottom of the slide be in contact with a 75°C surface to allow codenaturation of the specimen DNA and the probe.

10. We have left slides to incubate in a humidified chamber for several days with no problem as long as the box was kept moist.

11. The specimen can be damaged if force is needed to remove the cover slip. If the cover slip seems dried on, place the slide in a Coplin jar of 1X APK. Leave the slide submerged until the cover slip falls off the slide.

12. Verify that the 0.4X SSC is 70°C before placing slides in the Coplin jar. Placing additional slides into the Coplin jar can quench the temperature of the 0.4X SSC solution by 2°C per additional slide. The time submerged in 70°C 0.4X SSC may then need to be adjusted.

13. *Very important:* Make sure the Vectashield used does not contain DAPI. This altogether eliminates the benefit of the cIg staining, because all cellular nuclei will become positive. The rigors of the hybridization process can leave the tissue vulnerable to damage. Excessive pressure can lead to the cells looking shredded or ripped up.

14. If the AMCA staining is too intense or other non-PCs appear blue, one can decrease the concentration of the stain or skip **step 6** under **Subheading 3.1.** In addition, be sure to wash the slide for the appropriate time.

15. Here are some frequent problems and remedies:
    a. *All cells have no signal.* Make sure that the probe and hybridization buffer are at room temperature before measuring. Be sure tha the probe was added and mixed well before applying. Observe that there are no air bubbles after applying the cover slip before codenaturation. Double-check that the 0.4X SSC was made properly and that the temperature of the wash is 70°C.
    b. *Stained PCs have no signal but the non-PCs do.* The probe is having difficulty penetrating the cytoplasm of the PC. Utilize the enzyme treatment from **step 10** under **Subheading 3.1.**

c. *The signal is dim.* The probe and target are not adequately denatured. Increase the temperature to 77°C for 7 min. Be sure that the appropriate filters are used and that the mercury bulb has been used less than 200 h. Make sure that the slide hybridized at 37°C in a humidified chamber for a minimum of 12 h.

d. *The background is high.* High background with nonspecific signals all over the slide can be remedied with an increased time in the 70°C wash. Clean the slides with ethanol before making the cytospin.

e. *The morphology is poor.* The slides may have been too fresh to withstand the harsh conditions of the assay. Make sure that the slide is properly aged. Take great care when removing the rubber cement that the cover slip does not come off with it. When blotting the cover slip after applying the Vectashield, do not use extreme force.

Acknowledgments

This work was supported in part by Public Health Service grant R01 CA83724-01, The Mayo Foundation, and the "Fund to Cure Myeloma."

References

1. Dewald, G. W., Kyle, R. A., Hicks, G. A., and Greipp, P. R. (1985) The clinical significance of cytogenetic studies in 100 patients with multiple myeloma, plasma cell leukemia, or amyloidosis. *Blood* **66,** 380–390.

2. Sawyer, J. R., Waldron, J. A., Jagannath, S., and Barlogie, B. (1995) Cytogenetic findings in 200 patients with multiple myeloma. *Cancer Genet. Cytogenet.* **82,** 41–49.

3. Smadja, N. V., Fruchart, C., Isnard, F., et al. (1998) Chromosomal analysis in multiple myeloma: cytogenetic evidence of two different diseases. *Leukemia* **12,** 960–969.

4. Drach, J., Schuster, J., Nowotny, H., et al. (1995) Multiple myeloma: high incidence of chromosomal aneuploidy as detected by interphase fluorescence in situ hybridization. *Cancer Res.* **55,** 3854–3859.

5. Zandecki, M., Lai, J.L., and Facon, T. (1996) Multiple myeloma: almost all patients are cytogenetically abnormal. *Br. J. Haematol.* **94,** 217–227.

6. Fonseca, R., Ahmann, G. J., Juneau, A. L., et al. (1997) Cytogenetic abnormalities in multiple myeloma and related plasma cell disorders: a comparison of conventional cytogenetic analysis to fluorescent in-situ hybridization with simultaneous cytoplasmic immunoglobulin staining (meeting abstract). *Blood* **90,** 1558a, p1349.

7. Fonseca, R., Oken, M., Harrington, D., et al. (2001) Deletions of chromosome 13 in multiple myeloma identified by interphase FISH usually denote large deletions of the q-arm or monosomy. *Leukemia* **15,** 981–986.

8. Zojer, N., Konigsberg, R., Ackerman, J., et al. (2000) Deletion of 13q14 remains an independent adverse prognostic variable in multiple myeloma despite its frequent detection by interphase fluorescence in situ hybridization. *Blood* **95,** 1925–1930.

9. Facon, T., Avet-Loiseau, H., Guillerm, G., et al. (2001) Chromosome 13 abnormalities identified by FISH analysis and serum beta-2-microglobulin produce a powerful myeloma staging system for patients receiving high-dose therapy. *Blood* **97,** 1566–1571.

10. Avet-Loiseau, H., Daviet, A., Saunier, S., and Bataille, R. (2000) Chromosome 13 abnormalities in multiple myeloma are mostly monosomy 13. *Br. J. Haematol.* **111,** 1116–1117.

11. Fonseca, R., Harrington, D., Oken, M., et al. (2002) Biologic and prognostic significance of interphase FISH detection of chromosome 13 abnormalities (Δ13) in multiple myeloma: an Eastern Cooperative Oncology Group (ECOG) study. *Cancer Res.* **62,** 715–720.

12. Desikan, R., Barlogie, B., Sawyer, J., et al. (2000) Results of high-dose therapy for 1000 patients with multiple myeloma: durable complete remissions and superior survival in the absence of chromosome 13 abnormalities. *Blood 95,* 4008–4010.

13. Ahmann, G. J., Jalal, S. M., Juneau, A. L., et al. (1998) A novel three-color, clone-specific fluorescence in situ hybridization procedure for monoclonal gammopathies. *Cancer Genet. Cytogenet.* **101,** 7–11.

14. Fonseca, R. and Ahmann, G. J. (2003) Assays for neoplastic cell enrichment in bone marrow samples, in *Methods in Molecular Medicine, Vol. 85, Novel Anticancer Drug Protocols* (Buolamwini, J. and Adjei, A., eds.), Humana, Totowa, NJ, pp. 333–342.

7

Comparative Genomic Hybridization for Analysis of Changes in DNA Copy Number in Multiple Myeloma

Pulivarthi H. Rao

Summary

Multiple myeloma (MM) is a clonal neoplasm of terminally differentiated plasma cells (PCs). Conventional cytogenetic analysis is one of the widely accepted DNA genome-screening tools for identification of chromosomal aberrations in MM. The success rate of detection of abnormal karyotypes by conventional cytogenetic analysis in myeloma is very low because of the low mitotic activity and content of PCs in bone marrow. The advent of comparative genomic hybridization (CGH) has opened a new possibility for characterizing chromosomal aberrations in myeloma cells. CGH is one of the powerful global assays for detecting changes in DNA copy number in a given genomic complement. This method involves competitive hybridization of differentially labeled test DNA (tumor) and reference DNA (normal) to normal human metaphase chromosome spreads. Based on the relative intensity of the two fluorescent colors, regions of a chromosome with gain or loss can be identified in a single hybridization. One of the advantages of CGH is that it can make use of archival materials when frozen tissues are not available, thus greatly expanding the number of cases that can be analyzed. Prospective and retrospective application of CGH to tumor specimens would permit clinical correlative studies of changes in DNA copy number with a much greater power than conventional cytogenetic analysis. The detailed procedures for CGH, including DNA labeling, hybridization, fluorescence microscopy, digital image analysis, and data interpretation, as well as the limitations of CGH are discussed in this chapter.

Key Words

Multiple myeloma; genomic imbalances; comparative genomic hybridization.

1. Introduction

Conventional cytogenetic analysis is one of the widely accepted DNA genome-screening methods for identification of chromosomal aberrations in

From: *Methods in Molecular Medicine, Vol. 113: Multiple Myeloma: Methods and Protocols*
Edited by: R. D. Brown and P. J. Ho © Humana Press Inc., Totowa, NJ

multiple myeloma (MM) *(1–3)*. The success rate for detection of clonally abnormal karyotypes in short-term cultures of myeloma is limited because of the low mitotic activity of the plasma cells (PCs). Such a low rate of cytogenetic success introduces a bias in the representation of true genetic aberrations in the tumor genome. The molecular cytogenetic technique comparative genomic hybridization (CGH) enables identification of genomic imbalances in tumors without the need to perform conventional cytogenetic analysis. This approach has been utilized in MM to define changes in DNA copy number *(4–8)*.

CGH is one of the powerful global assays for detecting losses and gains in a given genomic complement in a single experiment *(9,10)*. This method involves competitive hybridization of differentially labeled test DNA (green) and reference DNA (red) to normal human metaphase chromosome spreads. The standard direct labeling protocol uses normal and tumor DNA that has been labeled by incorporation of fluorochrome-conjugated nucleotides. The alternative method involves a slightly different procedure using normal and tumor DNA that has been labeled with biotin or digoxigenin. This method requires additional steps for detecting these labels with fluorochrome-conjugated secondary agents. The repetitive sequences present in both genomes can be suppressed by adding an excess of unlabeled cot-1 DNA to the hybridization mixture or coprecipitating with the differentially labeled tumor and normal genomic DNA. Based on the relative intensity of the two fluorescent colors, regions of a chromosome with gain or loss can be identified in a single hybridization **(Fig. 1)**. If chromosomes or chromosomal subregions are present in identical copy numbers in reference and tumor genomes, the resulting fluorescence manifests as a mixture of equal red and green fluorescence intensities. If chromosomes are lost or chromosomal regions are deleted in the tumor genome, the resulting color is shifted to red. The increased green fluorescence on chromosomes indicates a gain of whole chromosome or chromosomal regions in the tumor genome. By this method, gains and losses in the tumor genomic complement ranging from entire chromosome or chromosomal bands can be detected, thereby providing a "DNA copy number" karyotype.

2. Materials

2.1. Human Lymphocyte Metaphase Chromosomes

1. RPMI-1640 medium (cat. no. 21870-050; Gibco-BRL, Gaithersburg, MD).
2. 200 m*M* L-Glutamine (cat. no. 25030-016; Gibco-BRL), 100 mL. Make 5-mL aliquots; add 5–500 mL of medium.
3. Penicillin/streptomycin (cat. no. 15070-014; Gibco-BRL). Make 5-mL aliquots; add 5–500 mL of medium.
4. Fetal bovine serum (FBS), qualified and heat inactivated (cat. no. 16140-022; Gibco-BRL).

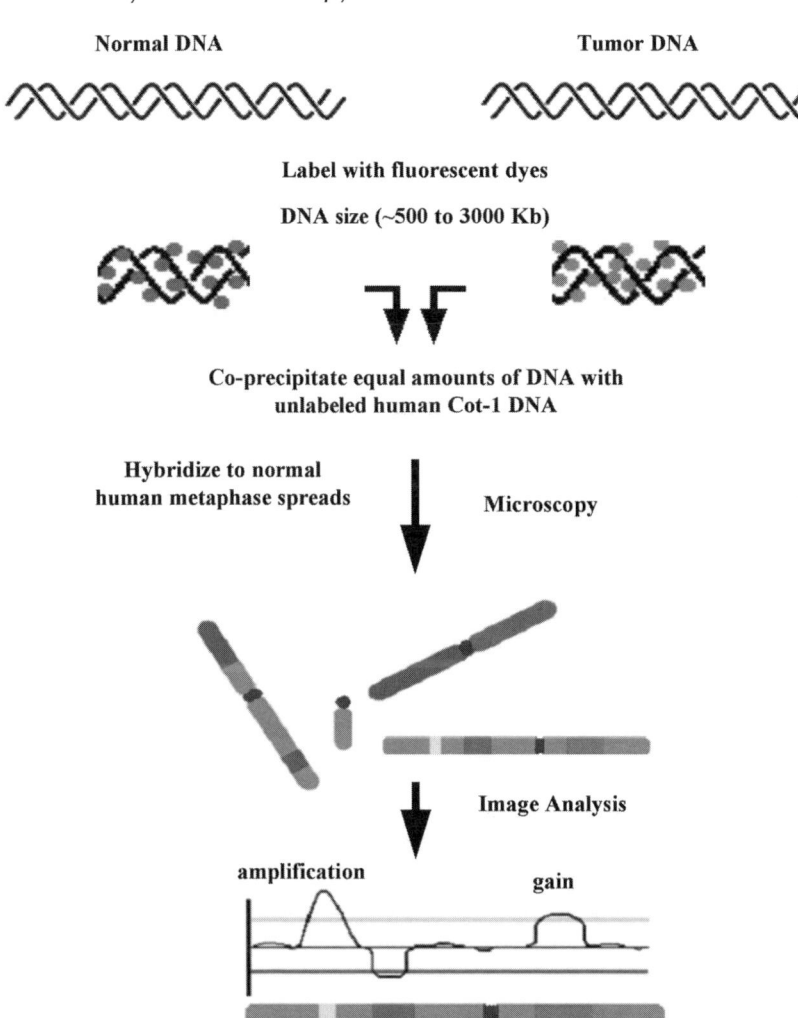

Fig. 1. Schematic outline of CGH method. Test and reference DNAs are labeled with green and red fluorochromes, respectively, and cohybridized to normal human metaphase chromosome spreads. Visualization of the chromosomes by fluorescent microscopy reveals differences in the fluorescent hybridization signals along the chromosomes representative of the abundance of the test DNA sequence. Analysis of these captured images can provide a color ratio profile indicative of changes in copy number in the test DNA relative to the reference DNA.

5. Phytohemagglutinin (PHA), lyophilized (cat. no. 10576-015; Gibco-BRL). Rehydrate 10 mL of sterile ddH$_2$O and store at –20°C.
6. Colcemid®, KaryoMAX Colcemid (10 µg/mL) (cat. no. 15210-016; Gibco-BRL).

2.2. Labeled DNA Probes for CGH

All solutions are prepared using standard conditions according to Sambrook et al. *(11)*.

1. 10X Nucleotide mix (*see* **Subheading 2.3., item 5**).
2. dTTP (25 µmol) (cat. no. 105 1482; Roche, Indianapolis, IN).
3. dATP (25 µmol) (cat. no. 105 1440; Roche).
4. dGTP (25 µmol) (cat. no. 105 1466; Roche).
5. dCTP (25 µmol) (cat. no. 105 1458; Roche).
6. Fluorescein 12-dUTP (cat. no. NEN-413; Dupont NEN, Boston, MA).
7. Texas Red 5-dUTP (cat. no. NEN-417; Dupont NEN).
8. DNA polymerase I (0.5 U/µL/0.4 mU/µL of DNase I) (cat. no. 18162016; Invitrogen, Carlsbad, CA).
9. DNA polymerase I (10 U/µL) (cat. no. 18010025; Invitrogen).
10. DNAse I type II (cat. no. D4527; Sigma, St. Louis, MO).
11. 2-Mercaptoethanol (cat. no. M6250; Sigma).
12. Agarose (cat. no. A9539; Sigma).
13. G-50 Sephadex columns (cat. no. 1523023; Roche).
14. Pepsin (cat. no. P6887; Sigma).
15. PN buffer (pH 8.0) (*see* **Subheading 2.3., item 6**).
16. Human Cot-1 DNA (cat. no. 15279-011; Invitrogen).
17. λ DNA/*Hind*III marker (cat. no. G1711; Promega, Madison, WI).
18. Formamide (cat. no. F 841; Fisher, Fairview, NJ).
19. 4′,6-Diamidino-2-phenylindole (DAPI) (cat. no. D-9542; Sigma).
20. Vectashield Mounting Medium (H-1000; Vector Laboratories, Burlingame, CA).
21. Diamond pencil.
22. Humidifier boxes.
23. Rubber Sealant.
24. Water baths (37, 45, and 75°C).
25. Circulating water bath (15°C) or polymerase chain reaction (PCR).
26. Glass slides (25 mm^2) and coverslips (24 × 50 mm).

2.3. Reagents and Solutions

1. DAPI:
   a. Stock solution (100 µg/µL): Dissolve 1 mg of DAPI in 10 mL in ddH$_2$O. Add a few drops of methanol to dissolve the DAPI before adding the ddH$_2$O. Store at –20°C.
   b. Working solution: Add 1 to 2 µL of DAPI stock solution to 1 mL of antifade mounting medium (Vectashield Mounting Medium). Aliquot into small brown tubes and store at –20°C.

2. Denaturation solution (pH 7.0): 350 mL of formamide, 50 mL of 20X saline sodium citrate (SSC), 100 mL of ddH$_2$O. Stir well and adjust pH to 7.0 if necessary with HCl. Store at 4°C.
3. DNase working solution (*see* **Note 1**):
   a. Stock solution: Dissolve 3 mg of DNase in 1 mL of 0.15 *M* NaCl and 50% glycerol. Aliquot 100 μL into small tubes and store at –20°C.
   b. Working solution: Add 1 μL of stock solution to ice-cold 500 μL of ddH$_2$O immediately before use; discard afterward.
4. Master hybridization buffer (pH 7.0): 5 mL of formamide, 1 mL of 20X SSC, 1 g of dextran sulfate. Make up to 10 mL with ddH$_2$O. Filter through a 0.22-μ filter and store at –20°C.
5. 10X Nucleotide mix: 100 μL of 10 m*M* dATP, 100 μL of 10 m*M* dGTP, 100 μL of 10 m*M* dCTP, 2.5 mL of Tris-HCl (pH 7.2), 250 μL of 1 *M* MgCl$_2$, 34 μL of 14.7 *M* 2-mercaptoethanol, 50 μL of 10 mg/mL of bovine serum albumin, and 1.866 mL of H$_2$O.
6. PN buffer (pH 8.0): 900 mL of distilled water, 1 g of sodium bicarbonate, 5 mL of Nonidet P-40. Stir well and store at 4°C.
7. Pepsin: A stock solution (10%) = 100 mg/mL. Dissolve in sterile water, make 50-μL aliquots, and store at –20°C. Mix 20 μL of pepsin in 100 mL of prewarmed 0.01 *M* HCl and adjust the pH to 2.0. Incubate slides at 37°C for 5–10 min and wash the slides in 1X phosphate-buffered saline (PBS) and 1X PBS/MgCl$_2$.
8. Washing solution (pH 7.0): 250 mL of formamide, 50 mL of 20X SSC, 200 mL of ddH$_2$O. Stir well and adjust the pH to 7.0 if necessary with HCl. Store at 4°C.

3. Method

3.1. Preparation of Human Lymphocyte Metaphase Chromosomes

The quality of metaphase spreads is crucial for CGH. The criteria for superior quality metaphase preparations include medium density, good spreading, slight or no cytoplasm, and little debris on the slide. It is better to avoid chromosomes that appear bright or hollow. Sometimes synchronized chromosome preparations will give granularity on the chromosomes, which can adversely affect the fluorescent ratios.

1. Prewarm 40 mL of RPMI-1640 medium containing 20% FBS, 1% L-glutamine, and 1% penicillin/streptomycin. Add 400 μL of PHA to the medium.
2. Collect 10 mL of whole blood in a heparin tube (green top).
3. Spin 10 mL of blood at 1500 rpm for 10 min or let sit at room temperature for 2 to 3 h.
4. Collect 2 mL of supernatant (lymphocyte layer/buffy coat), distribute to two to three T25 flasks or 10-mL tubes and culture for 72 h at 37°C (shake the flasks once a day).
5. Add 10 μg/mL of colcemid.
6. Transfer to 10-mL tubes immediately and centrifuge for 5 min at 1500 rpm.

7. Remove the supernatant and add 5 mL of prewarmed (37°C) 0.4% hypotonic solution (KCl) to each tube drop by drop, tapping the tubes, and add more 0.4% KCl to a total volume of 10 mL.
8. Incubate in a 37°C water bath for 15–20 min.
9. Centrifuge for 5 min at 1500 rpm and remove the supernatant.
10. Add 2 mL/tube of freshly prepared fixative (methanol:acetic acid [3:1]) drop by drop, tapping the tubes.
11. Add more fixative to total 10 mL/tube and let sit at room temperature for 1 to 2 h.
12. Centrifuge for 5 min at 1500 rpm and remove the supernatant. Repeat **steps 11** and **12** more than three times.
13. Resuspend in 1 to 2 mL of fixative per tube (depending on the size of the pellet).
14. Drop the suspension onto clean slides (dip the slides in ethanol and wipe with Kleenex tissue).
15. Check each batch of chromosome preparations for CGH and store at 4°C.

3.2. Preparation of Genomic DNA for CGH

High molecular weight genomic DNA from a normal donor (reference DNA) or from MM (test DNA) is required for CGH. Several DNA extraction kits are available commercially for genomic DNA preparation (Promega, Madison, WI; Qiagen, Valencia, CA). Degraded DNA should be avoided because it will yield probes that are too small on nick translation, thereby resulting in poor-quality CGH. The percentage of PCs in the bone marrow from a patient with MM is crucial for detecting genomic imbalances. If the PC count in the marrow is <40%, a normal CGH karyotype will result (*see* **Note 2**).

3.3. Labeling of Probe

1. To label test or reference DNA by nick translation, add the reagents in the following order: 1 µg of test DNA or reference DNA in 38 µL of ddH$_2$O, 5 µL of 10X dNTP mix, 1 µL of dTTP mix, 1 µL of fluorescein isothiocyanate (FITC) or Texas Red, 5 µL of enzyme mix containing DNA polymerase I/DNase I, and 1 µL of DNA polymerase I.
2. Mix the contents of the tubes well and incubate at 15°C for 1 h and 45 min (the nick translation time can be adjusted depending on the size of the genomic DNA).
3. Place the tubes on ice while keeping them protected from light.
4. Check the DNA fragment size by running a 1% agarose gel using a 3-µL aliquot of the reaction.
5. If the fragment size is in the appropriate range (500–3000 bp), heat the tubes at 75°C for 10 min, to inactivate the enzymes. If the fragment size is larger than 3000 bp, continue the incubation for another 15–20 min, adding 1 to 2 µL of DNase working solution if necessary.
6. Remove unincorporated nucleotides by running through a Sephadex G-50 column.

3.4. Purification of DNA

1. Allow a G-50 Sephadex column to warm up to room temperature. Gently invert it several times to resuspend the medium, while flicking it to remove any air bubbles.
2. Remove the top cap from the column, followed by the bottom tip. This sequence is absolutely necessary to avoid creating a vacuum and uneven flow of buffer. Place on a collection tube. Allow the buffer to drain by gravity and then discard the eluate.
3. Place the column and collection tube in a 15-mL centrifuge tube, and centrifuge for 3 min at 3000 rpm in a swinging-bucket rotor (*see* **Note 3**). Discard the eluted buffer.
4. Keeping the column in an upright position, carefully apply the DNA sample to the center of the column bed.
5. Place the column on a second collection tube while keeping it in an upright position. Centrifuge for 3 min at 3000 rpm.
6. Collect the eluate from the collection tube. This contains the purified DNA sample.

3.5. Precipitation of Probe DNA for Hybridization

1. Add 40 µL of FITC-labeled tumor DNA, 40 µL of Texas Red-labeled normal reference DNA, 20 µL of human Cot-1 DNA, 10 µL of 3 M sodium acetate, and 400 µL of cold absolute ethanol.
2. Mix the contents well and leave at –70°C for at least 1 h.
3. Centrifuge at 14,000 rpm for 30 min at 4°C.
4. Remove the supernatant. A good-size pellet should be visible at the bottom of the tube.
5. Wash the pellet with 500 µL of cold 70% ethanol.
6. Centrifuge at 14,000 rpm for 30 min at 4°C.
7. Remove the supernatant as thoroughly as possible. Air-dry the pellet in the dark for at least 2 h, until completely dry.
8. Resuspend the pellet in 10 µL of hybridization mixture. Mix thoroughly by tapping the bottom of the tube several times. Allow the pellet to dissolve over 2 to 3 h.

3.6. Pretreatment of Slides

1. Pretreat all slides before use for 1 h in 2X SSC at 37°C (*see* **Note 4**).
2. Rinse the slides in distilled water.
3. Treat the slides in an ethanol series (70, 80, and 100% absolute ethanol) for 2 min.
4. Air-dry the slides.

3.7. Denaturation of Slides

1. Place the slides in denaturation solution (70% formamide/2X SSC) for 2 min in a 74°C water bath. Denature two slides at a time.

2. After denaturation, immediately place the slides in ice-cold 70% ethanol. Wash the slides in 70, 80, and 100% ethanol for 2 min each.
3. Air-dry the slides.

3.8. Probe Denaturation and Hybridization to Target Chromosomes

1. Denature the probe in a 74°C water bath for 6 min.
2. On removal from the water bath, immediately apply the probe onto the slide and place a 25-mm^2 cover slip over the probe.
3. Seal the edges of the cover slip with rubber cement. Sealing the middle of the slide first will prevent the cover slip from moving when applying the rubber cement. Up to two probes can be applied onto the slide, using half the slide for each probe.
4. Place the slides in a humidified chamber (Tupperware with paper towels moistened with formamide solution). Incubate the slides at 37°C for 48 h.

3.9. Posthybridization Washes

1. Prewarm 50% formamide/2X SSC, 2X SSC, and 0.1% SSC in a 45°C water bath.
2. Remove the slides from the humidified chamber and carefully remove the rubber cement and cover slips from the slides.
3. Wash the slides in 50% formamide/2X SSC for 10 min.
4. Wash the slides twice in 2X SSC for 5 min each.
5. Wash the slides once in 0.1X SSC for 5 min.
6. Wash the slides once in 1X PN buffer for 5 min at room temperature.
7. Rinse the slides in distilled water.
8. Air-dry the slides in the darkness.
9. Apply 20 µL of DAPI/antifade across the slides.
10. Cover the slides with 24 × 50 mm cover slips.

3.10. Microscopy and Image Analysis for CGH

A fluorescence microscope equipped with a charge-coupled device and appropriate filters (DAPI, fluorescein, and Texas Red or rhodamine) is required to visualize metaphase spreads hybridized with differentially labeled test and reference DNA (**Fig. 2**). The differences in the relative intensities of the two fluorochromes can provide a color ratio profile indicative of changes in copy number in the test DNA relative to the reference DNA. The following criteria are essential for high-quality CGH:

1. Well-spread metaphase chromosomes with adequate length.
2. Uniform red and green hybridization (no granularity).
3. Red and green fluorescence distribution similar among two sister chromatids, two homologous chromosomes, and the same chromosome in all the metaphases.
4. Good DAPI banding for the identification of chromosomes.
5. Low and uniform background fluorescence level surrounding the chromosomes.

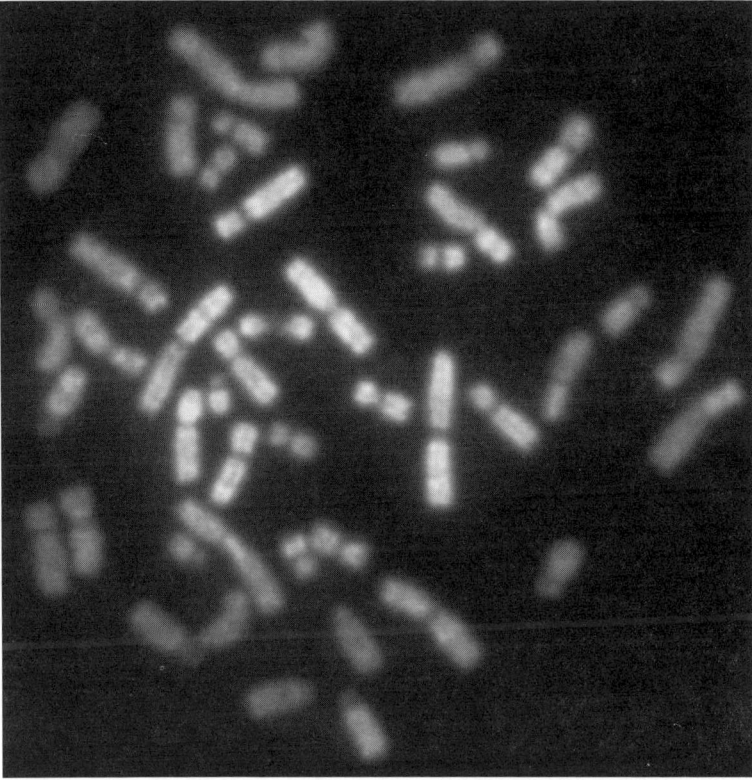

Fig. 2. Metaphase spread after simultaneous hybridization with differentially labeled normal (red) and myeloma DNA (green) by CGH. Chromosomal regions that were overrepresented in the tumor are visualized in green, whereas regions that were lost or deleted from the tumor are seen in red.

After the direct visual inspection, the metaphase chromosomes are subjected to quantitative analysis. This type of analysis can only be derived from digital imaging. Several digital imaging systems are available commercially for CGH analysis (Applied Imaging, San Jose, CA; Applied Spectral Imaging, Carlsbad, CA; Leica, Microsystems Inc., Bannockburn, IL; and Metasystems, Belmont, MA). By digital imaging, first individual chromosomes will be segmented, local background will be subtracted, and the median axes of the chromosome will be defined *(12,13)*. These chromosomes will then be normalized to standard length and combined in a minimum of 10 chromosomes to show statistically the mean and 95 or 99% confidence intervals of the red:green signal ratio. Control experiments (normal vs normal DNAs) are very helpful for interpretation of CGH results from tumor samples with a particular batch of slides and reagents. Only ratio changes that exceed the fluctuation seen in the control

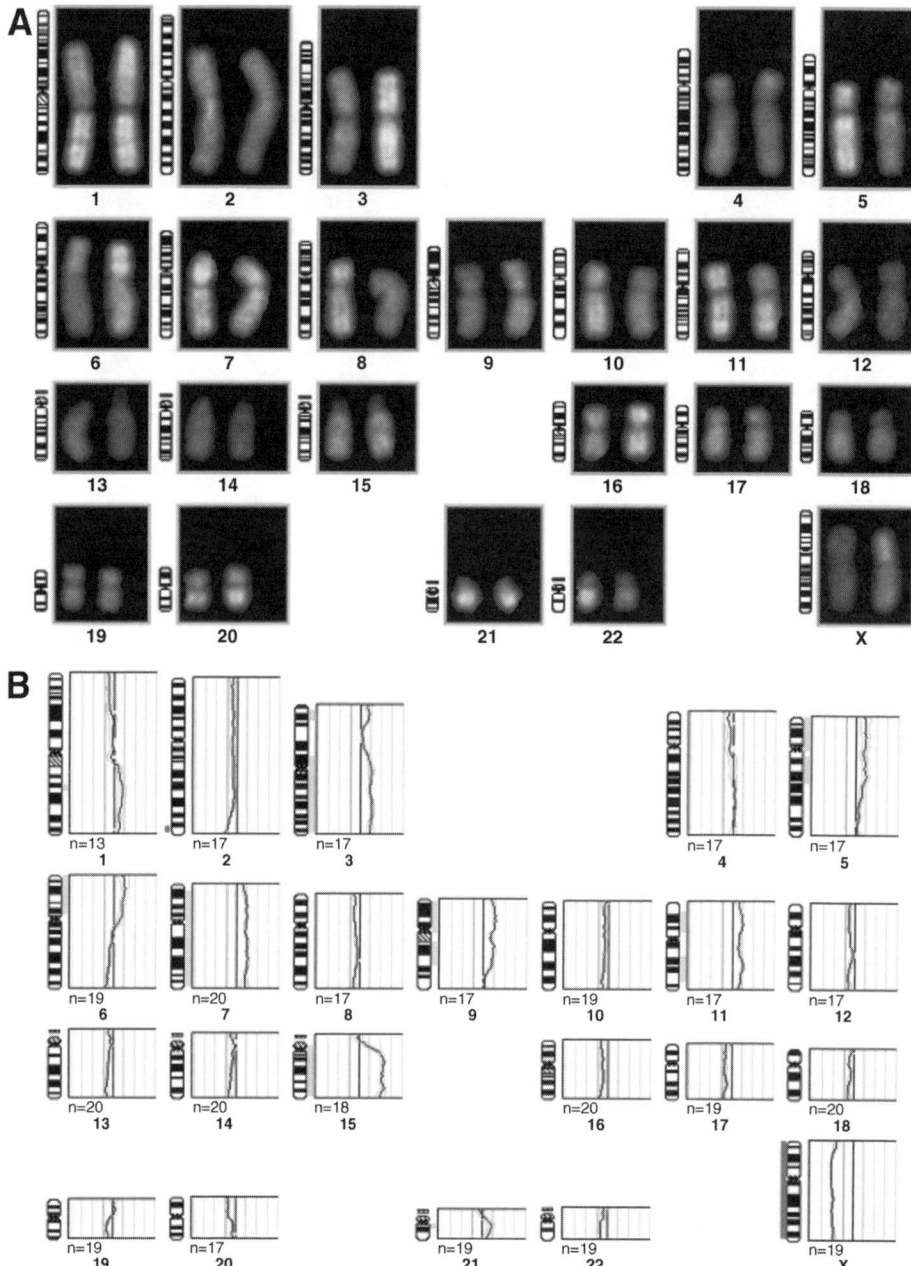

Fig. 3. Quantitative CGH analysis of myeloma. (A) Chromosomes from **Fig. 2** identified and karyotyped using quantitative imaging processing software (QUIPS; Applied Imaging). (B) Quantitative digital image analysis of fluorescence intensities ratios of MM (MM-14). Green-to-red fluorescence ratio profiles and shown for all

experiments are interpreted as evidence of real loss or gain in the tumor complement (**Fig. 3**). The normal variation in a given CGH experiment should not exceed ratios of 0.80 to 1.20 (±1 SD). In most cases, the telomeric, per-centromeric, or heterochromatic regions fall outside this range owing to low signal intensities. Therefore, these regions should be excluded from the analysis. In addition, caution should be exercised in interpreting ratio changes at 1p32-p36, 16p, 19, and 22 because of the high abnormal ratios in these regions (*see* **Note 5**). Gene or chromosomal amplifications (>10-fold) can be detected as strong localized FITC signal at the chromosomal site. For the precise assignment of amplification to chromosomal bands, the peak of the ratio profile should be compared with the corresponding DAPI band of the same chromosome.

4. Notes

1. Check the activity of DNase on normal DNA.
2. The PC count in the bone marrow is critical for detecting chromosomal changes in copy number in MM. If the PC count in the marrow is <40%, the resulting CGH karyotype will be normal. In those cases, the PCs can be separated using magnetic cell sorting against CD138 (syndecan-1) microbeads (Miltenyi Biotec, Aubwin, CA). The DNA extracted from sorted PCs can be used for CGH. However, the DNA isolated from sorted PCs may be insufficient for CGH analysis. Several whole genome amplification methods are currently available to generate the large quantities of DNA that are required for CGH and other genome-screening methods (*14*).
3. The speed and length of centrifugation should be calibrated for individual centrifuges.
4. Metaphase spreads that appear particularly cytoplasmic should undergo pepsin treatment.
5. Although CGH is a powerful genome-screening method, it has several limitations and complicating factors:
   a. Balanced translocations or inversions, point mutations, and intragenic rearrangements cannot be detected.
   b. Diploid and triploid/tetraploid tumors are not distinguishable.
   c. Changes in DNA copy number in pericentromeric, heterochromatic, and telomeric regions cannot be reliably detected.

Fig. 3. *(continued)* chromosomes. The mean ratio (blue line) and ±1 SD (black lines) of 13–20 measurements for each chromosome are shown. The ratio profiles for each chromosome are shown from pter to qter. The average value (1.0) representing the mean green-to-red ratio for the entire case (6–10 metaphases) and red and green lines indicate threshold values of 0.8 and 1.2 for loss and gain, respectively. Based on this analysis, the chromosomal regions that were overrepresented in myeloma case MM-14 were 3, 5pter-q15, 6p, 7, 9pter-q22, 11, and 15q, whereas X and 2q35-q37 were underrepresented.

d. Normal cell contamination in the tumor should be <40% to yield abnormal karyotype.

e. There is intratumor heterogeneity.

Another limitation of CGH is sensitivity, which is restricted to approx 10–15 megabases because of its dependence on the morphology of metaphase chromosomes. In addition, extensive follow-up work is required to identify candidate genes after regions of gain or loss have been identified. Recently, a new modification of CGH (array-based CGH) has been developed to replace normal metaphases as a platform with large stretches of human DNA (100–200 kb) packaged in replicable units called bacterial artificial chromosomes *(15)*. Although this method offers the promise of more power and sensitivity than CGH, the availability of high-quality arrays to investigators is still a limiting factor.

Acknowledgments

I thank Dr. Sheldon for critical reading of the manuscript and Charles P. Harris for excellent assistance with the artwork. This work was supported in part by Multiple Myeloma Research Foundation.

References

1. Sawyer, J. R., Waldron, J. A., Jagannath, S., and Barlogie, B. (1995) Cytogenetic findings in 200 patients with multiple myeloma. *Cancer Genet. Cytogenet.* **82,** 41–49.
2. Taniwaki, M., Nishida, K., Ueda, Y., and Takashima, T. (1996) Non-random chromosomal rearrangements and their clinical features and outcome of multiple myeloma and plasma cell leukemia. *Leuk. Lymphoma* **21,** 25–30.
3. Calasanz, M. J., Cigudosa, M. J., Odero, M. D., et al. (1997) Cytogenetic analysis of 280 patients with multiple myeloma and related disorders: primary breakpoints and clinical correlations. *Genes Chromosomes Cancer* **18,** 84–93.
4. Avet-Loiseau, H., Andree-Ashley, L. E., Moore, D., et al. (1997) Molecular cytogenetic abnormalities in multiple myeloma and plasma cell leukemia measured using comparative genomic hybridization. *Genes Chromosomes Cancer* **19,** 124–133.
5. Cigudosa, J. C., Rao, P. H., Calasanz, M. J., et al. (1998) Characterization of nonrandom chromosomal gains and losses in multiple myeloma by comparative genomic hybridization. *Blood* **91,** 3007–3010.
6. Gutierrez, N. C., Hernandez, J. M., Garcia, J. L., et al. (2001) Differences in genetic changes between multiple myeloma and plasma cell leukemia demonstrated by comparative genomic hybridization. *Leukemia* **15,** 840–845.
7. Nomdedeu, J. F., Lasa, A., Ubeda, J., et al. (2002) Interstitial deletions at the long arm of chromosome 13 may be as common as monosomies in multiple myeloma: a genotypic study. *Haematologica* **87,** 828–835.
8. Liebisch, P., Viardot, A., Bassermann, N., et al. (2003) Value of comparative genomic hybridization and fluorescence in situ hybridization for molecular diagnostics in multiple myeloma. *Br. J. Haematol.* **122,** 193–201.

9. Kallioniemi, A., Kallioniemi, O.-P., Sudar, D., et al. (1992) Comparative genomic hybridization for molecular cytogenetic analysis of solid tumors. *Science* **258,** 818–821.

10. Kallioniemi, O. P., Kallioniemi, A., Piper, J., et al. (1994) Optimizing comparative genomic hybridization for analysis of DNA sequence copy number changes in solid tumors. *Genes Chromosomes Cancer* **10,** 231–243.

11. Sambrook, J., Fritsch, E. F., and Maniatis, T. (1989) *Molecular Cloning: A Laboratory Manual*, 2nd ed., Cold Spring Harbor Laboratory Press, Cold Spring Harbor, NY.

12. du Manoir, S., Kallioniemi, O. P., Lichter, P., et al. (1995) Hardware and software requirements for quantitative analysis of comparative genomic hybridization. *Cytometry* **19,** 4–9.

13. Piper, J., Rutovitz, D., Sudar, D., et al. (1995) Computer image analysis of comparative genomic hybridization. *Cytometry* **19,** 10–26.

14. Lasken, R. S. and Egholm, M. (2003) Whole genome amplification: abundant supplies of DNA from precious samples or clinical specimens. *Trends Biotechnol.* **21,** 531–535.

15. Pinkel, D., Segraves, R., Sudar, D., et al. (1998) High resolution analysis of DNA copy number variation using comparative genomic hybridization to microarrays. *Nat. Genet.* **20,** 207–211.

8

Southern Blotting of IgH Rearrangements in B-Cell Disorders

Edna Yuen and Ross D. Brown

Summary

Southern blotting is a method whereby DNA fragments in the gel are denatured by soaking in an alkali solution, carried out of the gel, and transferred onto a membrane. After drying the membrane, the DNA is fixed irreversibly. The net result is a replica on the membrane of the DNA fragment pattern from the agarose gel. This technique is used to demonstrate B-cell clonality in blood and bone marrow down to the 1% level, though more reliably at the 5% level. The analysis is relatively nonselective and will detect novel rearrangements in relapse that were not seen at diagnosis. Modifications of the technique have been used to determine illegitimate switch recombinations and mutations of oncogenes.

Key Words

IgH; DNA extraction; gene rearrangement; Southern blot; B-cell.

1. Introduction

1.1. Principle of Southern Blotting (Fig. 1)

DNA is extracted from the tissue (blood, bone marrow tissue biopsies), digested with site-specific restriction enzymes, and the resulting fragments are separated by gel electrophoresis. The DNA is then denatured *in situ* and transferred and attached to a nylon membrane. A radio (or fluorescein)-labeled DNA probe specific for the gene in question is used to identify the appropriate DNA fragments by hybridization as detected by autoradiography or fluorescence. The size of bands complementary to the probe indicates the gene in question as germ line or rearranged. Deletions can also be recognized, as a reduced band size or as the absence of a signal, and may indicate the loss of DNA fragments. In this way, the Southern blot technique provides data on the

From: *Methods in Molecular Medicine, Vol. 113: Multiple Myeloma: Methods and Protocols*
Edited by: R. D. Brown and P. J. Ho © Humana Press Inc., Totowa, NJ

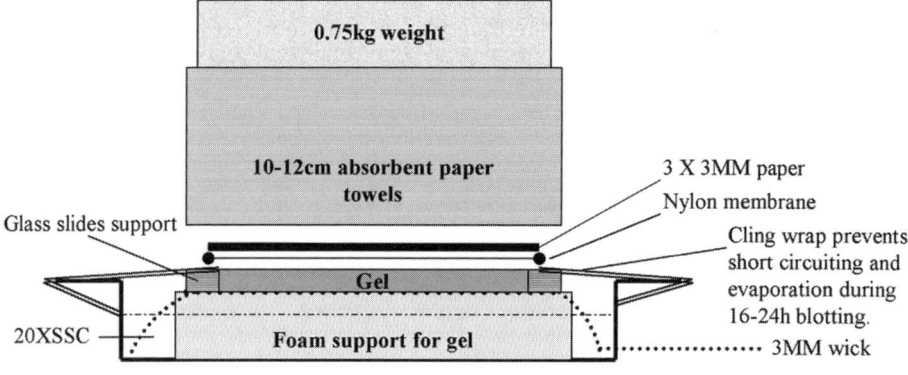

Fig. 1. Southern blot.

individual regions of a gene and will detect all copies of those genes present in a sample.

Southern *(1)* first described the basis of the Southern blot method in 1975. Restriction endonucleases are enzymes that recognize and cleave specific sequences within double-stranded DNA (dsDNA). These enzymes are mostly isolated from bacterial sources. A recognition site is a specific order of bases usually 4 (tetramer), 6 (hexamer), or 8 (octamer) bases in length. When a dsDNA molecule is cut with a restriction enzyme, smaller segments of DNA will be generated. For DNA hybridization to be performed, the dsDNA molecule must first be denatured. dsDNA is heated (>80°C) or alkalinized (pH >11.0) such that hydrogen bonds between nucleotide base pairs are broken and the two DNA strands separate. The solution now contains equal numbers of complementary single-stranded DNA molecules. This denaturation or melting of dsDNA is reversible. In appropriate conditions (e.g., slow cooling in the presence of NaCl at pH 7.0), the cDNA strands can reassociate by base pairing in the process of hybridization *(1–10)*. Over the past 10 yr, polymerase chain reaction technology has replaced the Southern blot method for routine detection of B-cell clonality; however, there are occasions when the Southern blot method is still more reliable *(11)*. Modifications of the technique have been used to determine illegitimate switch translocations in myeloma.

1.2. Clinical Significance

The sensitivity of the Southern blot technique used to detect clonality in residual disease is reported to be 1–5%. Although the method is laborious, the analysis is relatively nonselective and will detect novel rearrangements in relapse that are not seen at diagnosis *(4–6,8–10)*.

2. Materials

2.1. Solutions and Reagents

1. 5X ANE: 1.36 g of 0.5 M CH$_3$COONa 3H$_2$O, 5.84 g of 0.5 M NaCl, 0.372 g of 0.005 M Na$_2$EDTA, 5 g of 2.5% sodium dodecyl sulfate (SDS) (lauryl sulfate sodium salt, L5750; Sigma, St. Louis, MO). Make up to a 200-mL volume in H$_2$O. Aliquot to 20-mL tubes and store at –20°C. Once thawed, leave at room temperature.

2. B-cell IgH DNA probe: Dako IGHJ6 probe (1 µg/100 µL of TE buffer) code no. Y1420 (2003) or B-cell JH probe (400 ng/8 µL of TE buffer) Calbiochem cat. no. HLP02.

3. Chloroform-isoamyl alcohol (CIAA): Mix 20 mL of isoamyl alcohol (C$_5$H$_{11}$OH) + 480 mL of chloroform and store tightly capped at room temperature.

4. 100X Denhardt's: 2 g of Ficoll 400 (mol wt 400,000), 2 g of polyvinylpyrrolidine (mol wt 360,000), 2 g of bovine serum albumin (BSA) (product no. A2153, Fraction V, 96–99% albumin; Sigma). Make up to a 100-mL volume in H$_2$O. Dispense in 20-mL aliquots and store at –20°C.

5. 50% Dextran sulfate (sodium salt) (cat. no. D-8906; Sigma): Prepare in H$_2$O, warm, and continuously stir in a 250-mL glass beaker. Store at –20°C in 20-mL aliquots.

6. 500 mM Na$_2$EDTA: 18.61 g of Na$_2$EDTA in 100 mL of H$_2$O. Adjust the pH to approx 8.6 with concentrated NaOH so that the salt dissolves. Autoclave and store in 20-mL aliquots at 4°C.

7. 200 mM Na$_2$EDTA: 7.44 g/100 mL of H$_2$O. Store at 4°C.

8. 1% Ethidium bromide (EtBr) 10 mg/mL of H$_2$O. EtBr tablets (prepared for Sigma) (100 mg/tablet) (cat. no. E2515; Sigma).

9. EtBr destaining bags supplied by Continental Lab Products. Add one bag to EtBr solution overnight. One bag will remove 5 mg of EtBr from the solution. Pour the buffer down a sink and discard the used bag in decontaminated bins or incinerate.

10. Fetal calf serum (CSL Australia).

11. Ficoll-Paque (Amersham): a solution for the isolation of lymphocytes.

12. Ficoll/bromophenol blue, 100-mL stock solution: 15 g (15%) of Ficoll 400, 50 mg (0.05%) of bromophenol blue in 40 mM Tris buffer (0.48 g of Tris/100 mL of H$_2$O). Adjust the pH to 7.8 with 5 M HCl. Store stocks in 5- to 10-mL aliquots at –20°C.

13. Gel neutralization buffer (5-L volume): 876.5 g (3 M) of NaCl, 605.5 g (1 M) of Tris. Make to less than the required volume with H$_2$O, and then adjust the pH to 7.5 with 10 N HCl (about 300 mL). Make up to a 5-L volume, recheck the pH, and store at 4°C.

14. Genomic controls: normal controls from volunteers, positive controls from patients.

15. Hank's balanced salt solution (HBSS) without calcium and magnesium (cat. no. 11-100-0500V; Thermo Trace).

16. Lambda DNA-*Hind*III Digest (product no. 301-2S; New England Biolabs).

17. Lysing solution: 700 μL of 1 *M* Tris, pH 8.0; 182 μL of 4 *M* NaCl; 1.4 mL of 500 m*M* EDTA; 3.5 mL of 10% SDS; 0.0035 g of proteinase K (Boehringer Mannheim). Make up to a 70-mL volume with sterile H₂O. Immediately before use add proteinase K. Do not use a metal spatula to weigh proteinase K.

18. 1 *M* MgCl₂ stock solution: 10.17 g/50 mL of H₂O; autoclave and store at 4°C. To prepare 100 mL of 1 m*M* MgCl₂, take 100 μL of a 1 *M* stock solution and make up to 100 mL with H₂O.

19. Megaprime™ DNA labeling systems (cat. no. RPN 1606; Amersham). Check the manufacturer's table for relevant probe and prepare the dilutions as instructed.

20. 4 *M* NaCl: 23.38 g of NaCl/100 mL of H₂O. Autoclave and store in 20-mL aliquots at 4°C.

21. Nick translation kit (code no. 5000; Amersham).

22. Phenol saturated with Tris (*Caution:* Phenol burns, so handle with extreme care. Wear gloves and glasses. Burns should be treated with glycerol or polyethylene glycol solution, not water.)

   a. Dissolve phenol in an appropriate volume of H₂O. For 250 g of phenol add 27.5 mL of water. Stand the bottle of phenol in a basin of hot water to help dissolve the phenol. Keep the phenol in the dark and tightly capped to avoid oxidation and exposure to light. The basin of hot water may need to be changed. Cool before the next step.

   b. Add 125 mL of 0.5 *M* Tris, pH 8.0, and mix.

   c. Allow the phases to separate at room temperature and aspirate off the upper aqueous phase.

   d. Add 125 mL of 0.1 *M* Tris, pH 8.0, and mix.

   e. Allow the phases to separate at room temperature and aspirate off the upper aqueous phase.

   f. Repeat **steps d** and **e**.

   g. Wrap the tightly capped brown bottle in foil and store at 4°C. Prepared phenol should be clear. A pink tinge to phenol indicates oxidation, and, therefore, it should not be used.

23. α-³²P dCTP (Amersham or GeneWorks): check each batch for specific activity and concentration. The specific activity used in our laboratory is approx 3000 Ci/mmol (111 TBq/mmol). Also see ³²P Isoblue™ Nucleotides (ICN quote no. CRD030379).

24. Restriction enzymes: *Bam*HI, *Eco*RI, *Hin*dIII (Boehringer Mannheim).

25. Amersham BCS Biodegradable Counting Scintillant (code no. NBCS104).

26. Sonicated salmon sperm DNA (cat. no. 27-4565-01; Pharmacia Biotech) (100 U/5 g):

   a. Stock solution (concentration = 800 mg/mL): Add 6.25 mL of H₂O to a vial.

   b. Working solution (final concentration = 2 mg/mL): Add 0.1 mg of stock solution to 9.9 mL of H₂O (concentration = 8 mg/mL) and add all of this to 30 mL of H₂O to give a final concentration of 2 mg/mL. Before adding to hybridization buffer, boil for 5 min, chill on ice, and then add immediately to prewarmed buffer.

27. 20X saline sodium citrate (SSC): 876.5 g (3 *M*) of NaCl, 441 g (0.3 *M*) of Na₃ citrate. Make up to a 5-L volume in H₂O. Store in a cool atmosphere.

28. 2X SSC: 20 mL of 20X SSC in 200 mL of H_2O.
29. Sephadex™ G-50 fine (DNA grade) (code no. 17-0573-01; Pharmacia Biotech). Swell 2 g in 50 mL of TE buffer for 24 h before use. Store at 4°C.
30. 20 mM Spermidine solution (trihydrochloride crystalline) (S 2501; Sigma): Add 0.05 g of spermidine/10 mL of H_2O. Dispense in 2-mL aliquots and store at –20°C.
31. 10% SDS (lauryl dodecyl sulfate, sodium salt) (L 4390; Sigma): Wear a mask and protective glasses—causes eye and skin irritation. Place 10 g/100 mL of H_2O in a 250-mL glass beaker, warm, stir, and dispense in 20-mL aliquots. Store at room temperature or –20°C.
32. 1 M Tris $NH_2C(CH_2OH)_3$(hydroxymethyl) methylamine (BDH Analar 2-amino-2-[hydroxymethyl] propane-1,3-diol): 12.1 g/100 mL of H_2O, pH 8.0. Make up to less than full volume and adjust the pH with 5 M HCl. Make up to the required volume, recheck the pH, autoclave, and store in 20-mL aliquots at 4°C.
33. 10X TBE buffer (1-L volume): 108 g of Tris, 55 g of boric acid, 40 mL of 0.5 M EDTA, pH 8.0. Wrap in foil because 10X stock solution often precipitates out. It could be light sensitive, so store in the dark.
34. 0.5X TBE: Add 100 mL of 10X TBE stock solution to 2 L of H_2O.
35. TE (Tris-EDTA): 5 mL of 1 M Tris (pH 7.5–8.0), 1 mL of 500 mM Na_2EDTA. Make up to a 500-mL volume in H_2O. No further adjustment to the pH is required. Dispense in 20-mL aliquots and store at –20°C.

2.2. Equipment

1. Bio-Imaging Analyzer Bas-1000/1500 or equivalent, for faster results: The usual recommended exposure time is one-twentieth of the X-ray film exposure time.
2. Beckman LS 2800/LS5800 Series β Scintillation Counter Liquid Scintillation Systems: Consult the operating manual for details of the operating procedures.
3. 2X CRC Cassettes (35 × 43 cm) and 2X pair Dupont Cronex Intensifying screens (35 × 43 cm) (cat. no. 322202) (see later models).
4. Calibrated centrifuge, for column preparation: All centrifuges must be calibrated prior to use. The Sephadex columns are standardized so that the low-molecular-weight (LMW) labeled probe is collected into the microcentrifuge and the non-specific high-molecular-weight (HMW) unbound label is left in the column, which is discarded postcentrifugation. Calibrations should be done periodically. Recalibration must be carried out if the centrifuge is changed or if some other significant change in method occurs. To calibrate, follow these steps:
   a. Plug the base of a 1-mL syringe with a small amount of autoclaved glass wool. Stand the syringe in a 15-mL clear plastic tube.
   b. Add Sephadex G50 and pack to the top of the syringe. When packed, discard the TE buffer from the bottom of the 15-mL tube.
   c. Run 1 to 2 mL of TE buffer through the column to prime the column, and discard the TE buffer from the bottom of the 15-mL tube.
   d. Centrifuge at approx 2000 rpm (approx 550g) for approx 2 min; discard the TE buffer from the 15-mL tube.

e. Attach a 0.5-mL microcentrifuge tube to the base of the syringe and add 100 μL of TE buffer to the column. To establish the correct calibration, adjust the speed settings and time (use a stopwatch) until exactly 100 μL of TE is spun out into the microcentrifuge tube (usually about 550 g for 1.5–2 min). Repeat the procedure to validate the correct speed and time.

5. Sorvall Superspeed RC2-B centrifuge.
6. 3MM chromatography paper (cat. no. 3030917; Whatman).
7. Hybond-N Amersham nylon membrane (code RPN 203N) (store at ambient temperature).
8. Mesh (50 μ) supplied by Integrated Sciences (cat. no. HB-OV-RM).
9. Micro-4 Hybaid oven.
10. Hoefer Power Pack (model no. PS 500XT).
11. BRL horizontal systems tank for submerged gel electrophoresis (model no. H4-BRL cat. series 1025).
12. Hoefer HE33B Minnie gel tank horizontal agarose submarine unit. Insert an eight-well (1.5-mm well size) comb in the Minnie gel tank.
13. Ilford Anitec developing tray (27.9 × 33 cm).
14. Polypropylene tubes (30 mL and 50 mL).
15. Calibrated ultraviolet (UV) transilluminator (Ultra-Violet Products).
16. Certomat WR shaking water bath (type 886-441 DIN) or Labnet SW5050 shaking water bath.
17. Medical X-ray film (e.g., 35 × 43 cm Fuji New RX I.D. no. 036010).

2.3. Specimens

Specimens should be stored at 4°C and then processed within 3 d to buffy coat stage and stored at –20°C (*see* **Note 16**).

1. Peripheral blood: To obtain >100 μg of purified DNA, 2×10^8 mononuclear cells are needed *(10)*. If white cell count (WCC) is normal, 20–40 mL of whole blood is required and can be collected in EDTA, heparin, or acid citrate dextrose. Transport and storage should be at room temperature if processed within 24 h, or at 4°C if <72 h.
   a. Allow the specimens, normal saline, and Ficoll-Paque separating gradient to reach room temperature before proceeding.
   b. Dilute the blood samples 50:50 with room temperature saline.
   c. Gently place 20 mL of diluted blood over 15 mL of Ficoll-Paque solution in a 50-mL sterile polypropylene tube, avoiding disturbance of the blood/Ficoll-Paque interface.
   d. Spin at 400*g* for 25 min at room temperature.
   e. Pipet off the buffy coat layer into a 10-mL sterile tube. Wash the cells with cold saline and centrifuge at 550*g* for 10 min at 4°C; repeat three times. After the final wash, add just enough saline (~2 mm) to cover the cells, and store the buffy coat cells in a –20°C freezer.
2. Bone marrow (2×10^8 cells = 100 μg of purified DNA):
   a. Collect 2–5 mL of bone marrow in EDTA, heparin, or acid citrate dextrose or 2–5 mL of bone marrow into a sterile tube containing 0.1 mL of heparin

(1000 U/mL) and 0.9 mL of HBSS. The bone marrow sample must be prepared within 24 h of collection.

b. Wash the sample in 10 mL of room temperature saline, centrifuge at 550*g* for 5 min, discard the supernatant, and resuspend in 10 mL of room temperature saline.

c. Aspirate the bone marrow sample into a 10-mL syringe with an 18-gage drawing-up needle, and gently expel from the syringe through a 25-gage needle three times (this will break up the fragments).

d. Follow the procedure as for peripheral blood (**item 1, steps a–e**), except place the diluted bone marrow (10 mL) over 7 to 8 mL of Ficoll-Paque solution.

3. Methods

The major steps include preparation of samples for DNA extraction, extraction of DNA and quantitation of DNA by optical density (OD) measurements, restriction enzyme digestion of genomic DNA, preparation of agarose gels for electrophoresis, Southern blotting, column preparation for nick translation or megaprime DNA labeling using spun columns, prehybridization and hybridization, stringent washes, autoradiography, and interpretation of results. Gloves must be worn throughout the procedures (*see* **Note 1**). Store specimens/reagents on ice at all times.

3.1. Preparation of Specimens for DNA Extraction

Batching of specimens to be processed is encouraged. This depends on the centrifuge tube's capacity. Do not try to handle more than 10 tubes at any one time.

1. Take the frozen buffy coat and thaw slightly—do not allow the sample to warm up. Place on ice once thawed if there is to be a delay before the next step.
2. Wash with approx 10 mL of cold (4°C) 1 m*M* $MgCl_2$ to ensure complete lysis of red cells in the specimen. Centrifuge at 1200*g* for 20 min at 4°C to obtain a nuclear pellet.
3. Carefully aspirate the supernatant. Wash with approx 10 mL of cold (4°C) saline, shake vigorously, and centrifuge as in **step 2**.
4. Repeat **step 3**. Specimens may be stored at –20°C at this stage.
5. Prepare lysing solution immediately before use (*see* **item 17** under **Subheading 2.1.**).
6. Add 4 mL of lysing solution to the washed buffy coat, and disperse the material with a medium-width bore glass Pasteur pipet. Transfer to a clean 50-mL Erlenmeyer flask. Mix well by rotating but not inverting the flask.
7. Add another 4 mL of lysing solution to rinse out the tube, and then transfer this to the flask, giving a total volume of 8 mL of lysing solution per buffy coat, and mix again by rotation.
8. Incubate at 37°C overnight (4 h is sufficient; overnight is convenient).

3.2. DNA Extraction

1. Cool a Sorvall Superspeed RC2-B centrifuge to 4°C for at least 30 min before use. Add 0.20 vol of 5X ANE to the lysed buffy coat solution mixture and mix gently (i.e., for an 8-mL total volume, add 1.6 mL of 5X ANE). If 5X ANE is cloudy, put into a 37°C water bath for a few minutes. Wear protective eyeglasses and gloves, and working in a fume cupboard, do **steps 2–9**.

2. Add 4 mL of CIAA and gently mix. Then add 4 mL of Tris-saturated phenol, pH 8.0, and agitate for 3–5 min. Make sure the phenol and not the Tris is pipetted (*see* **Note 2**).

3. Transfer the material immediately to a 30-mL polypropylene tube. Centrifuge at 1350*g* for 20 min at 4°C.

4. Using a wide-bore Pasteur glass pipet, remove the upper phase (containing the DNA) to a clean 50-mL polypropylene tube. Dispose of the phenol/CIAA from each tube into an allocated waste bottle. Wash the tubes three times in tap water and three times in Milli-QUF PLUS H_2O (*see* **Note 3**) and drain (reuse these tubes for the next steps).

5. Repeat **steps 2–4** (i.e., a second extraction in CIAA/phenol).

6. Add 1 vol (8 mL) of CIAA and agitate for 3–5 min.

7. Transfer the material immediately to 30-mL tubes. Centrifuge at 1350*g* for 20 min at 4°C.

8. Using a wide-bore Pasteur glass pipet, remove the upper phase containing the DNA to a clean, sterile, new 50-mL polypropylene tube.

9. Repeat **steps 6** and **7** (i.e., a second extraction in CIAA alone) with clean, new tubes and remove the upper phase to clean, new 50-mL tubes.

10. Ethanol precipitate in 50-mL tubes: Add one-tenth vol of 4 *M* NaCl (800 µL) and a two times volume (i.e., 16 mL) of ice-cold –20°C 95–99% ethanol. Mix by gentle rotation, observe the DNA precipitation, and leave at –20°C for 1 to 2 h (may leave overnight at –20°C if necessary).

11. Transfer the precipitated DNA and ethanol to 30-mL tubes and centrifuge at 500–550*g* for 2 min at 4°C.

12. Carefully tip off the ethanol into a clean beaker (*see* **Note 4**).

13. Reconstitute the air-dried DNA in an aliquot of sterile H_2O, generally 200–500 µL, depending on the amount of DNA present. Refrigerate at 4°C overnight.

3.3. Reading OD of DNA

1. Use a medium-bore Pasteur glass pipet to transfer DNA from glass tubes to 1.5-mL polypropylene tubes for permanent storage in a freezer, if not required immediately. Otherwise, work the redissolved DNA to ensure a homogeneous DNA solution. More H_2O may be added if the DNA is too viscous.

2. Make a 1/100 dilution of DNA in H_2O in a polypropylene tube: i.e., 10 µL of DNA to 990 µL of H_2O. Lightly vortex to ensure a homogeneous DNA solution (*see* **Note 5**).

3. Read the OD at 260/280 nm (UV light, quartz cuvets) on a spectrophotometer.

4. Calculate as follows:

OD = $K \times C$ (concentration) $\times L$ (length of quartz cuvet) = 0.02 $\times C \times 1$ cm

For example, if OD = 0.108 = 0.02 $\times C \times 1$ cm, then

$$C = 0.108 \times 100 \div 0.02 = 540 \ \mu g/1000 \ \mu L$$

Therefore, for 10 μg,

$$10 \times 1000 \div 540 = 19 \ \mu L \ (\text{i.e.,} \ 10 \ \mu g \ \text{of DNA}/19 \ \mu L)$$

The ideal 260/280 OD reading is 0.08–0.12; ratio = >1.7 and <2.0. If >2.0 dilute with H_2O, if <1.7 repeat the ethanol precipitation steps but take into consideration the volume of the DNA, some of which is lost with every precipitation.

3.4. Restriction Enzymes BamHI, EcoRI, and HindIII: Digestion of Genomic DNA

The restriction of DNA is carried out in 1.5-mL microtubes. Wear gloves and store reagents on ice. Follow these steps to set up the digest:

1. For 1 μg of DNA, 2 U of restriction enzyme is required; that is, to 10 μg of DNA, add 20 U of enzyme. Ideally, the enzyme may be added in excess, say 30 U/10 μg of DNA, but enzyme volume should not be greater than one-tenth of total reaction.
2. Remove enzyme from the freezer for as short a time as possible and store on ice at all times. Always rinse enzyme into the mixture. Digests to which the enzyme has been added must begin incubation as soon as possible. One-tenth volume of 20 mM spermidine may be added to assist digestion.
3. When all the reagents are added, gently mix on vortex, or by flicking the tube with a finger.
4. Allow an appropriate time for restriction of DNA. Incubate the tubes at 37°C in a water bath overnight.

3.5. Preparation of Completed Digests for Electrophoresis

1. Remove the digests from the 37°C water bath and centrifuge briefly. Add 5 μL of stock Ficoll/bromophenol blue directly to the digest, gently mix, and microcentrifuge briefly. The samples are now ready for electrophoresis; store at 4°C if there is further delay.
2. Prepare a λ marker tube or a select suitable molecular weight marker for the expected size of the germ line and recombinant fragments.

3.6. Agarose Gel Electrophoresis

1. Prepare 0.5X TBE (100 mL of 10X TBE stock solution to 2 L of H_2O). For each BRL tank, prepare 300 mL of agarose; this gives a 6-mm depth (0.8% agarose = 2.4 g of agarose in 300 mL of 0.5X TBE in a 500-mL conical flask).

2. In a microwave oven, dissolve the agarose/TBE solution: high ≅ 5 to 6 min + defrost ≅ 4 min (settings for individual microwave ovens vary, predetermine for maximum effect). Ensure that the agarose is completely dissolved. Cool to <60°C by mixing gently with a magnetic stirrer on a hot plate. As the gel cools, 1% EtBr can be added.

3. Prepare a gel-former platform, and clean if necessary with dilute alcohol (10% ethanol). At both ends, press on a 250-mm-wide strip of masking tape to ensure a fluidtight seal. Set up in a level position with a medium-size (20 wells of 6.4 × 2 mm) comb in place. Gently pour the gel into the former platform. Remove any trapped air bubbles immediately with the point of a narrow plastic tip. Cover with aluminum foil for protection.

4. Allow the gel to set (1 h), wrap in plastic wrap, and store in a cool place. When possible, the gel should be prepared at least 2 h before use.

5. Fill the tank with 0.5X TBE, remove the masking tape from each end of the gel-former platform, and immerse in the tank toward the positive end. Notch the gel to mark lane one's position and carefully remove the comb (TBE buffer must completely cover the gel at a depth of 2 mm).

6. Load the samples carefully, making sure that the entire volume is added to the well (*see* **Note 6**).

7. Check that both the cathode and anode leads are correctly connected to the power pack.

8. Start electrophoresis immediately after loading the DNA samples. Electrophorese from the cathode end nearest to the wells to the anode end (nucleic acids migrate toward the anode end) at approx 40 mA, 30 V (constant voltage) for approx 18 h. Settings and time will vary according to the system in use.

9. Following electrophoresis, carefully remove the gel from the tank. Cut off the wells and excess gel at the anode end, ensure that the gel is notched for orientation, measure the gel, and record the measurement (*see* **Note 7**). Mix the buffer in the tank, and pour about two-thirds of it into a container. If EtBr was not added during the agar gel preparation stage, add 1 to 2 drops of 1% EtBr until reaching a faint orange. Stain the gel in EtBr solution for 5–10 min (no longer). EtBr may be reused for 3 mo. Take care with this carcinogen, avoiding all skin contact.

10. Wear a UV face shield to protect the face and eyes, and view the gel under a calibrated UV transilluminator (*see* **Note 8**). Place a ruler alongside the λ bands with the zero in line with the HMW edge of the gel from which an accurate assessment of DNA fragment size can be made.

3.7. Southern Blotting

3.7.1. Southern Blot Method

1. Place the gel in 1 *M* NaOH for 30 min to denature the DNA and shake gently, or for 60 min without shaking (20 g of NaOH in 500 mL of H$_2$O).

2. Place the gel in gel neutralization buffer for a minimum of 15 min to 1 h, and shake gently to bring the gel back toward a neutral pH.

3. Place the gel in 20X SSC for 5–15 min.
4. Choose a nylon membrane type according to the method used for Southern blot (*see* **Note 9**). Use a nylon membrane such as Hybond-N (Amersham).
5. Cut the nylon membrane to the size of the gel plus 5 mm. Cut three 3MM chromatography papers to the size of the gel less 5 mm. Cut a wick out of 3MM chromatography paper to the size of a tray plus extra length at the ends to overlap into the buffer.
6. Soak a sponge (medium-density foam) in a noncorrosive tray containing 20X SSC and carefully place the wick over the sponge. Gently press the wick over the edge of the sponge to reach below the surface of the buffer. Pour 20X SSC over the wick to wet it thoroughly. Ensure that there are no air bubbles or holes in the wick.
7. Carefully place the gel on top of the wick centrally positioned. Cover the gel and tray completely with cling wrap, and then slit carefully along three edges of the gel and peel back. The edges of the cling wrap must be closely butted against the gel edge on all four sides. This acts to prevent "short circuits" and evaporation.
8. Notch the nylon membrane to indicate lane one's position and label appropriately in pencil. Wet the nylon first in H_2O then in 2X SSC and place on top of the gel. All air bubbles must be excluded. Mark the membrane with a pencil along the HMW edge of the gel. The nylon should be moved as little as possible once contact has been made with the gel.
9. One by one, wet the three 3MM papers in 2X SSC, and then place these one at a time on top of the nylon. Place glass slides (equivalent to the height of the gel) around the gel edge for support.
10. Place approx 10–12 cm of paper towels on top of the 3MM paper plus a weight of approx 0.75 kg on top of the paper towels. Make sure that the weight is spread evenly. Check the level of buffer in the tray and that the 3MM wick is below the surface of the 20X SSC buffer.
11. Blot for 12–24 h.
12. After blotting, remove the membrane. Wash in 2X SSC for 10 s and air-dry for at least 30–45 min.
13. Wrap the membrane in cling wrap and place DNA side down on a UV transilluminator (calibrated for maximum time without damage to the DNA) to fix the DNA permanently onto the membrane. Store Hybond-N filters at 20°C.

3.7.2. Southern Blot by Alkali Method

1. Make a solution of 0.4 *M* NaOH: 32 g/2 L.
2. Place a medium-density piece of foam cut to 335×295 mm in a noncorrosive tray.
3. Fill the tray halfway with 0.4 *M* NaOH and soak the foam thoroughly, making sure that there are no air bubbles trapped in the foam.
4. Cut a wick out of 3MM chromatography paper the size of the tray plus enough to overlap the ends, and place on top of the foam in the tray containing the 0.4 *M* NaOH. Use a glass graduated pipet to remove any air bubbles by gently rolling over the 3MM paper wick.

5. Cut a positively charged membrane such as Hybond N+ (Amersham) the size of the gel plus 5 mm. Label with a pencil for orientation and cut a corner to mark lane one.
6. Cut three 3MM chromatography papers to the size of the gel (less 5 mm).
7. After photographing the gel for record purposes, place the gel on top of the foam, cover with cling wrap, and carefully cut the cling wrap around the gel. Butt the cling wrap around the gel so as to expose the top of the gel.
8. Wet the Hybond N+ transfer membrane thoroughly in 0.4 *M* NaOH and place on top of the gel, making sure that the orientation of the gel and the membrane match. Use a pipet to remove any air bubbles by gently rolling over the membrane.
9. Wet each of the 3MM papers separately before placing them one by one on top of the Hybond N+ membrane. Make sure that there are no air bubbles caught in between.
10. Place glass slides (the thickness of three slides) around the gel for support.
11. Place paper towels approx 10 cm thick on top and weigh down with an approx 0.75 kg weight. Do not move or bump once the blot is set up.
12. Leave 18 h overnight.
13. Wash the filters briefly ($\cong$10 s) in 2X SSC.
14. Blot off excess moisture and seal in plastic or wrap in cling wrap.
15. Store at 4 or –20°C. The filters are ready for the prehybridization step.

3.8. Probe Labeling

This procedure must be performed behind a Perspex shield (protects against exposure to β radiation).

3.8.1. Nick Translation Incubation Method

Nick translation buffer (NTB) and polymerase must be from the same batch.

1. Add in the following order:
   a. H_2O: XμL (sterile preferably).
   b. Tris buffer: 3 μL (nick translation buffer stored at –20°C).
   c. Ig JH probe: XμL =100 ng (stored at –20°C).
   d. α-^{32}P dCTP: 5 μL $\approx$3000 Ci/mmol (111 TBq/mmol).
   e. polymerase: 2 μL (polymerase in use is stored at –20°C; stock is stored at –65°C). The total volume = 20 μL. Set up the reaction in a 1.5-mL microtube and incubate at 16°C for 1.25 h exactly.
2. Stop the reaction with 10 μL of 500 m*M* Na$_2$ EDTA. Mix gently with a micropipet. Incubate at 65°C for 10 min, and store on ice. The probe is now ready for column preparation. Go to **step 4** under **Subheading 3.8.3.**

3.8.2. Megaprime Labeling System

1. In a 1.5-mL microtube, add in the following order 27.0 μL of H_2O + 1.0 μL of IGHJ6 JH Dako probe (50 ng) + 5 μL of primer for a total volume of 33.0 μL.

2. Boil the microtube for 10 min, chill immediately for 1 min on ice, mix, spin, and add in the following order 10.0 μL of labeling buffer + 5.0 μL of α-^{32}P dCTP (≈3000 Ci/mmol [111 TBq/mmol]) and 2.0 μL of enzyme for a total volume of 50.0 μL.
3. Incubate the megaprime-labeled probe in a 37°C water bath for a minimum of 60 min (overnight is convenient).
4. Stop the reaction by adding 5 μL of 200 m*M* Na$_2$EDTA. The probe is now ready for column preparation. Go to **step 4** under **Subheading 3.8.3.**

3.8.3. Column Preparation for Either Nick Translation or Megaprime DNA Labeling Using Spun Columns

1. Plug the base of a 1-mL disposable syringe with a small amount of autoclaved glass wool. Stand the syringe in a 15-mL clear plastic conical tube.
2. Add Sephadex G50 and pack to the top of the syringe.
3. When packed, discard the TE buffer from the 15-mL tube. Run 1- to 2-mL of TE buffer through the column.
4. Cover the top and bottom of the syringe with Parafilm™ and discard the TE buffer from the tube. Stop the procedure here, and proceed to probe labeling by either nick translation or megaprime methods. After probe labeling, continue on to **step 5**.
5. Remove the Parafilm from the top and bottom of the syringe, and centrifuge the column in a clear 15-mL tube in a designated centrifuge at a calibrated speed and time. Discard the 15-mL tube containing the TE buffer.
6. Attach a 0.5-mL microcentrifuge tube to the base of the syringe and add 100 μL of TE to the column. Centrifuge as in **step 5**. Repeat this step once (i.e., 2 × 100 μL of TE to prime the column). The column is now ready for the addition of nick translation or megaprime probe. Discard the microtube.
7. Label a new 0.5-mL microcentrifuge tube with the appropriate probe name, attach onto the base of the syringe, and place into a 20-mL Universal tube.
8. Behind the Perspex shield, make nick translation- or megaprime-labeled probe up to 100 μL with TE buffer, mix briefly with a micropipet, and immediately load all of the probe onto the column.
9. Centrifuge as in **step 5**. Check that the volume is 100 μL.
10. Check for two peaks; one is at the top of the column (containing the LMW non-specific bound ^{32}P + junk) with Geigy Counter set at IV. The second peak in the attached microtube contains the desired HMW specifically bound ^{32}P IgH probe. Carefully remove the microtube and place on ice. Discard the syringe (*see* **Note 10**).
11. Add 2 μL of probe in 10 mL of Amersham BCS Biodegradable Counting Scintillant. Use a β counter to estimate the counts per minute off of the column. To calculate the counts off of the column, use this formula: Volume off column × cpm ÷ volume added to scintillant. Ideally it should be approx 100 × 60,000 ÷ 2 = 31,000,000 = 32 × 10^6 cpm.
12. Store the labeled probe at −20°C if not used immediately. After removing from the freezer, immediately pierce the top of the microtube with a 21-gage needle, to

prevent pressure from building up in the tube and the lid popping off. Boil the probe for 5 min exactly and then immediately store on ice.

13. Add an appropriate amount of probe to an appropriate amount of hybridization buffer. Each filter requires $5–10 \times 10^6$ cpm in 2 mL of hybridization buffer. If the probe is used 1 wk later, add $10–15 \times 10^6$ cpm/filter.

3.9. Prehybridization

3.9.1. Prehybridization Mixture

To make the prehybridization mixture, *see* **Table 1**. Place at 65°C for a few minutes to remove the precipitate.

3.9.2. Prehybridization of Filters for Hybaid Oven

1. Prewarm cylinders to 65–67°C for 1 h prior to use. Each Hybaid cylinder will take two to three filters (20×20 cm²), holding a maximum of 20 mL of prehybridization solution:
   a. One filter: 5-mL small cylinder (HB-OV-BS) = 90 mL total volume.
   b. Two filters: 8- to 10-mL small cylinder (HB-OV-BS) = 90-mL total volume.
   c. Three filters: 10- to 15-mL medium cylinder (HB-OV-BM) = 150-mL total volume.

   This is a general guide and depends on the size of the filters.
2. Place filters, DNA side up on mesh in a shallow tray containing 2X SSC, and wet the filters and mesh well. Ensure that there are no air bubbles between the filters and the mesh, and then roll to form a cylinder (*see* **Note 11**).
3. Add 10–15 mL of 2X SSC to the cylinder, and allow the filters and mesh to unroll inside by gently rolling the cylinder horizontally. Pour out the SSC and replace with prewarmed prehybridization buffer (small cylinder: 5–10 mL of prehybridization buffer; medium cylinder: 10–20 mL of prehybridization buffer).
4. Add an extra 5–10 mL of prehybridization buffer for each filter.
5. Incubate for 4–24 h in a rotisserie oven.

3.10. Hybridization Using Hybaid Oven

1. Labeled probe is stored at –20°C. After removing from the freezer, immediately pierce the top of the microtube with a 21-gage needle to prevent pressure from building up in the tube and the lid popping off. Boil the probe for 5 min exactly and then immediately store on ice.
2. For a small cylinder, add the appropriate amount of probe to 3–5 mL of prewarmed hybridization buffer and mix. For a medium cylinder, add the appropriate amount of probe to 5–10 mL of prewarmed hybridization buffer and mix.
3. Pour in the probe/Hyb buffer mixture, and gently agitate the cylinder to ensure an even distribution of the probe in the hybridization buffer solution. Check that there are no air bubbles between the filter(s) and mesh.
4. Incubate overnight in the rotisserie oven.

Table 1
Prehybridization Mixture

Solution	Volume (mL)			Final concentration
20X SSC	15	or	30	6X SSC
100X Denhardt's	2.5	or	5	5X Denhardt's
10% SDS	2.5	or	5	0.5% SDS
Salmon sperm DNA (2 mg/mL)[a]	1	or	2	20 µg/mL
50% Dextran sulfate[b]	5	or	10	5% Dextran Sulfate[b]
Make up to final volume	50	or	100	Sterile H$_2$O

[a]Denature prior to adding to the mixture: Boil for 10 min, chill on ice, and add to the mixture at 65°C.
[b]Dextran sulfate is not used in some circumstances.

5. Carry out Hybaid oven stringency washes as follows using large volumes (approx 75 mL for a small cylinder, 100 mL for a medium cylinder) of the listed solutions prewarmed to the required temperature (*see* **Note 12**).
   a. 2 × 15 min with 2X SSC, 0.1% SDS at 65–67°C.
   b. 1 × 30 min with 1X SSC, 0.1% SDS at 65–67°C.
   c. 1 × 10 min with 0.1X SSC, 0.1% SDS at 65–67°C.
6. After the final wash, remove the filter(s) from the cylinder and blot off excess moisture but do not allow the filter(s) to dry completely.
7. Wrap in cling wrap before the next autoradiography step.

3.11. Autoradiography

Wear gloves at all stages, and prepare in a darkroom or use a phosphor imager for faster results (*see* **Note 13**). Disposable gloves, masking tape, scissors, a box of medical X-ray film (e.g., Fuji New RX I.D.), and cassettes are required. The following steps are for preparation in a darkroom:

1. Turn off the darkroom incandescent light and turn on the safe light (*see* **Note 14**). Remove two films from the box, notch both films for orientation, and place one on the bottom inside the cassette. Position the filters in the cassette (an intensifying screen is fitted one on each side inside the cassette). Record the orientation of the filters and film.
2. On the four corners of each filter, apply a small piece of masking tape, carefully place each filter on top of the bottom film, place the second film on top of the filters, and close the cassette.
3. Leave the filters in the cassette for 3–5 d at –65°C if β counts for the probe are normal. Different exposure times may need to be tried in order to obtain a suitable film for interpretation. Faint bands need >7–14 d, and heavy bands need <4 d.
4. Identify the films with the date, cassette, probe, and exposure time.

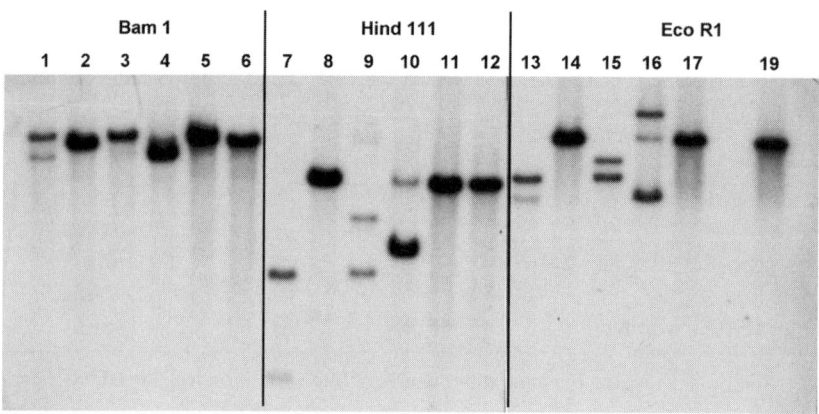

Fig. 2. Autoradiograph showing JH Ig gene rearrangements (r) and normal germ-line (g) controls. Plasmablastic cell line (MB2): lane 1 (*Bam*HI) = 2r; lane 7 (*Hin*dIII) = 1r; lane 13 (*Eco*RI) = 2r. Normal control: lane 2 (*Bam*HI) = g; lane 8 (*Hin*dIII) = g; lane 14 (*Eco*RI) = g. Plasmablastic cell line (SC5-F9): lane 3 (*Bam*HI) = 1r; lane 9 (*Hin*dIII) = 2r; lane 15 (*Eco*RI) = 2r. Patient 1 (prolymphocytic leukemia): lane 4 (*Bam*HI) = 1r; lane 10 (*Hin*dIII) = 1r; lane 16 (*Eco*RI) = 2r. Patient 2 (X-linked lymphoproliferative disorder): lane 5 (*Bam*HI) = g; lane 11 (*Hin*dIII) = g; lane 17 (*Eco*RI) = g. Patient 3 (B-cell non-Hodgkin lymphoma): lane 6 (*Bam*HI) = g; lane 12 (*Hin*dIII) = g; lane 19 (*Eco*RI) = g.

3.12. Interpretation of Autoradiographs (Fig. 2)

Results need to be interpreted in relation to other diagnostic tests such as flow cytometry, histopathology, cytochemistry, immunology, cytogenetics, and clinical circumstances. Clonal populations may be owing to reactive or transient populations that are not malignant. Only experienced personnel should interpret autoradiographs, albeit occasionally with some difficulty. The probe manufacturer's protocols and NCCLS guidelines are helpful in the analyses of results.

3.13. Stripping and Reprobing for Rehybridization (see Note 15)

1. Incubate the filter at 42–45°C for 30 min in 0.4 *M* NaOH.
2. Transfer to 500 mL of the following solution: 2.5 mL of 20X SSC + 5.0 mL of 10% SDS + 100 mL of 1 *M* Tris-HCl + H$_2$O. Incubate at 42–45°C for 30 min.
3. Proceed to prehybridization and hybridization or wrap in cling wrap and store at 4°C. To test for any traces of ^{32}P, follow the autoradiography procedure. It is preferable to prehybridize stripped filters before hybridization. Ideally, leave filters for 3 to 4 mo and do not rehybridize because DNA can be diminished, and remnants of probe used previously may interfere with interpretation of newly labeled probe.

4. Notes

1. Powderless disposable gloves must be worn at all times throughout the whole procedure.
2. When removing the upper phase, use the pipet gently to avoid disturbing and transferring the interphase. Care at this stage will ensure good-quality DNA.
3. Water = Milli-QUF PLUS water or equilavent.
4. DNA accidentally tipped off will then not be lost down the sink. If necessary, use a plastic tip to rescue DNA, *not* metal or wood applicators. Allow the DNA to air-dry for approx 20 min. It is important to remove carefully all traces of ethanol with a tissue from the sides of the test tube. Do not leave DNA longer than 30 min because human DNA becomes difficult to reconstitute if too dry.
5. Read the OD immediately, particularly if the DNA concentration is low. If the quantity of DNA is low (e.g., nanograms), add 10 μL directly to a cuvet containing 990 μL of H_2O and read the OD immediately (10–15% of the actual quantity of DNA may be lost if not read immediately). An ideal OD DNA reading should be between 0.8 and 0.12. A ratio of <2.0 is recommended. Otherwise, a partial digest may be present.
6. Occasionally, problems arise during gel loading when the DNA aliquot does not sink to the bottom of the well. This occurs when very high molecular weight DNA is present at the end of the digest and the digest is incomplete. Follow these steps to fix the problem:
   a. Run a small gel to test for incomplete digestion.
   b. Make a 0.8% agarose gel in 100 mL of 0.5X TBE buffer. Microwave to dissolve the agar. Cool to <50°C and gently pour into the unit, taking care to avoid bubbles. If bubbles are present, immediately use a narrow pipet tip end to remove the bubbles.
   c. If the DNA is stored at 4°C, heat to 56°C for 2 to 3 min before applying to the gel.
7. When handling gel, follow these steps:
   a. Cut off the wells as close to the well edges as possible. Be sure that the HMW bands are not accidentally removed. Remove excess agar from the LMW end of the gel. Bromophenol blue stain indicates the final position of migration; check under ultraviolet light.
   b. Handle fragile gel with extreme care. Spread both gloved hands under the gel for support while transporting the gel through each step.
8. Regarding the calibrated UV transilluminator, see the manufacturer's instructions.
9. Check manufacturers' guidelines for the most suitable types of membranes for use according to the method applied, and instructions regarding storage. After transfer of DNA from the gel to the nylon membrane, the gel may be restained with EtBr and checked under a UV transilluminator for completeness of the DNA transfer. Seal the cling-wrapped filters in plastic bags to prevent fungal/mold growth if stored in a refrigerator.
10. To dispose of α-^{32}P dCTP–labeled tubes, seal the Labeled probes in lead-lined cylinders, check every 6–12 mo for decay, and discard after the required safe level

is obtained. To dispose of nonsharp α-^{32}P dCTP wastes such as syringes and tips, place in a radioactive-labeled waste bag, keep for 6–12 mo in a Perspex box, check for remnants of radioactivity, and discard. To dispose of sharps, place in a designated plastic bottle, place in a Perspex box, and check for remnants of radioactivity as for nonsharps.

11. Multiple filters should be interleaved with more mesh, leaving the filter on top of the pile. Insert the roll in the cylinder in the right orientation, i.e., with the bottle opening facing front and the filter/mesh opening to the left.

12. An initial room temperature is not recommended and can cause background problems. The final wash is a high-stringency wash. In general terms, the stringency of hybridization and washing steps is increased by increasing the temperatures, or by decreasing the salt concentration. Hybridization should be carried out under relatively low-stringency conditions compared to the washing procedures. It is generally simpler and more effective to adjust the stringency during the washing steps by altering the salt concentration, rather than the temperature.

13. When using a phosphor imager, the usual recommended exposure time is one-twentieth that of X-ray film exposure time.

14. For medical X-ray films see the manufacturer's recommendations. To test the suitability of film, do the following:
    a. Turn off the darkroom light and turn on the safe light.
    b. Open the box of film and remove a sheet of film.
    c. Place a coin on the film emulsion side up.
    d. Expose the film for 2 min and process the film. If the outline of the coin is visible, then the safe light and/or darkroom conditions can be improved.

15. There are a number of methods for stripping and reprobing for rehybridization. We suggest using the method recommended by the manufacturer of the transfer nylon membrane.

16. DNA can be isolated from whole blood directly, but the heme group can interfere with some tests *(10)*.

References

1. Southern, E. M. (1975) Detection of specific sequences among DNA fragments separated by gel electrophoresis. *J. Mol. Biol.* **98,** 503–517.
2. Davis, L. G., Dibner, M. D., and Battey, T. F., eds. (1986) *Basic Methods in Molecular Biology*, Elsevier, New York.
3. Sambrook, J., Fritsch, E. F., and Maniatis, T., eds. (1989) *Molecular Cloning: A Laboratory Manual*, vol. 3, 2nd ed., Cold Spring Harbor Laboratory Press, Cold Spring Harbor, NY.
4. Warmington, J. (1990) *Molecular Biology in Medicine—A Workshop*, Curtin University of Technology, Perth, Australia.
5. Proctor, S. J., ed. (1991) Minimal residual disease in leukaemia, in *Ballière's Clinical Haematology*, Ballière Tindall, London.

6. van Dongen, J. and Wolvers-Tettero, I. (1991) Analysis of immunoglobulin and T cell receptor genes. Part I: basic and technical aspects. *Clin. Chim. Acta* **198,** 93–174.

7. Trent, R. J., ed. (1993) *Molecular Medicine*, Churchill Livingstone, Edinburgh.

8. Farkas, D. H., ed. (1993) *Molecular Biology and Pathology*, Academic, San Diego.

9. Farkas, D. H. (1993) Southern blot technology in the clinical laboratory: quality control and applications. *LabMedica Int.* **10,** 17–24.

10. National Committee for Clinical and Laboratory Standards (NCCLS). (1995) Immunoglobulin and T-cell receptor gene rearrangement assays; approved guideline. *MM2-A* Vol. 15, No. 18.

11. Bagg, A., Braziel, R. M., Arber, D. A., et al. (2002) Immunoglobulin heavy chain gene analysis in lymphomas: a multi center study demonstrating the heterogeneity of performance of polymerase chain reaction assays. *J. Mol. Diagn.* **4(2),** 81–89.

9

Identification and Assembly of V Genes as Idiotype-Specific DNA Fusion Vaccines in Multiple Myeloma

Surinder S. Sahota, Mark Townsend, and Freda K. Stevenson

Summary

Tumor-specific markers are important in identifying and tracking malignant cells. In this regard, functionally rearranged immunoglobulin variable (V) region genes in B-cell tumors fulfill and extend these criteria. V genes provide signature motifs in tumor cells and can delineate critical features of the clonal history of the cell of origin. They also define a tumor-specific antigen, which can be targeted for immunotherapy. Our focus has been on using novel DNA fusion vaccines to induce antitumor immunity. Here, we describe in detail the methods for identifying tumor-derived V genes at the nucleotide level in the malignant plasma cells of multiple myeloma. We further present the methodology for assembly of tumor V genes as single-chain variable region fragments (scFv), fused in frame with an immunopotentiating nontoxic bacterial sequence, Fragment C (FrC) of tetanus toxin. These scFv.FrC DNA vaccines provide protection in myeloma models and are currently in clinical trials. The vaccines are patient specific and can be rapidly assembled for clinical use.

Key Words

DNA vaccine; multiple myeloma; idiotype; immunoglobulion variable region.

1. Introduction

Immunoglobulin (Ig) variable (V) region gene use in B-cells underpins the generation of antibody diversity. At a primary level, this results from complex DNA rearrangement events in early B-cells. From a finite repertoire of germline gene elements, which are now mapped *(1–4)*, V genes are assembled by recombination among variable (V), diversity (D), and joining (J) gene segments *(3–5)*. A functional V-D-J transcription unit encodes the V_H gene and a V-J assembly the V_L gene, with expression driven by downstream enhancer

From: *Methods in Molecular Medicine, Vol. 113: Multiple Myeloma: Methods and Protocols*
Edited by: R. D. Brown and P. J. Ho © Humana Press Inc., Totowa, NJ

elements *(5)*. These transcriptional units encode core antigen-binding sites, which map to the complementarity-determining regions (CDRs), flanked by structurally important framework regions (FRs). Of these, the CDR3 is a signature motif for any given B-cell and its clonal progeny *(6)*.

The germ-line repertoire of V genes is now known, arranged at specific loci. The V_H gene segments are arranged as tandem clusters at the chromosome 14q32 locus *(1,2)*. There are 51 functional V_H gene segments that can be organized into seven families (V_H1–7) on the basis of nucleotide homology *(1,2)*. These map upstream of approx 27 D_H genes and 6 J_H genes *(7,8)*. Polymorphism in V_H gene segments is largely restricted, and known allelic variation can be accessed via available databases (*see* **Subheading 3.1.7.**). The V_L repertoire maps to distinct sites. For V_κ assembly, 32 functional V_κ segments can be grouped into six families (V_κI–VI), and together with five J_κ genes map to chromosome 2p11-12 *(3)*. V_λ gene rearrangement utilizes a pool of 37 V_λ gene segments that fall into 10 families (V_λ1–10) by homology, arranged upstream of seven J_λ-C_λ pairs on chromosome 22q11-2 *(4)*.

The singular combination of rearranged V_H and V_L genes defines specific epitopes that are recognized as idiotypes by induced antibodies. The V gene–encoded, functionally rearranged B-cell receptor allows the cell to enter the periphery. Here, antigen contact can lead to the initiation of somatic mutation, generally located in germinal centers (GCs) in secondary follicles of lymphoid organs *(9)*. At this site, T-cell help and associated cytokines are a prerequisite for maturation *(9,10)*. Somatic mutation alters the germ-line V(D)J elements of V genes in a highly specific manner, and these mutations, which occur at a high rate, can be readily tracked by immunogenetic analysis *(11,12)*. This potent mechanism provides the next tier of generating antibody diversity.

B-cell tumors arrest at multiple points along the differentiation pathway, and V gene sequence analysis can provide insight into the stage of arrest. It can identify whether the tumor is monoclonal or involves more than one clone. This analysis can also delineate any tumor-associated bias in V gene use and indicate whether the cell of origin has undergone any mutational events in the GC, and whether these events are ongoing. As a result, it is feasible to map B-cell tumors as having a pre-GC origin, as being located in the GC where tumors show intraclonal heterogeneity in V genes, or as being post-GC or postfollicular (reviewed in **ref. *13***). In multiple myeloma (MM), a disease of malignant plasma cells (PCs), V gene analysis has consistently revealed features indicative of a post-GC origin, in that V genes are mutated and show intraclonal homogeneity *(13)*. This indicates neoplastic arrest at a stage where somatic mutation has ceased. In the precondition to MM, monoclonal gammopathy of undetermined significance (MGUS), V_H genes have revealed that some cases display ongoing somatic mutation indicating a different clonal history of the cell of origin *(14)*. Other cases of MGUS reveal homogeneity of sequence *(14,15)*, but both presentations of disease can transform to MM *(15)*.

Defining V gene use in MM has delineated key aspects of ontogeny. It has also provided the basis for design of molecular probes to monitor minimal residual disease, and this is having an impact on evaluating outcome in the transplantation setting *(16)*. There has also been considerable interest in utilizing the idiotype in MM as a target for immunotherapeutic intervention. This is an attractive option because the idiotype is tumor-specific and obviates problems of nonspecificity. Our approach in this area has been to identify and utilize myeloma-derived V genes in a vaccine strategy, more specifically as DNA fusion vaccines *(17,18)*. DNA vaccines present an ease of manufacture in delivering a specific tumor-associated antigen and can activate multiple arms of the immune response, including innate mechanisms *(18)*. In our early experiments, we observed that idiotype delivery alone in a DNA vaccine format was weakly immunogenic *(19)*. By fusing idiotype genes to a foreign "danger" signal from fragment C (FrC) of tetanus toxin, we markedly potentiated the immune response, which proved protective against tumor challenge in a murine MM model *(19)*. FrC is critical in providing linked T-cell help in generating the immune response. These results then led to a clinical application of DNA fusion vaccines targeting idiotype in MM, and this trial is currently ongoing.

Given the range of potential applications of V gene analysis in MM, this chapter sets out to describe in detail the methodology required for an accurate identification of V_H and V_L genes in tumor cells. It also describes the protocols for assembly of these genes as single-chain variable gene fragments (scFv) in-frame with FrC to generate novel DNA fusion vaccines, for use in immunotherapeutic intervention strategies against MM.

2. Materials

2.1. Preparation of Mononuclear Cells

1. Lymphoprep (Robbins Scientific, Solihull UK).
2. RPMI-1640 (Invitrogen, Paisley, UK).
3. AB serum, batch tested (Sigma, Poole, UK).
4. Dimethylsulfoxide (DMSO) (Sigma).

2.2. Nucleic Acid Isolation and cDNA Synthesis

1. TRI reagent, chloroform, isopropanol, ethanol (molecular biology grade; Sigma).
2. Superscript II cDNA synthesis kit (Invitrogen).

2.3. Polymerase Chain Reaction Amplification

1. Oligonucleotide primers (Sigma-Genosys).
2. dNTPs (Promega, Southampton, UK).
3. HOT Start *Taq* enzyme and buffers (Qiagen, Crawley, UK).
4. Agarose (Sigma).
5. Sterile H_2O (clinical grade; hospital pharmacy).

2.4. Cloning of V Gene Polymerase Chain Reaction DNA Products

1. pGEM-T cloning kit (Promega).
2. Miniprep DNA extraction kit (Qiagen).
3. Luria-Bertani (LB) medium (Sigma).
4. Ampicillin (Penbritin, Uxbridge, UK).
4. Isopropyl-β-D-thiogalactopyranoside (IPTG), 5-bromo-4-chloro-3-indolyl-β-D-galactoside (X-gal) (Promega).
6. XL-1 Blue competent bacterial cells (Stratagene).

2.5. DNA Sequence Analysis

1. Big Dye Terminator v1.1 Cycle Sequencing Kit (Applied Biosystems, Warrington, UK).
2. 5X sequencing buffer (400 µL of 1 *M* Tris-HCl, 400 µL of 25 m*M* $MgCl_2$, 200 µL of dH_2O).

2.6. Assembly of Fusion DNA Vaccine

1. pVAC2 vector (modified from pcDNA3; Invitrogen).
2. Hi-Fidelity *Taq* enzyme with proof reading capacity (Roche, Welwyn Garden City, UK).
3. 10X PFU buffer (Roche).

2.7. Transcription Verification

1. TnT T7 IVTT (In Vitro Transcription and Translation) kit (Promega).
2. Full-range rainbow molecular size marker (Amersham, Little Chalfont, UK).
3. ^{35}S Methionine (Amersham).
4. Sodium dodecyl sulfate polyacrylamide gel electrophoresis (SDS-PAGE), gel-running equipment.
5. Ultraviolet light imaging equipment.

3. Methods

3.1. Identification of V Gene

3.1.1. Preparation of Bone Marrow Mononuclear Cells

Bone marrow aspirates are taken into lithium heparin or EDTA coagulant and processed as soon as possible without overnight storage. For PC leukemia, peripheral lymphocytes are suitable.

Bone marrow mononuclear cells are separated by standard gradient fractionation methods. Typically, bone marrow aspirates are diluted 1:4 using sterile cell culture medium (e.g., RPMI-1640) and layered (10 mL) over an equivolume of Lymphoprep and centrifuged at 2000 rpm at room temperature. Interphase cells are washed one to two times with medium before counting.

Bone marrow mononuclear cells can at this stage be directly lysed for total RNA or DNA or stored at –80°C prior to use. Cell storage medium comprises 50:40:10 (v/v/v) medium:stripped fetal calf serum:DMSO, and suspensions are typically frozen at concentrations of 1×10^6 to 1×10^7/mL. Storage requires a stepwise drop in temperature using cryopreservation protocols.

3.1.2. RNA Extraction

1. Rapidly thaw a vial of cells at 37°C, and spin down the cells (1300 rpm for 5 min). Wash once with sterile medium.
2. Resuspend the cells in a recommended volume of TRI reagent, and extract the RNA using the manufacturer's instructions in a triphasic separation. The DNA-containing interphase can be stored at 4°C for a separate extraction if required. Following a 75% ethanol wash, air-dry the RNA pellet for a few minutes and resuspend in RNase-free sterile H_2O. This can be stored at –80°C for long-term storage. Depending on yield, RNA is quantitated spectrophotometrically (A_{260}).

3.1.3. cDNA Synthesis

We employ the Invitrogen protocol for Superscript II for cDNA synthesis, but other suitable protocols can be used. RNA (up to 5 µg) is reverse transcribed using oligo-dT, the most consistent short-chain oligomer for cDNA synthesis in our hands, but random hexamers at 50 ng/µL and gene-specific primers (based on antisense C_H sequences) at 2 µM can also be used.

1. MIx RNA with oligo-dT and incubate at 65°C for 5 min. Then chill on ice for at least 1 min.
2. Add a mix of 10X reverse transcriptase (RT) buffer, 25 mM MgCl$_2$, 0.1 M dithiothreitol, and RNaseOUT-RNase inhibitor, and incubate at 42°C for 2 min prior to the addition of 50 U of Superscript II reverse transcriptase.
3. Incubate the reaction mixture at 42°C for a further 50 min, and terminate by heating to 70°C for 15 min, and place in ice (1 min).
4. Add 1 µL of RNaseH and incubate for 20 min at 37°C. The synthesized cDNA can be amplified immediately or stored at –20°C.

3.1.4. PCR Amplification of V Genes

Tumor-derived V_H and V_L genes are identified separately. For V_H, a mix of V_HLD 1–6 primers (**Table 1**) is utilized for identification of the full V_H sequence for scFv assembly. Additionally, an FR1 mix of V_H primers can be

Table 1
Oligomer Primers for Amplification of V$_H$ Genes

Primer	Sequence
V$_H$ sense (5′–3′)	
VHLD1	CTC ACC ATG GAC TGG ACC TGG AG
VHLD2	ATG GAC ATA CTT TGT TCC AGG CTC
VHLD3	CCA TGG AGT TTG GGC TGA GCT GG
VHLD4	ACA TGA AAC ANC TGT GGT TCT TCC
VHLD5	AGT GGG TCA ACC GCC ATC CTC G
VHLD6	ATG TCT GTC TCC TTC CTC ATC TTC
VH1FR1	CAG GTG CAG CTG GTG CAR YCT G
VH2FR1	CAG RTC ACC TTG AAG GAG TCT G
VH3FR1	GAG GTG CAG CTG GTG SAG TCY G
VH4aFR1	CAG STG CAG CTG CAG GAG TCS G
VH4bFR1	CAG GTG CAG CTA CAR CAG TGG G
VH5FR1	GAG GTG CAG CTG KTG CAG TCT G
VH6FR1	CAG GTA CAG CTG CAG CAG TCA
V$_H$ antisense (5′–3′)	
Cμ10	ACG AGG GGG AAA AGG GTT GG
Cμ100	GGA GAA AGT GAT GGA GTC GG
IgM	CGA GGG GGA AAA GGT
IgG 112	CTG AGT TCC ACG ACA CCG TCA
JHconsA	ACC TGA GGA GAC GGT GAC C
JHconsB	GTG ACC AGG GTN CCT TGG CCC CAG
JHconsC	TGA GGA GAC GGT GAC CAG GAT CCC TGG GCC CCA G

used if identification is for tracking the tumor clone. Downstream primer use will depend on the tumor isotype. J$_H$ consensus primers are also available and are obligatory if only DNA templates are used. For V$_κ$ gene identification, a mix of all sense primers is used with either constant region CK27 or CK69 (**Table 2**), and for V$_λ$ two separate mixtures of V$_L$1–4 and V$_L$5–10 are used simultaneously with either CL33 or CL85 downstream primers (**Table 2**).

Polymerase chain reaction (PCR) amplification is carried out for 30 cycles using 2–5 μL of template cDNA. PCR products are fractionated on a 1.2% agarose gel, and bands of predicted size are excised and amplified DNA eluted; agarose slices can be stored at –20°C prior to extraction of amplified DNA. We routinely use the Qiagen DNA elution protocol.

3.1.5. Cloning of V Gene-Amplified DNA

In cases in which the tumor burden is low, it is important to clone out V gene-amplified DNA in order to identify accurately the tumor-derived

Table 2
Oligomer Primers for Amplification of V$_L$ Genes[a]

Primer	Sequence
V$_K$ sense (5′–3′)	
VKL1 cons	ATR GAC ATG AGR GTS CYY GCT CAG CKC
VKL2 cons	ATG AGG CTC CYT GCT CAG CTY CTG GGG
VKL3 cons	ATG GAA ACC CCA GCG CAG CTT CTC TTC
VKL3.25	ATG GAA CCA TGG AAG CCC CAG CAC AGC
VKL4	ATG GTG TTG CAG ACC CAG GTC TTC ATT
VKL5	ATG GGG TCC CAG GTT CAC CTC CTC AGC
VKL6a	ATG TTG CCA TCA CAA CTC ATT GGG TTT
VKL6b	ATG GTG TCC CCG TTG CAA TTC CTG CGG
V$_K$ antisense (5′–3′)	
CK27	CAA CTG CTC ATC AGA TGG CGG GAA
CK69	AGT TAT TCA GCA GGC ACA CAA C
V$_λ$ sense (5′–3′)	
VL1 cons	ATGRCCDGSTYYCCTCTCYTCCTC
VL2 cons	ATGGCCTGGGCTCTGCTSCTCCTC
VL3 cons	ATGGCMTGGRYCVYWCTMYKBCTS
VL4a	ATGGCCTGGACCCAACTCCTCCTC
VL4b	ATGGCTTGGACCCCACTCCTCCTC
VL4c	ATGGCCTGGGTCTCCTTCTAC
VL5 cons	ATGGCCTGGACTCYTCTYCTYCTC
VL6	ATGGCCTGGGCTCCACTACTTCTC
VL7	ATGGCCTGGACTCCTCTCTTTCTG
VL8	ATGGCCTGGATGATGCTTCTCCTC
VL9	ATGGCCTGGGCTCCTCTGCTCCTG
VL10	ATGCCCTGGGCTCTGCTCCTCCTG
V$_λ$ antisense (5′–3′)	
CL33	GTTGGCTTGAAGCTCCTCAGAGGA
CL85	CACRGCTCCCGGGTAGAAGTCACT

[a]Primers should be diluted to a working concentration of 20 pmol/μL for heavy- or light-chain V gene amplification and diluted to 1.6 pmol/μL for DNA sequence cycle-sequencing reactions.

population. This method also allows an analysis of intraclonal variation in tumor-derived V gene clones, which is central to understanding ongoing somatic mutations.

Eluted PCR DNA is directly ligated into a vector such as pGEM-T for cloning in *Escherichia coli*. This vector allows the selection of cloned inserts using a chromogen-based (blue/white) substrate. Following ligation (1 h at room temperature using Promega 2X ligase buffer is sufficient), an aliquot is used to transform XL-1 Blue-competent bacterial cells (Stratagene), which are then plated on X-gal/0.1 *M* IPTG/LB agar + ampicillin (100 µg/mL) for overnight culture at 37°C. For each transformation, between 10 and 15 white colonies are picked and cultured individually in 2 mL of LB + ampicillin for approx 16–24 h.

Bacteria are harvested and extracted for plasmid DNA. We employ a column-based method for minipreps using Qiagen's protocol. Purified plasmid DNA is eluted in 60–100 µL of supplied resuspension buffer or sterile deionized H$_2$O. A small volume (2–4 µL) of plasmid is run on 0.8% agarose gels to check for purity and compare insert size. Plasmid DNA purified in this manner is suitable for cycle-sequencing protocols for analysis of DNA.

3.1.6. DNA Sequence Analysis

We employ an automated core DNA-sequencing facility, which uses the ABI PRISM 377 DNA Sequencer (Perkin-Elmer, CA) and the Big Dye Terminator v1.1 cycle-sequencing protocol (Applied Biosystems). For manual-based sequencing, standard molecular biology procedures are available utilizing radio-labeled dNTP and dideoxy NTPs *(20)*.

Cycle-sequencing reactions are carried using 3–5 µL of purified pDNA according to the supplied protocol in a 20-µL final volume for 25 cycles and then precipitated with 3 *M* sodium acetate, pH 5.2, and ethanol. Samples are resuspended in 1.2 µL of a 5:1 mix of formamide and dye-loading buffer for immediate analysis, or extended storage at –20°C.

Data files of nucleotide sequence and elution profiles are imported into relevant software for analysis. We utilize the MacVector 7.1.1 software for DNA sequence analysis, and the Edit View program for correlating elution profiles.

3.1.7. Analysis of V Genes

Proliferation and clonal expansion of a tumor clone will yield a dominant clonal V gene sequence, with a low degree of individual V gene sequences derived from copurified normal B-cells. The clonal, tumor-derived V gene is identified by a unique signature CDR3 motif in both V$_H$ and V$_L$ (**Fig. 1**).

Extensive databases exist for accessing human germ-line sequences of V$_H$ and V$_L$ genes. Two of the most robust on-line databanks available for real-time Blast comparisons are at http://www.mrc-cpe.cam.ac.uk/dnaplot and http://www.nlm.nih.gov/IGBLAST. These Blast comparisons will identify individual V(D)J gene segments.

Each sequence derived from cloned plasmid DNA is compared with the V gene database and verified as an Ig gene. Using CDR3 motifs, the dominant tumor-derived V$_H$ and V$_L$ genes are identified. Each sequence is translated to verify potential functionality of tumor V gene.

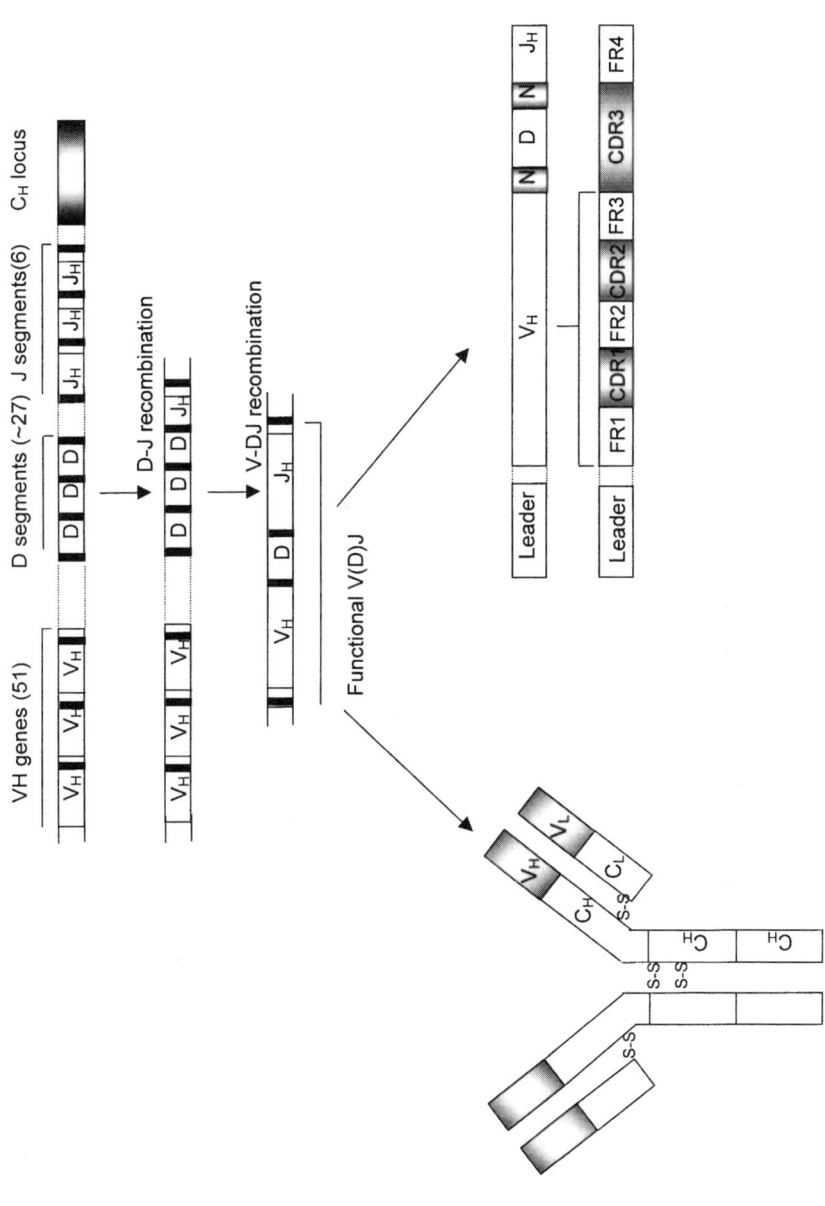

Fig. 1. Schematic representation of V, D, and J gene segments as arranged on chromosome 14q32 locus, representing available germ-line gene repertoire. Derivation of specific domains in the functionally rearranged V(D)J unit, encoding the V_H region, from individual gene segments is further delineated.

The Blast searches will readily determine whether the tumor V genes are somatically mutated or unmutated. It should be borne in mind that although a 98% homology to germ-line V genes can be of diagnostic relevance in B-cell tumors *(21,22)*, low levels (<2% deviation from germ line) may also be functionally relevant *(23)*. For myeloma, V genes are invariably mutated (reviewed in **ref. *13***).

Intraclonal variation among tumor-derived clones is assessed by aligning all clones with the donor germ-line V gene. Mutational variation within tumor clones requires verification in 2 or more clones and/or in replicate PCRs.

3.2. Assembly of Idiotype-Specific DNA Fusion Vaccines

3.2.1. Expression Vector

The expression plasmid is a modified form of pcDNA3 (Invitrogen) generated in-house, called pVAC2. The alterations are excision of the neomycin resistance gene, excision of the SV40 origin of replication, and addition of a V_H1 leader sequence as well as the gene for full-length FrC of tetanus toxin (1.4 kb) (unpublished data). The vector is engineered for cloning scFv inserts using *Sfi*I and *Not*I sites upstream of FrC.

3.2.2. Strategy for scFv.FrC Assembly by PCR Synthesis-by-Overlap-Extension (SOE)-ing

The objective of PCR SOEing is to fuse V_H and V_L tumor-derived genes in frame with a 45-nucleotide (nt) linker to generate the scFv for cloning into pVAC2. Specific restriction enzyme sites at the 5′ and 3′ ends of the assembled scFv allow positional cloning.

Primer design is based on the following format, shown schematically in **Fig. 2**:

1. Primer incorporating the *Sfi*I restriction enzyme site and the 5′ FR1 region of the V_H gene.
2. Primer incorporating the 3′ end of V_H and 5′ of linker (two-thirds of its length). Primer incorporating 3′ of linker (2/3 of its length) fused to the 5′ FR1 region of the V_L gene.
3. Primer incorporating the 3′ end of V_L and the *Not*I restriction enzyme site.

3.2.3. Assembly of ScFv

Plasmid templates for tumor V_H and V_L genes with verified sequence are utilized.

1. Amplify each V_H and V_L gene with extended primers (a + b1 and b2 + c). A high-fidelity *Taq* is essential, such as *Pfu* with a minimum number of PCR cycles (=25).
2. Check each PCR product on an agarose gel (1 to 2%), with an expected size of ≈450 bp.

1. V$_H$ + V$_L$ amplification

a. *Sfi* I FR1 (F)

b1+b2. Linker primers

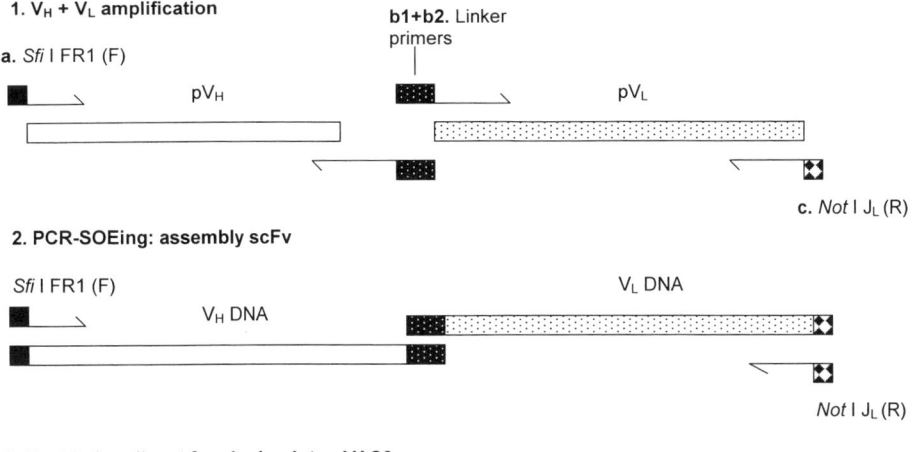

pV$_H$

pV$_L$

c. *Not* I J$_L$ (R)

2. PCR-SOEing: assembly scFv

Sfi I FR1 (F)

V$_H$ DNA

V$_L$ DNA

Not I J$_L$ (R)

3. Restriction digest for cloning into pVAC2

Assembled scFv

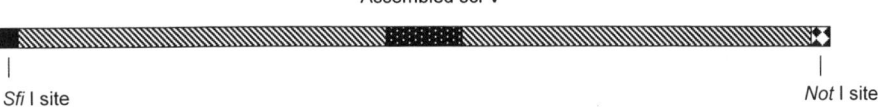

Sfi I site

Not I site

Fig. 2. Outline of stepwise protocol for assembly of an scFv from tumor-derived V$_H$ and V$_L$ genes. Forward and reverse primers with incorporated restriction enzyme sites (*Sfi*I and *Not*I) or linker sequences (b1 and b2) for overlap extension are utilized as shown.

3. Excise the amplified DNA and elute in an appropriate volume of buffer. This can be stored at −20°C.
4. Assemble the extended V genes by PCR SOEing using equivolumes of template DNA and high-fidelity *Taq*. An initial phase of five PCR cycles at low annealing temperatures may assist in obtaining optimal yields.
5. Run out assembled products on an agarose gel (1.2%) to check an expected size of approx 800 bp.
6. Excise the correctly amplified product and elute in an appropriate volume of buffer.

3.2.4. Cloning of scFv in pVAC2

Purified scFv DNA is sequentially digested to allow positional cloning. Between 7 and 10 μL of eluted DNA is digested first with *Sfi*I (2 h at 50°C), and *Not*I can be added subsequently (3 h at 37°C). Digested product is separated on a 1% agarose gel and eluted. The digest can now be ligated into the pVAC2 vector, linearized with the same restriction enzymes. Ligation and cloning in *E. coli* follows standard protocols (*see* **Subheading 3.1.5.**). Between

5 and 10 colonies are randomly selected and amplified by overnight culture using ampicillin selection. Plasmid DNA is purified by the miniprep method.

It is important to sequence the complete insert, and sequence integrity needs to be verified across the cloning sites as being in frame with the upstream V_H leader and downstream FrC gene segments. For sequencing, both T7 and SP6 vector primers, and primers based on the linker sequence, are utilized. An FrC 92 REV primer (5′-TCGTTGTTGATGTCCAAG) is also useful.

A transcriptionally functional assembly of scFv.FrC will need to be determined. We utilize the Promega TnT T7 IVTT Kit to verify the correct size of the expressed protein resulting from transcription of the scFv.FrC fusion gene. This procedure uses radiolabeled methionine (^{35}S) incorporation. For template, 1 μL of p[scFv.FrC] is used. Following the IVTT reaction, synthesized protein is denatured at 100°C for 5 min and resolved together with size markers on a 4–12% SDS-PAGE precast gel (200 V for 50 min). The gel is dried and exposed for autoradiographic detection overnight. For a correctly translated scFv.FrC construct, the protein size should be between 75 and 85 kDa, based on an average 2.2 kb for the construct and 110 Daltons for each amino acid.

In vivo responses to the assembled scFv.FrC DNA fusion vaccine are also assessed using wild-type mice, and we have reported this methodology elsewhere *(24)*. Antibody responses to both scFv and FrC are measured *(24)*.

Following these quality controls, the construct is ready for clinical use. The DNA fusion vaccine must then be produced under stringent good manufacturing procedures prior to vaccination in MM patients, or healthy donors of allogeneic transplants *(18)*.

4. Notes

1. An aliquot of bone marrow mononuclear cells, typically 1×10^6 to 1×10^7, resuspended in 1 mL of TRI-reagent for RNA/DNA extraction can be directly stored at –80°C for subsequent extraction. This suspension is also amenable to shipment in order to minimize loss of RNA integrity.

2. To identify the tumor-derived clonal sequence, >3/10 clones sequenced must display the same CDR3 V gene sequence, and this will require confirmation by replicate PCR and cloning analysis.

3. The validity of using the CDR3 motif-based procedure to identify the tumor-derived idiotype has been demonstrated by analysis of xenogeneic murine anti-Id antibody responses to human myeloma p[scFv.FrC] vaccines *(24)*. Notably, anti-Id antibodies were highly specific and were focused largely on private Id determinants of the corresponding natural human tumor-derived Ig, purified from serum.

4. When using an FR1 mix of PCR primers, care must be taken in excluding primer sequences from calculating homologies to germ-line donor V genes. Mutations

in the last codon in FR3 can be included in assessments of the percentage of homology to germ line if followed by a 2-nt match to donor gene. For patient-specific scFv.FrC assembly, the complete sequence should ideally be assessed using leader primers with downstream constant region primers.

5. Identification of D segment use follows the criteria delineated by Corbett et al. *(7)*. An accurate determination of intraclonal sequence heterogeneity in tumor-derived clones is based on the same mutation being identified in 2 or more clones and/or from separate PCRs.

6. A cutoff value of ≥98% homology has been used to determine mutational status in leukemic cells, to allow for unknown allelic differences, and this has been of prognostic importance in chronic lymphocytic leukemia *(21,22)*. However, a low level of mutation, <2% in deviation from germ line, and verified by replicate analysis may also be significant to ascribe a mutational status *(25)*.

7. For PCR SOEing, primers must be high-performance liquid chromatography purified to prevent erroneous incorporation, which will affect the coding sequence or restriction enzyme sites. Optional primers can also be designed in V_H or V_L to assist in sequence verification of the insert, especially across flanking restriction sites.

Acknowledgments

This work was funded by the Leukaemia Research Fund (UK), and the Multiple Myeloma Research Foundation (US). SSS is an LRF senior scientist.

References

1. Cook, G. P. and Tomlinson, I. M. (1995) The human immunoglobulin V_H repertoire. *Immunol. Today* **16,** 237–242.

2. Matsuda, F., Ishii, K., Bourvagnet, P., et al. (1998) The complete nucleotide sequence of the human immunoglobulin heavy chain variable region locus. *J. Exp. Med.* **188,** 2151–2162.

3. Zachau, H. G. (1995) The human immunoglobulin κ genes, in *Immunoglobulin Genes* (Honjo, T. and Alt, F. W., eds.), Academic, San Diego, pp. 173–191.

4. Williams, S. C., Frippiat, J.-P., Tomlinson, I. M., Ignatovich, O., Lefranc, M.-P., and Winter, G. (1996) Sequence and evolution of the human germline Vλ repertoire. *J. Mol. Biol.* **264,** 220–232.

5. Okada, A. and Alt, F. W. (1994) Mechanisms that control antigen receptor variable region gene assembly. *Semin. Immunol.* **6,** 185–196.

6. Kirkham, P. M. and Schroeder, H. W., Jr. (1994) Antibody structure and the evolution of immunoglobulin V gene segments. *Semin. Immunol.* **6,** 347–360.

7. Corbett, S. J., Tomlinson, I. M., Sonnhammer, E. L. L., Buck, D., and Winter, G. (1997) Sequence of the human immunoglobulin diversity (D) segment locus: a systematic analysis provides no evidence for the use of DIR segment, inverted D segments, "minor" D segments or D-D recombination. *J. Mol. Biol.* **270,** 587–597.

8. Ravetch, J. V., Siebenlist, U., Korsmeyer, S., Waldmann, T., and Leder, P. (1981) Structure of the human immunoglobulin mu locus: characteristics of embryonic and rearranged J and D genes. *Cell* **27,** 583–591.

9. Berek, C. (1992) The development of B cells and the B-cell repertoire in the microenvironment of the germinal center. *Immunol. Rev.* **126,** 5–19.

10. MacLennan, I. C. (1994) Germinal centers. *Annu. Rev. Immunol.* **12,** 117–139.

11. Dorner, T., Foster, S. J., Brezinschek, H. P., and Lipsky, P. E. (1998) Analysis of the targeting of the hypermutational machinery and the impact of subsequent selection on the distribution of nucleotide changes in human VHDJH rearrangements. *Immunol. Rev.* **162,** 161–171.

12. Goossens, T., Klein, U., and Kuppers, R. (1998) Frequent occurrence of deletions and duplications during somatic hypermutation: implications for oncogene translocations and heavy chain disease. *Proc. Natl. Acad. Sci. USA* **95,** 2463–2468.

13. Stevenson, F. K., Sahota, S. S., Ottensmeier, C. H., Zhu, D., Forconi, F., and Hamblin, T. J. (2001) The occurrence and significance of V gene mutations in B cell–derived human malignancy. *Adv. Cancer Res.* **83,** 81–116.

14. Sahota, S. S., Leo, R., Hamblin, T. J., and Stevenson, F. K. (1996) Ig V$_H$ gene mutational patterns indicate different tumor cell status in human myeloma and monoclonal gammopathy of undetermined significance. *Blood* **87,** 746–755.

15. Zojer, N., Ludwig, H., Fiegl, M., Stevenson, F. K., and Sahota, S. S. (2003) Patterns of somatic mutations in VH genes reveal pathways of clonal transformation from MGUS to multiple myeloma. *Blood* **101,** 4137–4139.

16. Voena, C., Malnati, M., Majolino, I., et al. (2003) Detection of minimal residual disease by real-time PCR can be used as a surrogate marker to evaluate the graft-versus-myeloma effect after allogeneic stem cell transplantation. *Bone Marrow Transplant.* **32,** 791–793.

17. Hawkins, R. E., Zhu, D., Ovecka, M., et al. (1994) Idiotypic vaccination against human B-cell lymphoma: rescue of variable region gene sequences from biopsy material for assembly as single-chain Fv personal vaccines. *Blood* **83,** 3279–3288.

18. Zhu, D., Rice, J., Savelyeva, N., and Stevenson, F. K. (2001) DNA fusion vaccines against B-cell tumors. *Trends Mol. Med.* **12,** 566–572.

19. King, C. A., Spellerberg, M. B., Zhu, D., et al. (1998) DNA vaccines with single-chain Fv fused to fragment C of tetanus toxin induce protective immunity against lymphoma and myeloma. *Nat. Med.* **4,** 1281–1286.

20. Sambrook, J., Fritsch, E. F., and Maniatis, T. (1989) *Molecular Cloning: A Laboratory Manual*, 2nd ed. Cold Spring Harbor Laboratory Press, Cold Spring Harbor, NY.

21. Hamblin, T. J., Davis, Z., Gardiner, A., Oscier, D. G., and Stevenson, F. K. (1999) Unmutated Ig V(H) genes are associated with a more aggressive form of chronic lymphocytic leukemia. *Blood* **94,**1848–1854.

22. Damle, R. N., Wasil, T., Fais, F., et al. (1999) Ig V gene mutation status and CD38 expression as novel prognostic indicators in chronic lymphocytic leukemia. *Blood* **94,** 1840–1847.

23. Cook, W. D., Rudikoff, S., Giusti, A. M., and Scharff, M. D. (1982) Somatic mutations in a cultured mouse myeloma cell affects antigen binding. *Proc. Natl. Acad. Sci. USA* **79,** 1240–1244.

24. Forconi, F., King, C. A., Sahota, S. S., Kennaway, C. K., Russell, N. H., and Stevenson, F. K. (2002) Insight into the potential for DNA idiotypic fusion vaccines designed for patients by analysing xenogeneic anti-idiotypic antibody responses. *Immunology* **107,** 39–45.

25. Forconi, F., Sahota, S. S., Lauria, F., and Stevenson, F. K. (2004) Revisiting the definition of somatic mutational status in B-cell tumors: does 98% homology mean that a V_H gene is unmutated? *Leukemia* **18,** 882–883.

10

Identification of Clonotypic IgH VDJ Sequences in Multiple Myeloma

Brian J. Taylor, Jitra Kriangkum, Erin R. Strachan, Juanita Wizniak, and Linda M. Pilarski

Summary

In multiple myeloma (MM) the rearranged immunoglobulin heavy chain (IgH) variable, diversity, and joining (VDJ) DNA sequence of malignant plasma cells (PCs) serves as a marker for cells in the MM clone. This clonotypic sequence can be isolated from MM PCs by reverse transcriptase polymerase chain reaction (RT-PCR) with consensus primers that amplify the rearranged IgH repertoire. This chapter focuses on the key steps in determining patient-specific clonotypic sequences, including bulk RT-PCR using purified bone marrow mononuclear cell (BMMC) RNA, single-cell RT-PCR using RNA from PCs sorted by flow cytometry, IgH sequence alignments using IMGT or V BASE, and patient-specific primer design. In a test panel of several MM patient BMMCs, primers specific for the proposed sequence must amplify IgH from only the original patient. Furthermore, the proposed IgH sequence is not confirmed as clonotypic until these primers generate positive amplifications in the majority of single PCs from the original patient. This two-part test ensures that the proposed IgH sequence satisfies the definition of the clonotypic sequence as the most frequent, unique IgH sequence in an MM patient PC sample. With this patient-specific MM marker, a better understanding of transformed PCs and their B-lineage predecessors can be developed.

Key Words

Multiple myeloma; immunoglobulin heavy chain; complementarity-determining region; framework; constant region; V_H family; reverse transcription; flow cytometry; consensus primers.

1. Introduction

1.1. The Clonotypic IgH Sequence Is a Marker of the Multiple Myeloma Clone

In multiple myeloma (MM), transformation of a single B-lineage cell leads to an accumulation of malignant plasma cells (PCs) in the bone marrow (*1*). These

From: *Methods in Molecular Medicine, Vol. 113: Multiple Myeloma: Methods and Protocols*
Edited by: R. D. Brown and P. J. Ho © Humana Press Inc., Totowa, NJ

PCs share the same rearranged immunoglobulin heavy chain (IgH) DNA sequence as their transformed B-cell progenitor *(2,3)*. This is a *clonotypic* sequence because it is present in all the members of the MM clone. In normal bone marrow, clones of PCs with different IgH sequences coexist, reflecting the normal development of polyclonal B-cells in response to antigen. In MM, clonotypic PCs greatly outnumber normal PCs, disrupting the normal function of the bone marrow. The clonotypic sequence is thus the most frequently occurring Ig sequence isolated from MM PCs, greatly exceeding the frequency of any normal Ig sequence. The clonotypic sequence can be isolated from MM bone marrow samples by reverse transcriptase polymerase chain reaction (RT-PCR) using consensus primers that amplify the entire repertoire of Ig sequences *(4–9)*. It is the most frequent IgH sequence isolated from MM bone marrow samples; in many samples, it is the only IgH sequence that is observed. A PCR assay with primers specific for the clonotypic IgH sequence can be designed to distinguish members of the MM clone from their normal counterparts. This enables sensitive and specific monitoring of tumor cells, correlation of gene expression with transformation, and identification of pretransformed B-cell clones *(8,10–16)*. This chapter focuses on the methods used to determine the clonotypic IgH sequence and the design of specific primers to study the MM clone.

1.2. Amplification of Diverse IgH Sequences: Strategies and Challenges

The diversity of the IgH repertoire allows researchers to use rearranged IgH sequences as tumor-specific markers in MM. IgH is made up of variable (V_H) and constant domains (C_H) involved in antigen recognition and effector functions, respectively. The V_H domain consists of three separate, germ-line-encoded segments—the V (variable), D (diversity), and J (joining) segments—which come together to form a contiguous V-D-J open reading frame by sequential recombination *(17–19)*. Diversity of antigen recognition is generated by the existence of many distinct V, D, and J segments with the potential to form the VDJ unit: 123–129 V segments (seven different families based on sequence homology), 27 D segments, and 9 J segments *(20,21)*. Sequence variability at the VDJ junctions *(22,23)* and somatic hypermutation *(24)* further contribute to the diversity. The VDJ region is subdivided into the V_H leader region, encoding a conserved signal peptide sequence; three hypervariable complementarity-determining regions (CDRs) that are involved in antigen recognition; and four conserved framework regions (FRs) that maintain structural integrity of the molecule **(Fig. 1)**. The strategy for amplifying IgH VDJ is to use primers specific for conserved sequences in the V_H leader, FR, and constant regions. The biggest challenge is that the sequence diversity frequently extends into the conserved regions, disrupting primer hybridization. For this reason, it

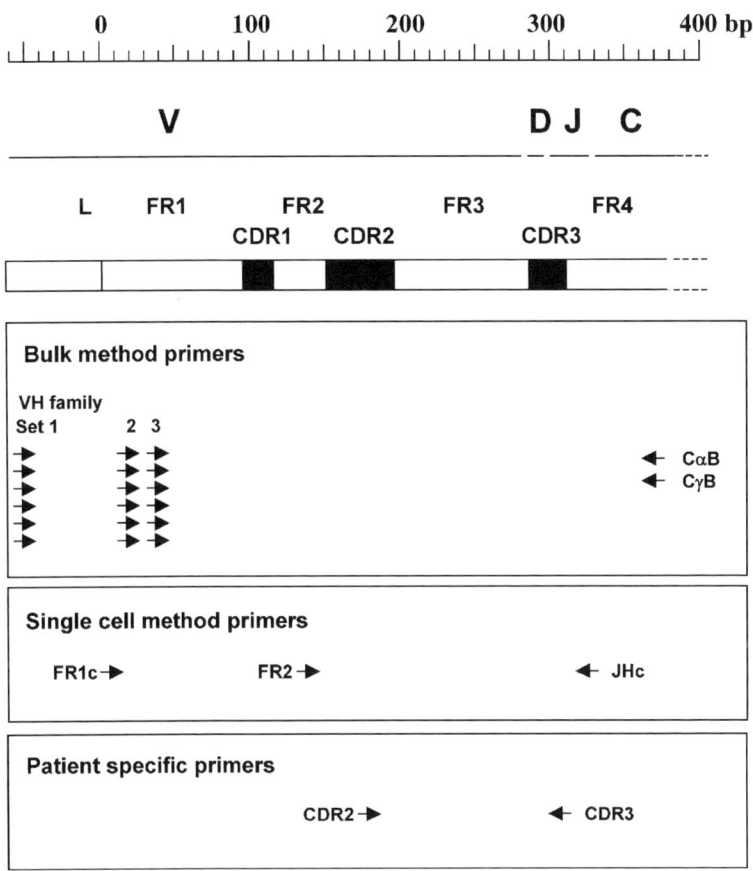

Fig. 1. Diagram of primer target regions in rearranged IgH locus: V, variable; D, diversity; J, joining; C, constant region; L, leader; FR framework region; CDR, complementarity-determining region (shown as black boxes). The position of each primer set is shown relative to the VDJ region. The scale is based on the numbering system by Kabat et al. *(30)*, which starts at –60 bp with the leader region. Right arrows are sense primers, and left arrows are antisense primers.

is necessary to have several sets of primers that target different conserved sequences (**Table 1**).

1.3. Experimental Overview

Two PCR methods, bulk (*see* **Subheading 3.1.**) and single-cell RT-PCR (*see* **Subheading 3.2.**), are used to identify clonotypic IgH sequences and design patient-specific primers in the CDR2 and CDR3 regions. The bulk RT-PCR uses V_H family-specific primer sets and constant region primers to amplify an

Table 1
Nucleotide Sequences of Primers Used in PCR Experiments

Primer	Nucleotide sequence, $5' \to 3'$ orientation	References
Sense primers		
V_H1-1, Set 1	CC ATG GAC TGG ACC TGG A	5
V_H2-1	ATG GAC ATA CTT TGT TCC AC	5
V_H3-1	CCA TGG AGT TTG GGC TGA GC	5
V_H4-1	ATG AAA CAC CTG TGG TTC TTC	5
V_H5-1	ATG GGG TCA ACC GCC ATC CT	5
V_H6-1	ATG TCT GTC TCC TTC CTC ATC	5
V_H1-2, Set 2	CAG TCT GG(A/G) GCT GAG GT(A/G) AA	*
V_H2-2	ATC ACC TTG AAG GAG TCT GGT CC	*
V_H3-2	GGT GCA GCT GGT GGA G(A/T)C	*
V_H4-2	GCT GCA GGA GT(C/G) (C/G)GG C	*
V_H5-2	TGC AGC TGG TGC AGT CTG	*
V_H6-2	CAG GTG CAG CTG CAG GAG	*
V_H1-3, Set 3	CTC AGT GAA GGT (C/T)TC CTG CAA GG	4
V_H2-3	GAC CCT CAC (A/G)CT GAC CTG C	*
V_H3-3	GTC CCT GAG ACT CTC CT(G/T) TGC AG	4
V_H4-3	TTC GG(A/G) GAC CCT GTC CCT CAC	4
V_H5-3	CTG AGG TGA A(A/G)A AGC C(C/T)G G	*
V_H6-3	GGG CCC AGG ACT GGT G	*
FR1c	AGG TGC AGC TG(C/G)(AT) G(C/G)A GTC (A/G/T) GG	6
FR2	TAT GAA TTC GGA AAG GGC CTG GAG TGG	8
$5'$ β2M	CCA GCA GAG AAT GGA AAG TC	31
$5'$ β2M int	TGT CTT TCA GCA AGG ACT GG	*
Antisense primers		
CαB	GAG GCT CAG CGG GAA GAC CTT	10
CδB	CCC AGT TAT CAA GCA TGC CAG GAC	10
CγB	GGG GAA GAC CGA TGG GCC CT	10
CμB	GAC GGA ATT CTC ACA GGA GAC	10
JHc	ACC TGA GGA GAC GGT GAC C(A/G)(G/T)(G/T)GT	6
$3'$ β2M	GAT GCT GCT TAC ATG TCT CG	31

[a]An asterisk indicates primers designed in our laboratory for IgH and β2M amplification.

IgH segment containing CDR1, 2, and 3 (*see* **Subheading 3.1.2.**). The template for the PCR is total RNA isolated from purified patient bone marrow mononuclear cells (BMMCs) (*see* **Subheading 3.1.1.**). Positive PCR products are resolved by gel electrophoresis and directly sequenced.

DNA products obtained by the bulk RT-PCR method are sequenced and aligned with known IgH sequences in repositories such as IMGT *(21)* or V BASE (*see* **Subheadings 2.7.** and **3.1.4.**). Patient-specific IgH primers are designed based on this alignment, which highlights the regions of the clonotypic sequence that differentiate it from the database IgH sequences. To obtain the best specificity, two primers are designed for each clonotypic sequence: a sense primer specific for CDR2 and an antisense primer specific for CDR3 (*see* **Fig. 2**). The patient specificity and clonotypic specificity of these primers is tested by PCR on (1) a panel of bulk BMMC cDNA from several patients with MM (*see* **Subheading 3.1.5.**), and (2) single-cell cDNA from the original patient (*see* **Subheading 3.1.6.**). A specific amplification of the original patient's cDNA in (1), and the majority (>75%) of single cells in (2) confirms the specificity of the primers for the clonotypic IgH sequence.

The single-cell method is performed in parallel to the bulk method, providing cDNA template that is used to (1) confirm the specificity of the CDR2 and CDR3 primers designed in the bulk method or (2) directly determine the IgH sequence, should the bulk method fail (*see* **Subheading 3.2.**). PCs are distinguished from other BMMCs by immunostaining with fluorochrome-conjugated anti-CD38, anti-CD138, and anti-CD56 monoclonal antibodies (MAbs) *(25–27)*. Single CD38^{++}/138^{+}/56^{+} cells are sorted by fluorescence-activated cell sorting (FACS) into individual tubes (*see* **Subheading 3.2.1.**) *(13)* and reverse transcribed by the direct lysis reverse transcription procedure (*see* **Subheading 3.2.2.** and **Table 2**). IgH VDJ sequences are amplified in a heminested PCR. In the first stage, FR1c consensus primers hybridizing to all V$_{H}$ segments and JHc consensus primers hybridizing to the J region are used. In the second-stage reaction, a similar FR2 consensus primer is used with JHc (*see* **Subheading 3.2.3.**). Positive PCR products from this reaction are sequenced, and the most frequent sequence is used to design CDR2 and CDR3 primers. The primer confirmation is the same as for the bulk PCR (*see* **Subheadings 3.1.5.** and **3.1.6.**). By combining two amplification strategies with distinct template and primer sets, the clonotypic IgH sequence is determined, and tumor-specific PCR primers are designed.

2. Materials

2.1. Purification of BMMCs

1. Ficoll-Paque (Amersham, Piscataway, NJ), to purify BMMCs by density gradient centrifugation.
2. Hemocytometer for counting cells.

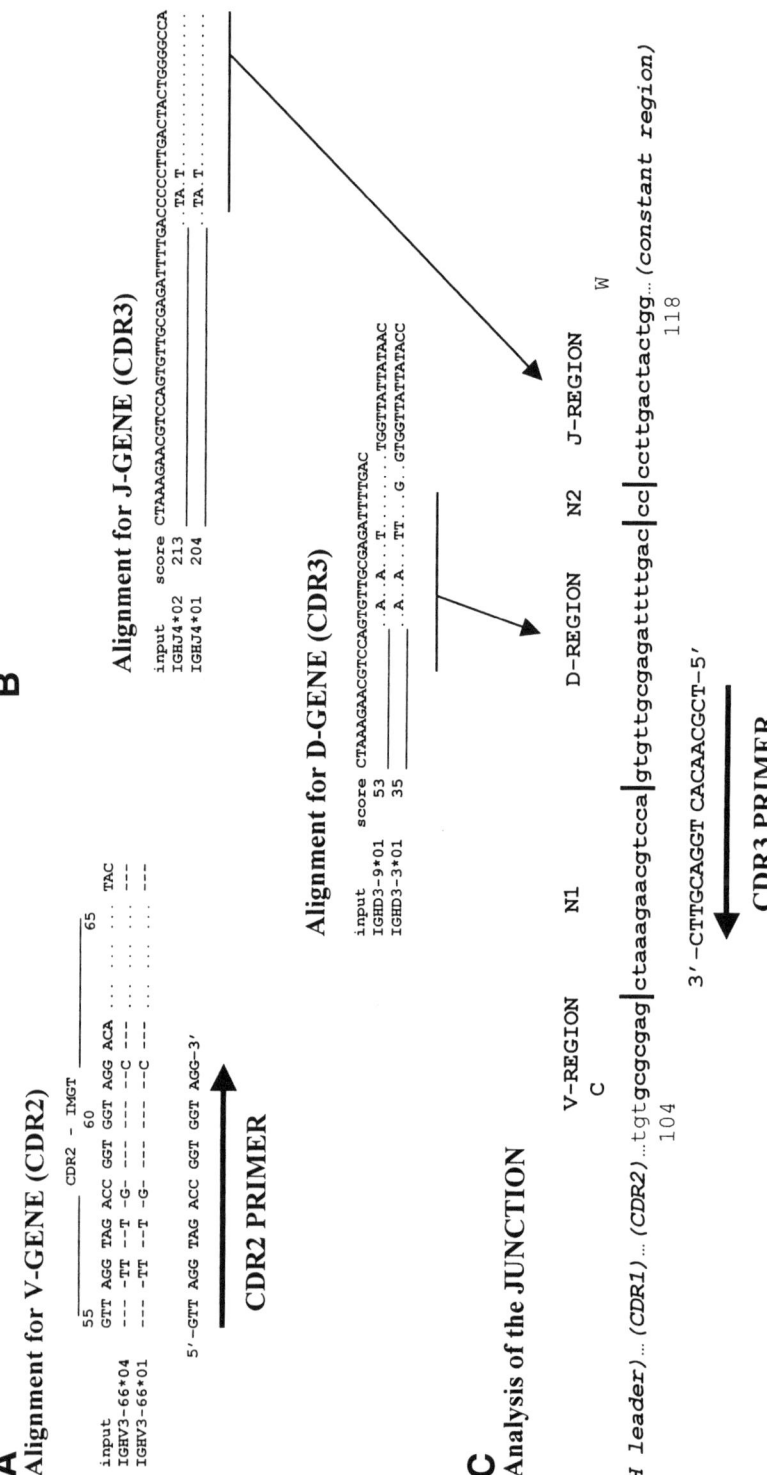

Table 2
Direct Lysis Reverse Transcription Protocol

Reagent	Single-tube volume (µL)	Master mix volume for 400 tubes (µL)
0.1% DEPC H$_2$O	3.9	1560
5X First-strand buffer	2	800
0.1 *M* DTT	1	400
10 m*M* dT15	0.5	200
10 m*M* dNTPs	0.5	200
IGEPAL CA-630 detergent	0.05	20

2.2. Bulk Reverse Transcription Reaction

1. Trizol (Invitrogen, Carlsbad, CA), to isolate RNA from purified BMMCs.
2. Superscript RT (200 U/µL) (Invitrogen).
3. 5X buffer: 250 m*M* Tris-HCl (pH 8.3), 375 m*M* KCl, 15 m*M* MgCl$_2$.
4. 0.1 *M* Dithiothreitol (DTT).
5. 10 µ*M* Oligo(dT)$_{15}$ primer.
6. 10 m*M* dNTPs: 10 m*M* of dATP, dCTP, dGTP, dTTP (Roche, Indianapolis IN).
7. 0.1% Diethylpyrocarbonate (DEPC) H$_2$O (Sigma, St. Louis, MO) (*see* **Note 1**).
8. Thermocycler or incubator.

2.3. Additional Reagents and Equipment for Single-Cell Direct Lysis Reverse Transcription Reaction

1. IGEPAL CA-630 detergent (Sigma).
2. RNaseOUT (40 U/µL) (Invitrogen).
3. Ultraviolet (UV) transilluminator.

Fig. 2. *(see facing page)* Design of patient-specific primers using IMGT/V-QUEST. **(A)** Alignments of clonotypic sequence and two database sequences for V, D, and J genes (*see* **Subheading 3.1.4.**). Only the CDR2 portion of the V gene alignment is shown; dashes indicate sequence identity, and dots indicate CDR2 gaps according to the IMGT unique numbering *(29)*. A CDR2 primer, chosen in a region with five unique nucleotides is presented under the alignment. **(B)** V, D, and J junction with N1 and N2 nucleotide insertions. The D and J gene alignments start at the right of the underscored region; dots indicate sequence identity. **(C)** The V$_H$ leader, CDR1, CDR2, and constant regions are indicated in italics for orientation of the VDJ junction. The boundaries of the VDJ junction by IMGT numbering are C (Cys) 104 and W (Trp) 118. An antisense CDR3 primer is designed that hybridizes to the N1/D region, the most unique part of this VDJ junction. Only the relevant portions of the total IMGT/V-QUEST output are shown here.

2.4. Bulk, Single-Cell, and Primer Confirmation PCR Reagents and Equipment

1. Platinum Taq High Fidelity DNA polymerase (5 U/μL) (Invitrogen).
2. 10X Platinum Taq High Fidelity PCR buffer: 600 mM Tris-SO$_4$ (pH 8.9), 180 mM (NH$_4$)$_2$ SO$_4$.
3. 50 mM MgSO$_4$ salts for Platinum Taq High Fidelity.
4. Platinum Taq DNA polymerase (5 U/μL) (Invitrogen).
5. 10X Platinum Taq PCR buffer: 200 mM Tris-HCl (pH 8.4), 500 mM KCl.
6. 50 mM MgCl$_2$ for Platinum Taq.
7. 10 mM dNTPs (10 mM of dATP, dCTP, dGTP, dTTP).
8. 10 μM 5′ Sense primer (*see* **Table 1**).
9. 10 μM 3′ Antisense primer *(see* **Table 1**).
10. Thermocycler.

2.5. Nucleotide Sequences of Primers Used in PCR Experiments

See **Table 1** for a listing of sequences.

2.6. Sequencing of PCR Products

1. ExoSAP-IT (US Biochemicals, Cleveland, OH).
2. Reagents for automated fluorescent cycle sequencing such as a Big Dye terminator kit (Applied Biosystems, Foster City, CA).

2.7. IgH Sequence Databases and Primer Design Programs

1. IMGT, the international ImMunoGeneTics information system® (http://imgt.cines.fr:8104/).
2. IMGT/V-QUEST Ig sequence alignment program (http://imgt.cines.fr:8104/textes/vquest/).
3. V BASE database of human Ig variable region genes (www.mrc-cpe.cam.ac.uk/).
4. DNAPLOT Ig sequence alignment program (http://www.mrc-cpe.cam.ac.uk/DNAPLOT.php?menu=901).
5. DNA analysis program such as Genetool 2.0 (BioTools, Edmonton, Alberta, Canada).
6. Primer design program such as Primer3 (www.frodo.wi.mit.edu/cgi-bin/primer3/primer3_www.cgi).

2.8. Reagents for Immunostaining BMMCs and Flow Cytometry

1. Anti-CD38 PE (Becton Dickinson, San Jose, CA).
2. Anti-CD138 Pc5 (Beckman Coulter/Immunotech, Miami, FL).
3. Anti-CD56 FITC (Serotec, Raleigh, NC).
4. Phosphate-buffered saline (PBS) (pH 7.4).
5. Flow-check fluorospheres (Beckman Coulter).

2.9. Other Equipment

1. Reagents and apparatus for agarose gel electrophoresis, DNA sequencing, flow cytometry, automated cell sorting, and primer synthesis.

2.10. Other Methods

BMMC purification, RNA isolation, gel electrophoresis, DNA sequencing, and flow cytometry are not covered in detail in this chapter. The first four are commonly used laboratory techniques *(28)*. The operation of the flow cytometer is conducted by trained personnel according to the manufacturer's protocols. In **Subheading 3.2.1.**, we describe a general protocol for alignment of the flow cytometer Autoclone cell deposition unit.

3. Methods

3.1. Identification of Clonotypic IgH VDJ by Bulk RT-PCR (Fig. 3)

3.1.1. Reverse Transcription of Bulk BMMC RNA (see **Notes 1–3**)

This reverse transcription of the total RNA of the entire BMMC population ("bulk" RNA) provides cDNA template for PCR in **Subheadings 3.1.2.** and **3.1.5.**

1. In a 0.2-mL thin-walled PCR tube, combine 1 µg of RNA from purified patient BMMCs, 1 µL of 10 µ*M* dT15 primer, 1 µL of 10 m*M* dNTPs, and 0.1% DEPC H_2O to a total volume of 12 µL.
2. Incubate the reaction at 70°C for 10 min, and then cool to 4°C.
3. To this tube add 4 µL of 5X first-strand buffer, 2 µL of 0.1 *M* DTT, and 1 µL of Superscript enzyme (200 U/µL).
4. Incubate at 42°C for 60 min, followed by 99°C for 3 min to inactivate the enzyme. Cool to 4°C and use immediately in a PCR or store at –80°C.

3.1.2. Amplification of IgH VDJ With V_H Family Primer Sets (see **Notes 4–6**)

This standard PCR protocol uses three distinct primer sets that provide the best coverage of the VDJ region. For PCR reagents and thermocycling conditions, *see* **Table 3**.

1. Set up 12 PCRs per patient using the following:
   a. V_H family set 1 (V_H1-1 to 6-1) with CαB primers in tubes 1–6 (*see* **Table 1** and **Fig. 1**).
   b. V_H family set 1 (V_H1-1 to 6-1) with CγB in tubes 7–12.
   c. 1 µL of patient BMMC cDNA template diluted 1/10 with sterile distilled water (*see* **Subheading 3.1.1.**).
2. Set up 12 matching negative control reactions replacing the cDNA template with sterile distilled H_2O.
3. Set up one positive control PCR using the following:
   a. 5'β2M and 3'β2M primers (*see* **Table 1** and **Fig. 1**).
   b. 1 µL of patient BMMC cDNA template diluted 1 : 10 with sterile distilled water (*see* **Subheading 3.1.1.**).

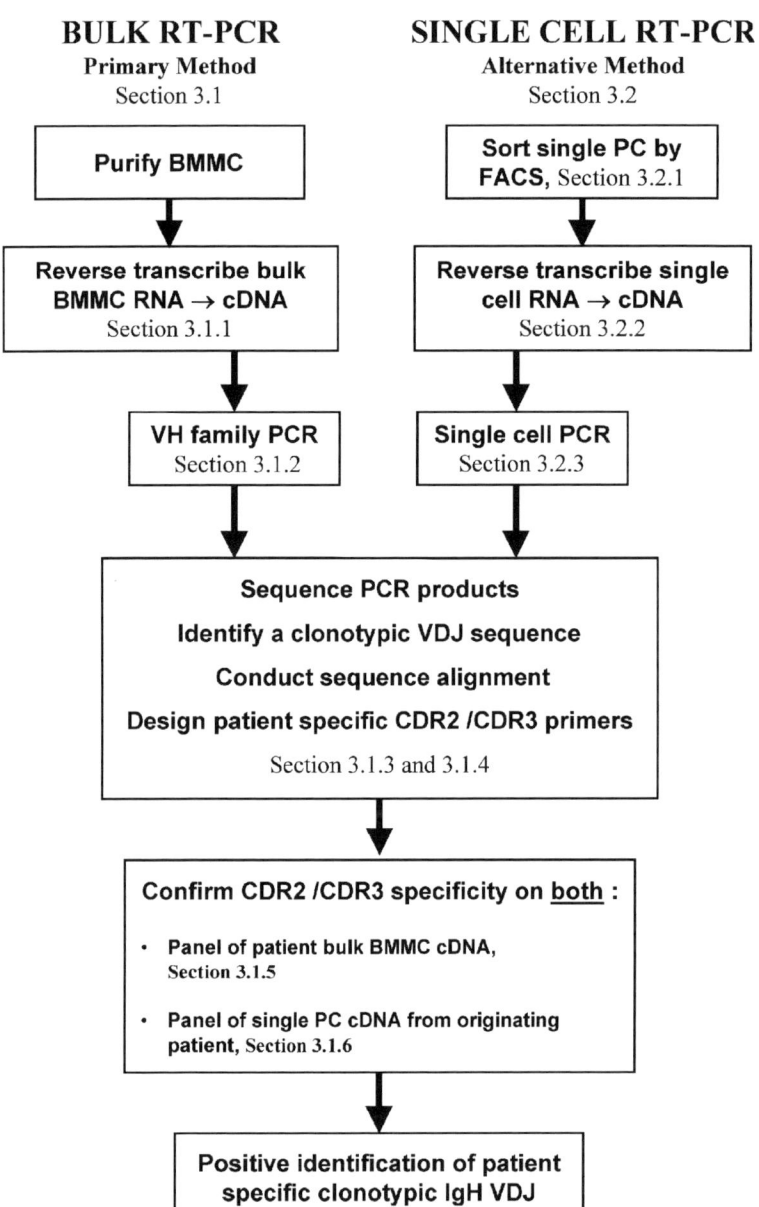

Fig. 3. Flow diagram of experimental procedures in identifying and confirming a clonotypic IgH sequence.

Table 3
IgH VDJ Bulk PCR Protocol[a]

Reagent	Volume (μL)
10X Platinum Taq High Fidelity buffer	2.5
50 m*M* MgSO$_4$	1.0
10 m*M* dNTPs	0.5
10 μM Sense primer	0.5
10 μM Antisense primer	0.5
cDNA template	1.0
Platinum Taq High Fidelity polymerase (5 U/μL), sterile distilled H$_2$O to 25-μL total volume	0.1

[a]Run the PCR program as follows: 94°C for 2 min; 30 cycles of 94°C for 30 s; 60°C for 30 s; and 68°C for 30 s; 68°C for 7 min; and 4°C hold.

4. Mix the reactions, centrifuge at 400*g* for 2 min, and run the thermocycling program described in **Table 3**.
5. Resolve the products by agarose gel electrophoresis. The expected product size is approx 400 bp for the V$_H$ family set 1 PCR, 150 bp for the β2M PCR (*see* **Fig. 4A**).
6. If no positive PCR products are observed, repeat this PCR with V$_H$ sets 2 and 3 (*see* **Table 1** and **Fig. 4A**) and the same constant region primers. The expected product size is approx 300 bp.

3.1.3. Preparation of PCR Products for Sequencing (see **Note 7**)

Exonuclease I/shrimp alkaline phosphatase (ExoSAP-IT) is an enzyme combination that degrades PCR primers and nucleotides, respectively, which can interfere with downstream sequencing reactions.

1. For each reaction, add 5 μL of PCR product from **Subheading 3.1.2.** or **3.2.3.** and 2 μL of ExoSAP-IT.
2. Incubate the reaction at 37°C for 15 min, followed by 80°C for 15 min to inactivate the enzymes.
3. Dilute this reaction up to 1:10 in sterile distilled water, and use as the template in a sequencing reaction (10–100 ng of template).

3.1.4. Design and Synthesis of Patient-Specific CDR2 and CDR3 Primers (see **Note 8**)

The sequences of PCR products in **Subheading 3.1.3.** are analyzed using DNA software packages such as Genetool (*see* **Subheading 2.7.**), which will analyze electropherograms from automated fluorescent cycle sequencing, convert them to DNA sequence files, and export them to alignment programs.

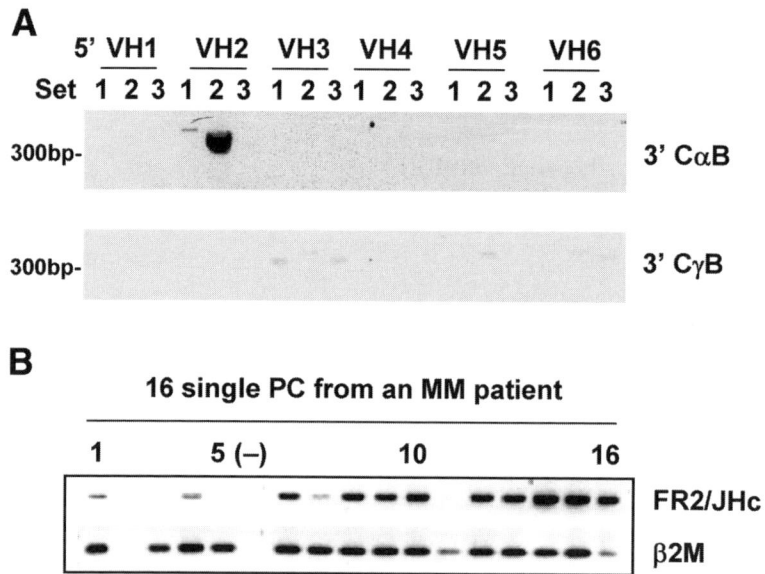

Fig. 4. Bulk and single cell methods of IgH VDJ amplification. PCR products from each method were resolved by agarose gel electrophoresis. **(A)** PCRs with V_H family (V_H1–6, sets 1–3), constant region primers (CαB, CγB), and bulk BMMC cDNA template from an IgA MM patient (*see* **Subheading 3.1.2.**). Weak and strong positive bands are observed for V_H2-1 and V_H2-2, respectively. **(B)** Second-stage FR2/JHc and β2M PCR products from a single-cell RT-PCR experiment (*see* **Subheading 3.2.3.**). Lane 2: a tube that did not receive a PC; lanes 3, 5, and 11: tubes that received a PC, but no IgH VDJ product could be amplified; (–): negative control.

Comparisons of the clonotypic sequence with IgH sequences are conducted using Web-based alignment programs such as IMGT/V-QUEST or DNAPLOT (V BASE) (*see* **Subheading 2.7.**). These programs align a query sequence with a number of database sequences to determine the positions of hypervariable regions V_H (CDR1 and 2), and the VDJ junction (CDR3), according to Ig numbering schemes *(29,30)*.

CDR2 and CDR3 primers are designed based on these alignments, targeting unique sequences within the respective CDR region (*see* **Fig. 2**). Parameters such as primer size (18–30 bp) and melting temperature (55–60°C) are further refined with Genetool or Primer3 (*see* **Subheading 2.7.**), a web-based program for designing primers.

3.1.5. Confirmation of Patient CDR2/CDR3 Primer Specificity Using Bulk BMMC cDNA as Template (see **Note 9**)

In this primer test, a panel of patient bulk BMMC cDNA including the original patient is assembled. At least 10 patients of the same V_H family are chosen

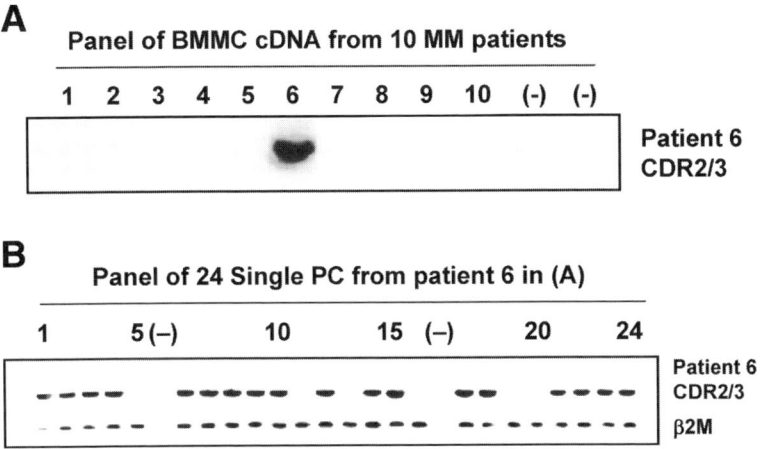

Fig. 5. Primer confirmation PCRs resolved by agarose gel electrophoresis: **(A)** PCRs with CDR2/CDR3 primers and cDNA samples from patient bulk BMMCs including original patient in lane 6 (*see* **Subheading 3.1.5.**); **(B)** nested PCR on 24 single PCs from original patient with first-stage FR1c/JHc and second-stage CDR2/CDR3 primers indicating that 18/24 PC cells are positive (*see* **Subheading 3.1.6.**). (–), negative controls; β2M, positive controls to confirm the presence of cDNA.

so that the CDR2 and CDR3 primers must distinguish the clonotypic IgH sequence of the original patient from closely related sequences.

1. Assemble 12 PCRs using the bulk PCR protocol (*see* **Table 3**) with the following exceptions:
   a. Use Platinum Taq enzyme, 10X buffer, and Mg^{2+} salts instead of the Platinum Taq High Fidelity reagents in **Subheading 3.1.2.**
   b. Use 72 instead of 68°C for extension in the thermocycling program (this is the "Platinum Taq thermocycling program").
   c. Add CDR2 and CDR3 primers to each tube (*see* **Subheading 3.1.4.**).
   d. Add 1 μL of each of the 10 patient cDNA templates diluted 1:10 with sterile distilled water to 10 tubes.
   e. Add 1 μL of sterile distilled water to the remaining two tubes as negative controls.
2. Assemble a matching set of 12 positive control reactions using 5'β2M and 3'β2M (*see* **Table 1**) instead of CDR2 and CDR3 primers.
3. Mix the reactions, centrifuge the tubes at 400*g* for 2 min, and run the Platinum Taq thermocycling program.
4. Resolve the amplification products by gel electrophoresis as in **Subheading 3.1.2.** The reaction with the cDNA template from the original patient (reaction six in **Fig. 5A**) should generate a positive band of 150–200 bp, whereas the other tubes should be negative. The β2M controls should be positive.

3.1.6. Confirmation of Patient CDR2/CDR3 Primer Specificity
by Single-Cell RT-PCR (see **Note 10**)

This test verifies that the predicted clonotypic IgH sequence is detectable in the majority of single PCs of the original patient. The first-stage product from the single-cell heminested PCR (*see* **Subheading 3.2.3.**) is used as a template for this second-stage PCR. The same β2M control reactions in **Subheading 3.2.3.** are used in this experiment.

1. Assemble 24 second-stage PCRs (*see* **Table 3**) using Platinum Taq and its appropriate 10X buffer, Mg^{2+} salts, and conditions (*see* **Subheading 3.1.5.**).
   a. Add patient-specific CDR2 and CDR3 primers (*see* **Subheading 3.1.5.**).
   b. Transfer 1 μL of product from the first-stage FR1c/JHc reaction to each of the corresponding second-stage tubes (*see* **Subheading 3.2.3.**).
2. Run the Platinum Taq thermocycling program (*see* **Subheading 3.1.5.**), and resolve the nested PCR products by gel electrophoresis (*see* **Fig. 5B**).
3. Calculate the frequency of PCs expressing the clonotypic IgH sequence as the number of CDR2/CDR3 positives divided by the number of β2M positives in **Subheading 3.2.3.** If the frequency is 75% or greater, the proposed IgH sequence is considered clonotypic. If the frequency is 20–75%, a second test on a new set of cells is recommended. If intermediate or low frequencies persist, the sequence is not clonotypic, or the sample itself may be in question (*see* **Note 10**). If the frequency is 0–20%, the proposed IgH sequence is rejected as clonotypic, and a new sequence must be proposed (either from the alternative single-cell method in **Subheading 3.2.**, or from a new sample).

3.2. Single-Cell Heminested RT-PCR: A Strategy for Amplifying Clonotypic IgH Transcripts Directly From Individual Patient PCs (see **Fig. 3** and **Notes 11–14**)

This protocol provides single cells for the completion of primer confirmation in the bulk PCR (*see* **Subheading 3.1.6.**). These single cells are also used as an alternative method for determining the clonotypic IgH sequence, should the bulk method fail. Single PCs sorted by flow cytometry provide a source of RNA in a heminested PCR. The first-stage FR1c/JHc product is the template for the single-cell primer confirmation PCR (*see* **Subheading 3.1.6.**); the second-stage FR2/JHc product is used in the alternative method to determine IgH sequence directly from each single-sorted PC. The most frequently observed sequence is designated clonotypic and tested in the same manner as sequence isolated by the bulk PCR method (*see* **Subheadings 3.1.4.–3.1.6.**).

3.2.1. Sorting Single PCs by Flow Cytometry (see **Note 11** and **Fig. 6**)

Single cells are sorted into individual tubes using a flow cytometer with a cell deposition unit (e.g., Beckman Coulter Epics Altra with Autoclone sort

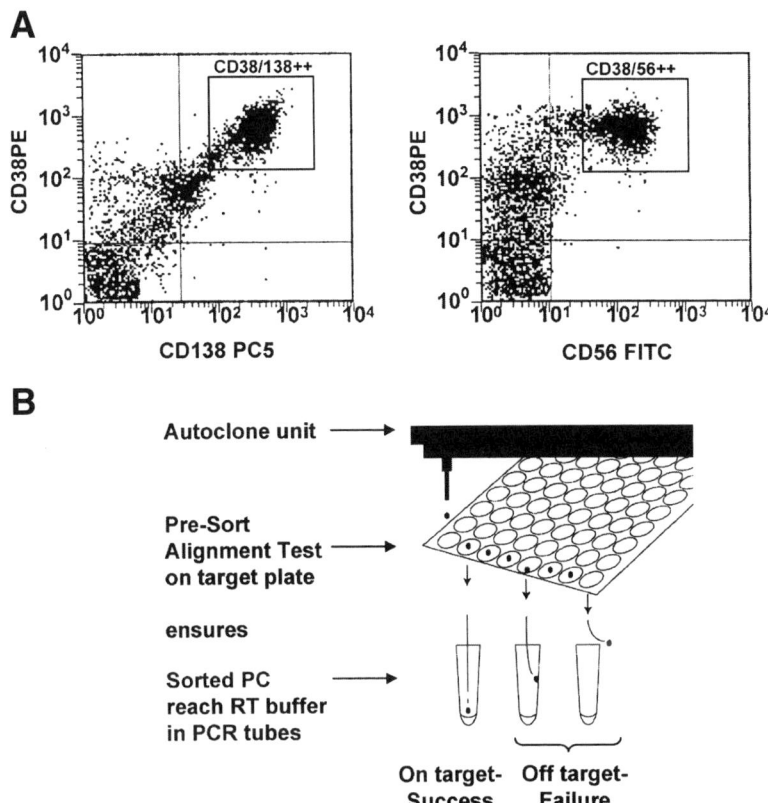

Fig. 6. Sorting of single PC by flow cytometry. (**A**) Dot plots of fluorescence intensity of BMMCs stained with CD38 PE, CD138 Pc5, and CD56 FITC, as analyzed by flow cytometry. Sorting gates set to acquire PCs are indicated by a square. These PCs are sorted into RT buffer in individual tubes. (**B**) The Autoclone unit is aligned before each sort as described in **Subheading 3.2.1.** The consequences of poor alignment on RT-PCRs are shown in the downstream PC sort.

option) equipped to hold a 96-position rack for 0.2-mL PCR tubes. Alignment tests are conducted before each single-cell sort, to ensure that cells are delivered directly into the buffer at the bottom of the tube.

1. Conduct the testing of cell deposition on the lid of a 96-well enzyme-linked immunosorbent assay plate, where the accuracy of sorting is easily assessed.
2. Deliver 20 Flow-Check fluorospheres to each of the 96 positions in a volume visible to the naked eye (1 µL).
3. Visually assess the accuracy of sorting for the center of each position, and make changes in Autoclone unit alignment until the best accuracy is achieved. It is

important to hit the exact center of the 96-well lid targets, because the 0.2-mL PCR tubes used for cell sorting are a smaller target.

4. Set the stringency of the Autoclone unit to deliver at most one fluorosphere per target. Conduct a stringency test on three 96-well plates. On average, 99% of targets receive a single bead, 1% receive no beads, and none of the targets receive two beads. This is important because the single-cell RT-PCR method is based on the premise that only one IgH sequence is present in each tube.

5. For each single-cell experiment, stain BMMCs as follows:
   a. Incubate 10×10^6 purified BMMCs in 500 µL of PBS/2% fetal bovine serum (FBS) with the MAbs CD38-PE, CD138-Pc5, and CD56-FITC combined in one reaction at the manufacturer's suggested concentrations.
   b. Prepare one control reaction for each antibody with 1×10^6 BMMCs in 50 µL of PBS/2% FBS. An identical single reaction combining the three isotype-matched control antibodies and a reaction with no antibody serve as further controls.
   c. Incubate these six reactions at 4°C for 30 min, centrifuge at 400g for 2 min, wash two times with PBS/0.5 mM EDTA, and send to the flow cytometer.
   d. Measure the immunofluorescence intensity of the labeled cells, and use the control reactions to define the parameters for sorting CD38^{++}/138$^+$/56$^+$ cells (*see* **Fig. 6A**).

6. Before the cells are sorted, complete the alignment and stringency quality control tests. Then replace the 96-well lid with a 96-position rack with 0.2-mL PCR tubes containing direct lysis RT buffer, and deliver a single CD38^{++}/CD138$^+$/CD56$^+$ PC into each tube. During the sorting process, monitor flow cytometry parameters such as stream stability and cell flow rate. This procedure ensures that a single cell is directly deposited into the RT buffer of almost every tube (*see* **Fig. 6B**).

3.2.2. Direct Lysis Reverse Transcription of Single Cells (see **Note 12**)

In this protocol, RNA from single-sorted PCs is reverse transcribed into cDNA template for heminested PCRs. A heminested PCR is necessary because of the small amount of cDNA template generated from the direct lysis reverse transcription reaction. Mix the following reagents together in order:

1. Place the master mix components in a clear polypropylene tube on a UV transilluminator (254-nm wavelength), and irradiate for 5 min to inactivate any contaminating DNA fragments.
2. Add 20 µL of RNaseOUT (40 U/µL) to the master mix tube.
3. Aliquot 8 µL of master mix to individual 0.2-mL PCR tubes. Perform 24 reactions per patient, and set up an additional two reactions as negative controls. Store the remainder of the master mix at –80°C for up to 1 mo.
4. Add a single-sorted PC in 1 µL of PBS to each individual tube, except the negative controls. Then set the flow cytometer to deliver 1 µL of PBS alone as a negative control.
5. Centrifuge the tubes at 400g for 2 min to ensure that the cell is immersed in the buffer.

6. Incubate the reaction at 70°C for 10 min and then cool to 4°C.
7. Add 1 µL of Superscript diluted 1:8 in 0.1% DEPC H_2O. The total volume of the reverse transcription reaction should be 10 µL.
8. Incubate the reaction at 42°C for 60 min, followed by 99°C for 3 min to inactivate Superscript. Cool to 4°C and proceed with the PCR, or store at −80°C.

3.2.3. Heminested Amplification of IgH VDJ
From Single-Cell cDNA (see Notes 13 and 14)

3.2.3.1. FIRST-STAGE PCRs

1. Assemble 24 PCRs (*see* **Table 3**) using Platinum Taq polymerase and its appropriate 10X buffer, Mg^{2+} salts, and conditions (*see* **Subheading 3.1.5.**).
   a. To set 1, add the FR1c and JHc primers (*see* **Table 1**).
   b. Add 3 µL of single-cell cDNA (*see* **Subheading 3.2.2.**) to 24 of the PCRs. Add sterile distilled water to make the total reaction volume 25 µL.
   c. Add sterile distilled water to the remaining two reactions as negative controls.
2. Assemble a matching set of 24 positive control reactions using 5′β2M and 3′β2M primers (*see* **Table 1**). Each positive control reaction should receive cDNA from the same single cell as its corresponding FR1c/JHc reaction.
3. Mix the reactions, centrifuge the tubes at 400*g* for 2 min, and run the Platinum Taq thermocycling program (*see* **Subheading 3.1.5.**).

3.2.3.2. SECOND-STAGE PCRs

1. Assemble 24 PCRs (*see* **Table 3**) using Platinum Taq and its appropriate 10X buffer, Mg^{2+} salts, and conditions (*see* **Subheading 3.1.5.**).
   a. Add FR2 and JHc primers (*see* **Table 1**).
   b. Transfer 1 µL of product from the first-stage FR1c/JHc reaction to each of the corresponding second-stage tubes.
2. Assemble a matching set of positive control reactions using 5′β2Mint and 3′β2M primers (*see* **Table 1**). Transfer 1 µL of product from the first-stage β2M PCR to each of the corresponding second-stage tubes.
3. Mix the reactions, centrifuge the tubes at 400*g* for 2 min, and run the Platinum Taq thermocycling program (*see* **Subheading 3.1.5.**).
4. Resolve the second-stage PCR products by gel electrophoresis (*see* **Fig. 5B**). The expected FR2/JHc product size is approx 200 bp. The integrity of the single-cell cDNA is determined by the β2M reactions. Prepare the FR2/JHc PCRs with positive amplifications for sequencing (*see* **Subheading 3.1.3.**). Use only FR2/JHc reactions that have a positive amplification in the corresponding β2M positive control.
5. After sequencing, choose the most frequent IgH sequence as the proposed clonotypic sequence.
6. Design CDR2 and CDR3 primers (*see* **Subheading 3.1.4.**) and confirm them as in **Subheadings 3.1.5.** and **3.1.6.**

4. Notes

1. Superscript is the enzyme used to reverse transcribe IgH mRNA into cDNA. It is the last reagent added to the reverse transcription reaction. After the other reagents

have been added, Superscript should be removed from −20°C storage on ice, added to the reaction, then promptly returned to storage. DEPC H_2O and RNaseOUT RNase inhibitor are used in the single-cell direct lysis protocol to reduce RNA degradation as much as possible. DEPC H_2O is prepared by adding DEPC to 1 L of water to a final concentration of 0.1%, shaking to mix the DEPC and water completely, incubating overnight at room temperature, and autoclaving on a standard liquids cycle the following day.

2. A separate low-traffic area should be designated for reverse transcription experiments such as a sterile laminar flow hood. Strict adherence to standard protocol is essential to avoid RNA degradation by RNases. This includes the use of dedicated RNA reagents, plasticware, pipettors, gloves, and regular cleaning of all areas with a 10% bleach solution. This is of utmost importance for experiments with single cells, which have small amounts of RNA compared to the bulk RT-PCR experiments. It is also important to keep PCRs and associated reagents out of the reverse transcription area. Exogenous DNA from PCRs is a major source of contamination, especially in single cell experiments that use a two-stage PCR capable of amplifying extremely small amounts of target DNA.

3. A high-quality sample is essential to the success of these experiments. Samples should be processed within 30 min of collection and purified within 2–3 h of collection for reliable results. Samples should not be stored overnight. Purified cells are resuspended in Trizol, and total RNA is isolated according to the manufacturer's protocol. Typically, 10–30 μg of total RNA is obtained from 1×10^7 BMMCs. Additional factors can contribute to the failure to amplify a clonotypic sequence, even in promptly processed samples. The distribution of PCs in the bone marrow can be heterogeneous, such that some bone marrow aspirates may not contain a good sampling of PCs ("bad pull" aspirate). It may be necessary to test two or three separate bone marrow aspirates before a clonotypic sequence is determined. Furthermore, the number of bone marrow PCs varies from patient to patient (10–100% BMMCs). In patients with fewer PCs, it is more difficult to amplify IgH sequences.

4. Two different thermostable polymerases are used in PCRs in this chapter. High Fidelity Platinum Taq polymerase contains a mixture of Taq polymerase and a thermostable proofreading enzyme along with an anti-Taq antibody to prevent nonspecific template amplification before the thermocycling reaction begins. This enzyme mixture minimizes nucleotide misincorporation errors in the bulk PCR, which is used to determine the clonotypic IgH sequence. In the single-cell method, the Platinum Taq/antibody mix (without the proofreading enzyme) is used because it gives higher yields than the high-fidelity polymerase mix. This is important because of the small amounts of starting template in the single-cell reaction. The Platinum Taq/antibody mix is also used in the primer confirmation PCR because only the primer specificity is being tested; an IgH sequence is not isolated from these PCRs.

5. The V_H family primer sets can be used in stages or can be put together in one 36-tube PCR experiment as shown in **Fig. 4A**. CγB and CαB primers are used because in the majority of patients with MM clonotypic VDJ is joined with either

Cγ (55%) or Cα (20%) constant regions. If clinical data are available, the patient "clinical isotype" (i.e., the isotype of the monoclonal paraprotein, the antibody encoded by the clonotypic IgH sequence) indicates which constant region primer will successfully amplify the clonotypic IgH sequence. In rare cases when the clinical isotype is IgM or IgD, CμB or CδB primers (**Table 1**) can be used, respectively. In the case of light-chain patients, light-chain consensus primers may be needed to amplify a clonotypic IgL sequence (*9*); in the case of nonsecretors, neither IgH nor IgL transcripts may be present at detectable levels. The bulk PCR generates a single band of 300–400 bp; rarely are multiple bands seen in a single lane. One of three profiles is normally observed in MM patient PCR experiments: a band in 1 of the 12 V_H family reactions, several bands in separate V_H family reactions, or no bands. In the first and second cases, the band is almost always a single IgH VDJ species on direct sequencing. Although the V_H primers are family specific, some crossreactivity is occasionally observed as these primers target conserved regions with some sequence homology between families. Single bands that generate an overlapping sequence readout, suggestive of polyclonal IgH VDJ amplification, occur infrequently. These can be cloned and sequenced to test whether a predominant clonotypic sequence exists among the polyclonal sequences. In cases in which only polyclonal sequences are detected, or no bands are generated at all, the patient's diagnosis may be incorrect, the sample quality may be poor, or the clonotypic IgH sequence may be mutated in the primer target regions. For most patients, the use of three separate V_H sets results in a successful amplification of clonotypic IgH.

6. It is tempting to use consensus primers such as FR1c if the V_H family sets fail to amplify clonotypic IgH. However, we have observed that using FR1c primer instead of the V_H family primers in the bulk PCR leads to identification of an IgH sequence that often fails the single-cell confirmation PCR test in **Subheading 3.1.6.** This suggests that the FR1c primer disproportionately amplifies IgH VDJ from a bulk population, preferentially hybridizing to certain infrequent sequences over the predominant clonotypic sequence. Primers specific for the infrequent sequence may pass the bulk primer confirmation test in **Subheading 3.1.5.**, but fail in **Subheading 3.1.6.** where the frequency of the sequence in the PC population is tested. The FR1c primer is better suited for single-cell PCR because there is no competition between different IgH sequences for primer binding.

7. Bulk or single-cell PCR products are sequenced directly without cloning. These products are first treated with the ExoSAP-IT reagent to prepare them for sequencing and then are sequenced by automated fluorescent cycle sequencing. Both V_H family and constant region primers are used as sequencing primers for bulk PCR products, and the FR2 and JHc primers can be used to sequence single-cell PCR products. The use of two different primers generates sequence data for both DNA strands, which can be compared.

8. IMGT/V-QUEST and DNAPLOT (V BASE) Ig sequence alignment programs are invaluable tools in primer design. The V-QUEST program offers the option of analyzing the VDJ junction, indicating the positions of N nucleotide insertions.

These programs align the V, D, and J regions separately, as opposed to one contiguous sequence (*see* **Fig. 2** for the V-QUEST alignment). These programs also indicate whether the VDJ unit is an in-frame rearrangement (i.e., a functional rearrangement). If the sequence is not in frame, there is a sequencing error (either in the sequence readout or in the actual sequencing reaction) such as a base insertion or deletion, or a nonfunctional VDJ has been amplified. Even with good sequence data and unique CDR target sequences, it may be necessary to design two or three different primer sets before the bulk and single-cell primer confirmation tests can be passed.

9. The bulk primer confirmation PCR tests the specificity of the CDR2 and CDR3 primers for the clonotypic sequence of the original patient. Positive amplifications in the reactions containing other patient cDNA indicate a lack of specificity for the clonotypic sequence. Absence of clonotypic IgH amplification in the original patient cDNA reaction indicates poor cDNA integrity, miscalled bases on sequencing leading to incorrect primer design, poor primer design using the correct sequence, transposed PCRs or primers, or exogenous DNA contamination in the V_H family or single-cell PCR.

10. This is the definitive test for identifying a clonotypic sequence. The majority (75%) of single-cell reactions should be positive in the CDR2/CDR3 PCR; and at least 16, preferably 24, β2M positive reactions must be counted. Most proposed clonotypic sequences from the bulk PCR that are confirmed in **Subheading 3.1.5.**, either predominate (confirmed as clonotypic) or are undetectable (rejected as clonotypic) in single-sorted PCs (*see* **Subheading 3.2.**). When intermediate IgH sequence frequencies (25–75% of PCs) are observed, a second test on a new set of cells is performed. If the same results are observed in the second set, a new sample may be required to confirm the clonotypic sequence. The first sample may have been a "bad pull" bone marrow biopsy (*see* **Note 3**), in which insufficient quality or quantity of BMMCs is obtained. If low IgH sequence frequencies are observed (0–25%), the proposed sequence is not clonotypic. If the failed sequence originated from the bulk method, another PCR using the bulk method can be performed, but this will most likely amplify the same sequence. The best alternative is to complete the single-cell PCR (*see* **Subheading 3.6.**), and sequence the IgH VDJ of individual PCs.

11. In **Subheading 3.2.1.**, BMMCs are stained with anti-CD38 and anti-CD138 to specifically label PCs. Other MAbs, such as anti-CD19 and anti-CD56, can also be included to distinguish malignant PCs from normal PCs *(27)*. Immunostained cells are washed with PBS/0.5 m*M* EDTA to prevent cell clumps that can clog the flow cytometer. These cells must never be exposed to fixatives such as formalin, which sequesters RNA in aggregates of fixed proteins, making it unavailable for reverse transcription in the direct lysis reverse transcription protocol. The most important aspect of single-cell sorting is aligning the Autoclone unit to deposit cells directly into the RT buffer. The challenge is to align the Autoclone unit so that it moves parallel to the strip of PCR tubes, along a line through the center of

each tube. In practical terms, small rotational adjustments of the rack holder can be made using the touch-screen controls of most flow cytometers to optimize the alignment. Cells deposited on the side of the tube in a misaligned sort are quickly dehydrated by evaporation and are resistant to centrifugation into the buffer. Inaccurate targeting of cells can lead to negative results in sorting experiments in which other parameters such as stream stability and cell flow rate were within acceptable ranges. At least 96 PCs should be sorted per patient to have enough material for single-cell primer confirmation (*see* **Subheading 3.1.6.**) and the alternative method of determining the IgH sequence (*see* **Subheading 3.2.**). Sorted PCs can be stored at –80°C for up to 6 mo before performing the reverse transcription reaction. Conversely, B-cells, which are often sorted into different populations and studied for coexpression of specific genes and clonotypic IgH, should be reverse transcribed immediately after sorting. MM B-cell IgH transcripts, which are relatively low in abundance compared with PC IgH transcripts, are difficult to detect even with prompt processing and amplification.

12. Direct lysis RT buffer is prepared and aliquoted in a sterile designated area as discussed in **Note 2**. Batches of RT buffer are prepared without Superscript enzyme, aliquoted into 12-strip 0.2-mL PCR tubes in groups of 96, capped, and stored at –80°C for up to 1 mo. Quality control tests on samples from the batch can be conducted with a standard cDNA and β2M primers. Having large high-quality batches of RT buffer minimizes variation in sample yield and contamination.

13. This is the most direct method for determining the clonotypic IgH sequence from individual cells. Although the yield from the second-stage FR2/JHc reaction is relatively low in many cases, direct sequencing using both FR2 and JHc as sequencing primers is usually successful for all but the weakest bands. In some cases, the FR1c/JHc amplification may continue in the second-stage reaction, leading to multiple bands in a single lane. When both FR2/JHc and β2M reactions are negative, the quality of the sort is implicated. When FR2/JHc is negative and β2M is positive, the IgH sequence may not be recognized by the consensus primers or the flow cytometer may have sorted non-PCs. It may be necessary to perform single-cell PCR on a number of samples taken at different times before the clonotypic sequence can be determined. When FR2/JHc is positive but the corresponding β2M reaction is negative, contamination of the reaction with FR2/JHc PCR product (exogenous DNA from pipettors or tips, or cross-contamination between reactions) is likely.

14. Contamination of samples with exogenous DNA or cross-contamination between tubes is a significant problem in single-cell nested PCR reactions. Although negative controls are good indicators of contamination, often the exogenous DNA is present in such small amounts that contamination is sporadic yet significant. The level of DNA contamination can be assessed by performing 24 heminested β2M reactions (described in **Subheading 3.2.3.**) using water as a template. From this a "percentage contamination" value is determined, and cleanup procedures (decontamination with 10% bleach; new reagents and plasticware and clean pipettors) can be initiated.

References

1. Pilarski, L. M., Masellis-Smith, A., Szczepek, A., Mant, M. J., and Belch, A. R. (1996) Circulating clonotypic B cells in the biology of multiple myeloma: speculations on the origin of myeloma. *Leukoc. Lymphoma* **22,** 375–383.
2. Billadeau, D., Blackstadt, M., Greipp, P., et al. (1991) Analysis of B-lymphoid malignancies using allele-specific polymerase chain reaction: a technique for sequential quantitation of residual disease. *Blood* **78,** 3021–3029.
3. Bakkus, M. H., Heirman, C., Van Riet, I., Van Camp, B., and Thielemans, K. (1992) Evidence that multiple myeloma Ig heavy chain VDJ genes contain somatic mutations but show no intraclonal variation. *Blood* **80,** 2326–2335.
4. Deane, M. and Norton, J. D. (1991) Immunoglobulin gene 'fingerprinting': an approach to analysis of B lymphoid clonality in lymphoproliferative disorders. *Br. J. Haematol.* **77,** 274–281.
5. Campbell, M. J., Zelenetz, A. D., Levy, S., and Levy, R. (1992) Use of family specific leader region primers for PCR amplification of the human heavy chain variable region gene repertoire. *Mol. Immunol.* **29,** 193–203.
6. Aubin, J., Davi, F., Nguyen-Salomon, F., et al. (1995) Description of a novel FR1 IgH PCR strategy and its comparison with three other strategies for the detection of clonality in B cell malignancies. *Leukemia* **9,** 471–479.
7. Owen, R. G., Johnson, R. J., Rawstron, A. C., et al. (1996) Assessment of IgH PCR strategies in multiple myeloma. *J. Clin. Pathol.* **49,** 672–675.
8. Bergsagel, P. L., Smith, A. M., Szczepek, A., Mant, M. J., Belch, A. R., and Pilarski, L. (1995) In multiple myeloma, clonotypic B lymphocytes are detectable among CD19+ peripheral blood cells expressing CD38, CD56, and monotypic Ig light chain. *Blood* **85,** 436–447.
9. van Dongen, J. J., Langerak, A. W., Bruggemann, M., et al. (2003) Design and standardization of PCR primers and protocols for detection of clonal immunoglobulin and T-cell receptor gene recombinations in suspect lymphoproliferations: report of the BIOMED-2 Concerted Action BMH4-CT98-3936. *Leukemia* **17,** 2257–2317.
10. Billadeau, D., Ahmann, G., Greipp, P., and Van Ness, B. (1993) The bone marrow of multiple myeloma patients contains B cell populations at different stages of differentiation that are clonally related to the malignant plasma cell. *J. Exp. Med.* **178,** 1023–1031.
11. Bakkus, M. H., Van Riet, I., Van Camp, B., and Thielemans, K. (1994) Evidence that the clonogenic cell in multiple myeloma originates from a pre-switched but somatically mutated B cell. *Br. J. Haematol.* **87,** 68–74.
12. Szczepek, A. J., Bergsagel, P. L., Axelsson, L., Brown, C. B., Belch, A. R., and Pilarski, L. M. (1997) CD34+ cells in the blood of patients with multiple myeloma express CD19 and IgH mRNA and have patient-specific IgH VDJ gene rearrangements. *Blood* **89,** 1824–1833.
13. Szczepek, A. J., Seeberger, K., Wizniak, J., Mant, M. J., Belch, A. R., and Pilarski, L. M. (1998) A high frequency of circulating B cells share clonotypic Ig heavy-chain VDJ rearrangements with autologous bone marrow plasma cells in multiple

myeloma, as measured by single-cell and in situ reverse transcriptase-polymerase chain reaction. *Blood* **92**, 2844–2855.

14. Reiman, T., Seeberger, K., Taylor, B. J., et al. (2001) Persistent preswitch clonotypic myeloma cells correlate with decreased survival: evidence for isotype switching within the myeloma clone. *Blood* **98**, 2791–2799.

15. Taylor, B. J., Pittman, J. A., Seeberger, K., et al. (2002) Intraclonal homogeneity of clonotypic immunoglobulin M and diversity of nonclinical post-switch isotypes in multiple myeloma: insights into the evolution of the myeloma clone. *Clin. Cancer Res.* **8**, 502–513.

16. Kriangkum, J., Taylor, B. J., Mant, M. J., Treon, S. P., Belch, A. R., and Pilarski, L. M. (2003) The malignant clone in Waldenstrom's macroglobulinemia. *Semin. Oncol.* **30**, 132–135.

17. Tonegawa, S. (1983) Somatic generation of antibody diversity. *Nature* **302**, 575–581.

18. Alt, F. W., Oltz, E. M., Young, F., Gorman, J., Taccioli, G., and Chen, J. (1992) VDJ recombination. *Immunol. Today* **13**, 306–314.

19. Bassing, C. H., Swat, W., and Alt, F. W. (2002) The mechanism and regulation of chromosomal V(D)J recombination. *Cell* **109(Suppl.)**, S45–S55.

20. Matsuda, F., Ishii, K., Bourvagnet, P., et al. (1998) The complete nucleotide sequence of the human immunoglobulin heavy chain variable region locus. *J. Exp. Med.* **188**, 2151–2162.

21. Lefranc, M. P. (2003) IMGT databases, web resouces and tools for immunoglobulin and T cell receptor sequence analysis, http://imgt.cines.fr. *Leukemia* **17**, 260–266.

22. Alt, F. W. and Baltimore, D. (1982) Joining of immunoglobulin heavy chain segments: implications from a chromosome with evidence of three D–J$_H$ fusions. *Proc. Natl. Acad. Sci. USA* **79**, 4118–4122.

23. Komori, T., Okada, A., Stewart, V., and Alt, F. W. (1993) Lack of N regions in antigen receptor variable region genes of TdT-deficient lymphocytes. *Science* **261**, 1171–1175.

24. Papavasiliou, F. N. and Schatz, D. G. (2002) Somatic hypermutation of immunoglobulin genes: merging mechanisms for genetic diversity. *Cell* **109(Suppl.)**, S35–S44.

25. Pellat-Deceunynck, C., Bataille, R., Robillard, N., et al. (1994) Expression of CD28 and CD40 in human myeloma cells: a comparative study with normal plasma cells. *Blood* **84**, 2597–2603.

26. Wijdenes, J., Vooijs, W. C., Clement, C., et al. (1996) A plasmocyte selective monoclonal antibody (B-B4) recognizes syndecan-1. *Br. J. Haematol.* **94**, 318–323.

27. Harada, H., Kawano, M. M., Huang, N., et al. (1993) Phenotypic difference of normal plasma cells from mature myeloma cells. *Blood* **81**, 2658–2663.

28. Ausubel, F. M., Brent, R., Kingston, R. E., et al. (eds.) (1994–1998) *Current Protocols in Molecular Biology*, 2nd ed., 4 vols. John Wiley & Sons.

29. Lefranc, M. P., Pommie, C., Ruiz, M., et al. (2003) IMGT unique numbering for immunoglobulin and T cell receptor variable domains and Ig superfamily V-like domains. *Dev. Comp. Immunol.* **27**, 55–77.

30. Kabat, E. A., Wu, T. T., Perry, H. M., Gottesmann, K. S., and Foeller, C. (1991) *Sequences of Proteins of Immunological Interest*, 5th ed., NIH Publication no. 91-3242, U.S. Department of Health and Human Services, Washington, DC.
31. Keats, J. J., Reiman, T., Maxwell, C. A., et al. (2003) In multiple myeloma, t(4;14)(p16; q32) is an adverse prognostic factor irrespective of FGFR3 expression. *Blood* **101,** 1520–1529.

11

Real-Time Polymerase Chain Reaction of Immunoglobulin Rearrangements for Quantitative Evaluation of Minimal Residual Disease in Myeloma

Mara Compagno, Barbara Mantoan, Monica Astolfi, Mario Boccadoro, and Marco Ladetto

Summary

The evaluation of minimal residual disease (MRD) is critical in the evaluation of treatments aimed at maximal cytoreduction in multiple myeloma (MM). Qualitative evaluation of MRD now has a 10-yr-long history, but it remains a relatively sophisticated procedure. More recently, real-time quantitative approaches have also been developed. These approaches allow a very effective monitoring of disease but introduce additional complexity and costs to the procedure. This chapter describes how we currently perform real-time polymerase chain reaction (PCR) in MM. Compared to the first description of the assay in June 2000, significant improvements have been made. Although real-time PCR is the main focus of the chapter, most of the information suitable for a proper setup of a qualitative approach is also provided.

Key Words

Real-time polymerase chain reaction; immunoglobulin genes; minimal residual disease; lymphoid tumors; multiple myeloma.

1. Introduction

The evaluation of minimal residual disease (MRD) through polymerase chain reaction (PCR)-based approaches plays a major role in assessing current efforts of achieving maximal tumor reduction in multiple myeloma (MM), particularly in the transplantation field *(1)*. Because long-lasting molecular remission following standard myeloablative allogeneic transplantation is frequently achieved, PCR negativity is now considered a preliminary step for any innovative treatment delivered with a curative intent *(2–4)*. In recent years, the value

From: *Methods in Molecular Medicine, Vol. 113: Multiple Myeloma: Methods and Protocols*
Edited by: R. D. Brown and P. J. Ho © Humana Press Inc., Totowa, NJ

of PCR analysis has been further increased, by developing effective real-time PCR strategies that allow robust and reproducible quantitative evaluation of tumor burden *(5–11)*.

Despite these results, PCR analysis is still not a widespread approach in MM, and several large institutions do not routinely evaluate MRD in their patients. This underlines a number of drawbacks associated with this approach, including the need for sequencing of the myeloma-specific immunoglobulin heavy chain (IgH) to develop clone-specific primers, sequencing failure in approx 30% of patients, a lack of definite and standardized procedures for primer and probe design, a lack of extensive evaluation of intercenter reproducibility, and the cost and complexity of the procedure.

Efforts toward the resolution of these problems are ongoing *(8,12)*. Although the evaluation of MRD is still far from becoming a routine technique, we expect to witness its rapid and widespread use, as already observed in acute and chronic myeloid leukemias. This will allow the majority of patients to take advantage of it for effective monitoring of their disease. In this chapter, we summarize current knowledge on the use of real-time PCR for the evaluation of MRD. The chapter is organized as a practical guide that should help scientists to develop and perform this procedure on their own even if they work in mid-size or small laboratories. Basic structural requirements, instruments, reagents, experimental protocols, and practical recommendations are provided. We hope that our effort might be useful to our colleagues and deeply appreciate any feedback that might come from those who try to set up IgH-based real-time PCR following some of our recommendations.

2. Materials

2.1. Structural Requirements

1. RNA-dedicated area: In a small laboratory, one might choose to have a common area for RNA preparation and pre-PCR processing. However, this might be problematic, especially if some operators perform only PCR and are not well trained in RNase-free procedures.
2. Pre-PCR area: Keep away from this area any PCR product or anything related to the cloning procedure. Bring only very diluted plasmid aliquots to set up the reaction.
3. Post-PCR area: Cloning and bacterial handling can be performed here.

2.2. Instruments

1. Spectrophotometer.
2. Thermal cycler dedicated to qualitative PCR. Reactions may be run in an analytical thermal cycler, but a dedicated instrument is preferred.
3. DNA electrophoresis apparatus and power supply.

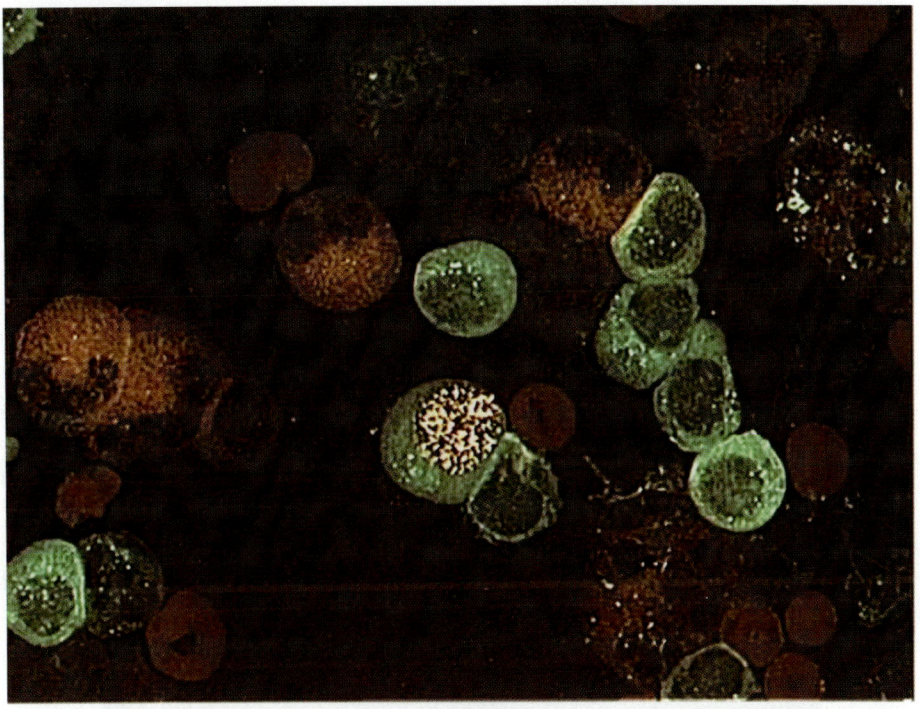

Color Plate 1, Fig. 1. (*see* discussion in Ch. 3 and caption on p. 33). Note the brightly labeled nucleus and the eccentric placement of the nucleus in the labeled PC. Also seen are nonlabeled PCs with similar morphology.

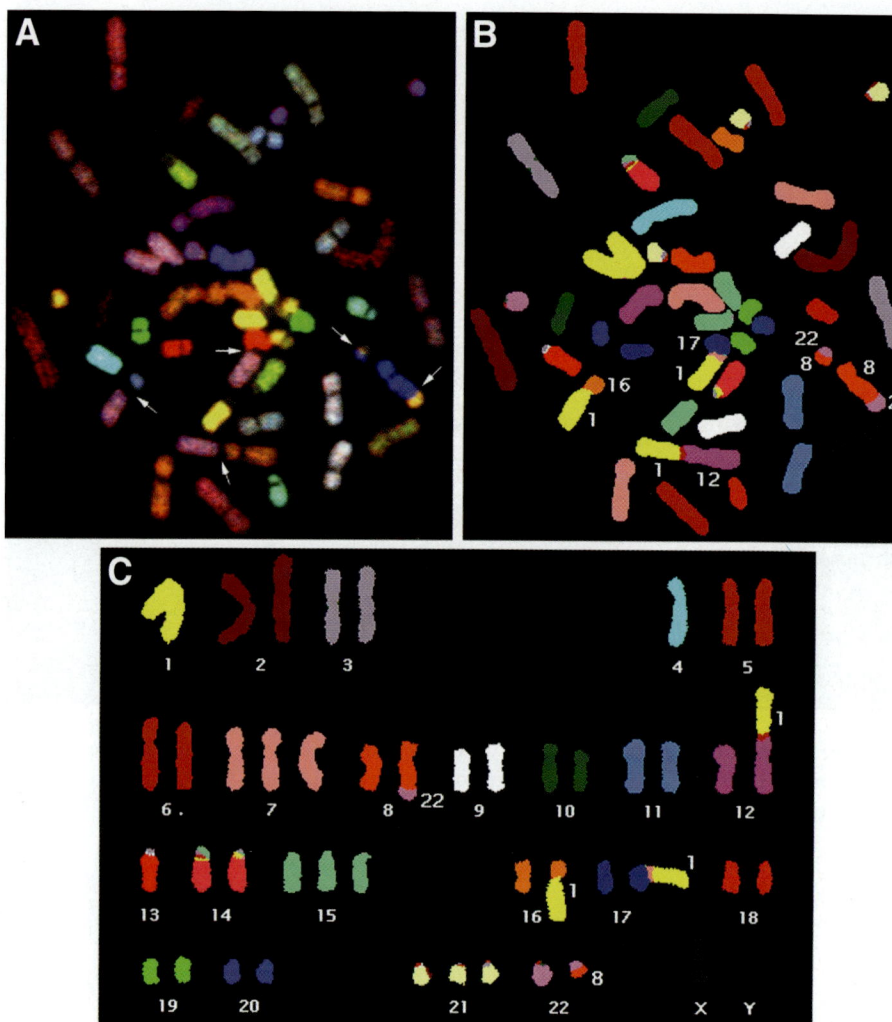

Color Plate 2, Fig. 1. (*see* discussion in Ch. 5 and caption on p. 51). Spectral karyotyping of bone marrow sample of a patient with MM. The simultaneous hybridization of 24 combinatorially labeled chromosome painting probes is demonstrated. **(A)** Metaphase shown in display colors as seen through microscope; **(B)** same metaphase cell shown in classification colors after spectral classification of chromosomes in pseudocolors; **(C)** spectral karyotype of same metaphase shown in classification colors. Note that multiple translocations are identified by changes in color patterns.

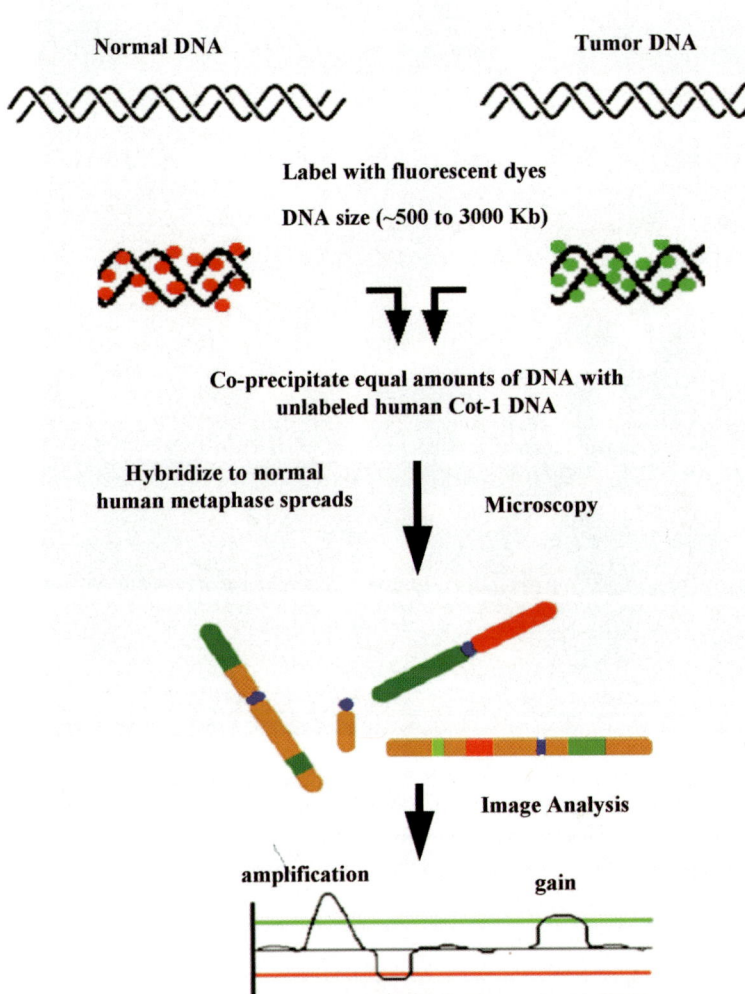

Color Plate 3, Fig. 1. (*see* discussion in Ch. 7 and caption on p. 73). Schematic outline of CGH method. Test and reference DNAs are labeled with green and redfluorochromes, respectively, and cohybridized to normal human metaphase chromosome spreads. Visualization of the chromosomes by fluorescent microscopy reveals differences in the fluorescent hybridization signals along the chromosomes representative of the abundance of the test DNA sequence. Analysis of these captured images can provide a color ratio profile indicative of changes in copy number in the test DNA relative to the reference DNA.

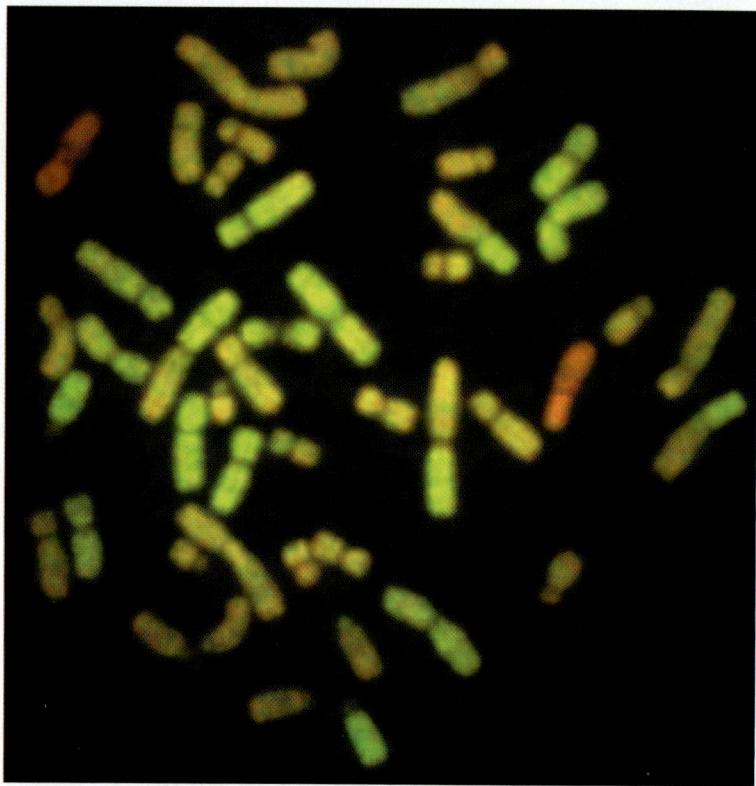

Color Plate 4, Fig. 2. (*see* discussion in Ch. 7 and caption on p. 79). Metaphase spread after simultaneous hybridization with differentially labeled normal (red) and myeloma DNA (green) by CGH. Chromosomal regions that were overrepresented in the tumor are visualized in green, whereas regions that were lost or deleted from the tumor are seen in red.

Color Plate 5, Fig. 3. [opposite page](*see* discussion in Ch. 7 and caption on p. 80). Quantitative CGH analysis of myeloma. **(A)** Chromosomes from Fig. 2 identified and karyotyped using quantitative imaging processing software (QUIPS; Applied Imaging). **(B)** Quantitative digital image analysis of fluorescence intensities ratios of MM (MM-14). Green-to-red fluorescence ratio profiles and shown for all chromosomes. The mean ratio (blue line) and ±1 SD (black lines) of 13-20 measurements for each chromosomeare shown. The ratio profiles for each chro-

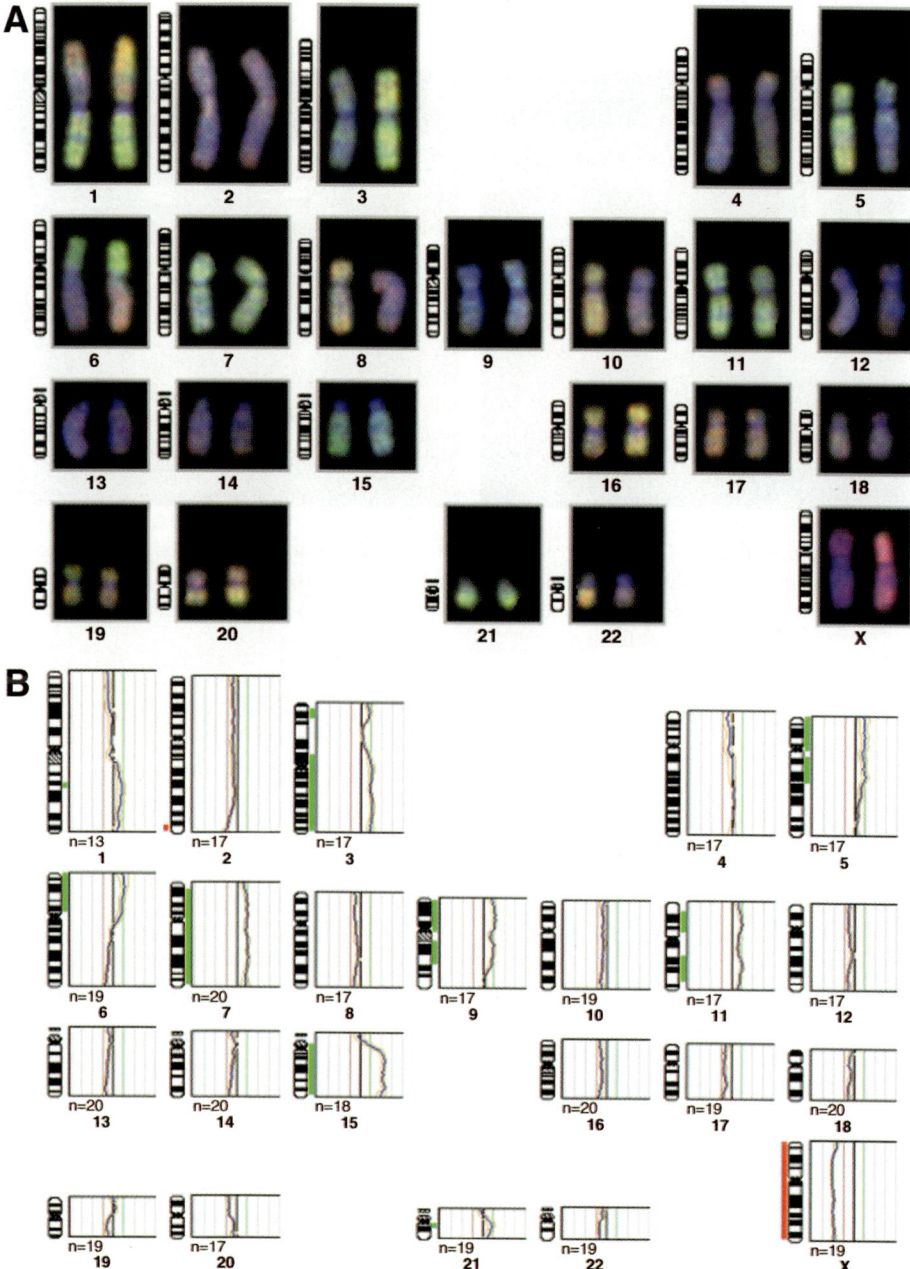

mosome are shown from pter to qter. The average value (1.0) representing the mean green-to-red ratio for the entire case (6-10 metaphases) and red and green lines indicate threshold values of 0.8 and 1.2 for loss and gain, respectively. Based on this analysis, the chromosomal regions that were overrepresented in myeloma case MM-14 were 3, 5pter- q15, 6p, 7, 9pter-q22, 11, and 15q, whereas X and 2q35-q37 were underrepresented.

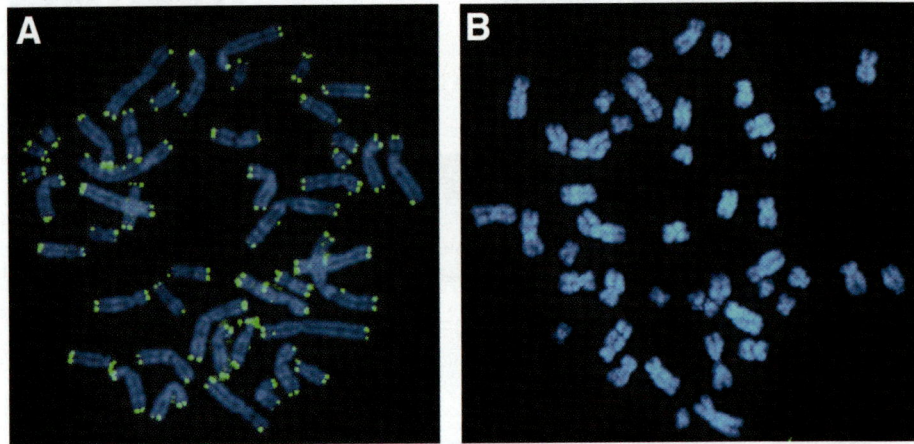

Color Plate 6, Fig. 4. (*see* discussion in Ch. 16 and caption on p. 221). Q-FISH assay. **(A)** Normal peripheral blood mononuclear cells and **(B)** SKO-007 myeloma cell telomeres were visualized using FITC-labeled peptide nucleic acid (CCCTAA)$_3$ telomere probe.

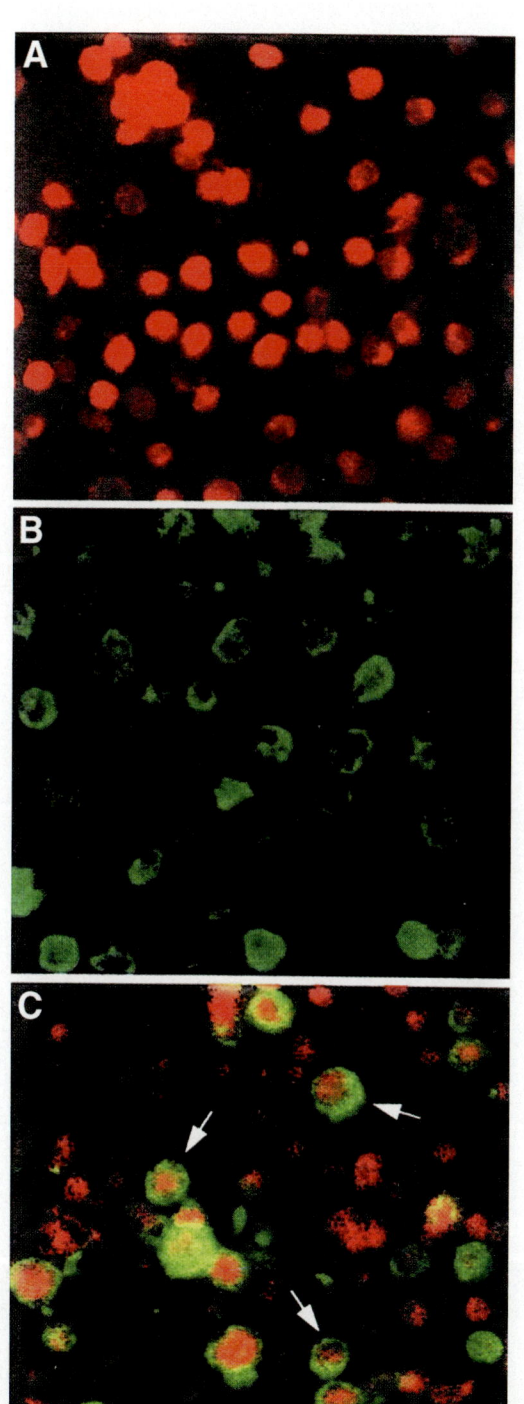

Color Plate 7, Fig. 1. (*see* discussion in Ch. 17 and caption on p. 231). Fluorescence photomicrographs of J558-IL-4 and DC fusion preparations. (**A**) J558-IL-4 cells were stained with TRITC. The TRITC-labeled J558-IL-4 cells were fused with DCs using PEG. (**B**) DCs and (**C**) DC/J558-IL-4 fusion preparation were then stained with rat anti-CD11c antibody followed by goat anti-rat IgG-FITC antibody. Arrows represent the fusion hybrids (DC/J558-IL-4) (magnification: ×400).

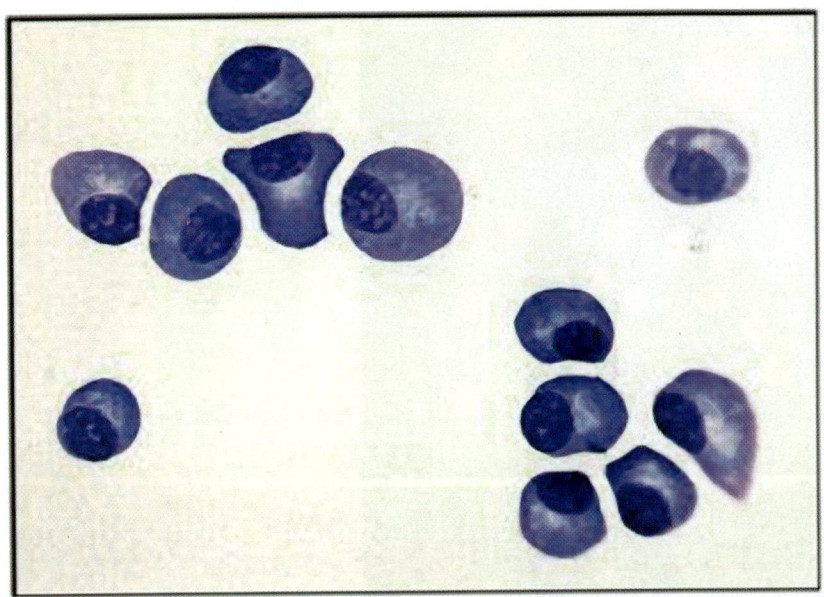

Color Plate 8, Fig. 1. (*see* discussion in Ch. 21 and caption on p. 272). MGG-stained cytospin preparation of PCs purified from a diagnostic bone marrow aspirate of a patient with myeloma using CD138 magnetic microbeads.

4. Scientific camera.
5. Sequencing facilities (can be performed externally).
6. Thermomixer: A perfect temperature is critical for cloning when *Escherichia coli*-competent cells are heat-shocked, so revise it frequently.
7. Bacterial incubator with shaking.
8. Analytical thermal cycler, to make quantitative analysis of genomic DNA samples. We have always used the ABI Prism 7700 and, more recently, the ABI Prism 7900. However, several investigators have also been satisfied also with nonlaser-based thermal cyclers, which are smaller and less expensive.
9. PCR Ampliwax 100 (PE Biosystem).
10. Chemical hood.

2.3. Reagents and Kits

1. Ficoll-Hypaque (Amersham Pharmacia Biotech AB, Uppsala, Sweden) for separation of white blood cells (stable at room temperature, light sensitive).
2. Trizol, for RNA extraction (Invitrogen, Carlsbad, CA) (store at 4°C, toxic); Dnazol ($\geq 5 \times 10^6$ cells) (stable at room temperature, toxic) (Life Technologies, Grand Island, NY); or GenomicPrep Cells and Tissue DNA Isolation Kit ($<5 \times 10^6$ cells) (Amersham, Piscataway, NJ), for DNA extraction (store at 4°C).
3. Reagents for cDNA: DNase (Boehringer Mannheim, GmbH, Germany), Rnasin (Promega, Madison, WI), 10 mM MgCl$_2$ (Gibco-BRL, Gaithersburg MD), random examers (PE Applied Biosystems, Roche, NJ), 0.1 M DDT (dithiothreitol) (Gibco-BRL), 10 nM dNTP (Amersham), 5X buffer (Gibco-BRL), reverse transcriptase (PE Applied Biosystems, Roche) (all reagents must be stored at –20°C).
4. PCR reagents for IgH sequencing and cloning: 15 or 20 mM MgCl$_2$ (Promega), 10X MgCl$_2$-free buffer (Promega), Taq DNA polymerase (Promega), 20 p/λ primers (Sigma-Genosys Aldrich House, UK), sequencing-grade solution 2 mM dNTPs (Amersham Biosciences) (all reagents must be stored at –20°C).
5. Materials for gel preparation: agarose, regular and low melting point (for preparation of 2% agarose gel, stable at room temperature) (Promega), 1X TAE buffer (40 mM Tris-acetate; 1 mM EDTA, pH 8.0; stable at room temperature), ethidium bromide (light sensitive, stable at room temperature, toxic).
6. QIAquick Gel Extraction Kit (Qiagen GmbH, Germany) (stable at room temperature).
7. TOPO-TA Cloning Kit (Invitrogen) (store at –70°C).
8. Solid and liquid Luria-Bertani (LB) medium (Invitrogen) and plates (store at 4°C).
9. Wizard Plus Minipreps resin and minicolumns DNA Purification System (Promega) (stable at room temperature).
10. TaqMan PCR Core Reagent Kit reagents (PE Applied Biosystems, Roche) (store at −20°C) and TaqMan Universal Master Mix (PE Applied Biosystems, Roche) (store at 2–8°C).
11. Probes for real-time PCR (PE Applied Biosystems, Roche) (store at –20°C).
12. Primers for real-time PCR (Sigma-Genosys Aldrich House) (store at –20°C).

3. Methods

3.1. Sample Selection, Nucleic Acid Extraction and Storage, and DNA Synthesis and Analysis

3.1.1. Samples for IgH Sequencing

A bone marrow sample containing a high amount of tumor cells is required. The rate of success of IgH sequencing falls dramatically if attempted on samples displaying <5% tumor contamination.

3.1.2. Nucleic Acid Extraction (see **Note 1**)

Bone marrow samples are collected in heparin-containing tubes. We usually perform cell separation through a Ficoll-Hypaque density gradient *(5)*. Cells are then stored as pellets at –70°C. For DNA extraction, these samples can be used indefinitely. For RNA extraction, we noticed a reduced efficiency for samples older than 24 mo (unpublished observation). RNA extraction is usually performed on samples at diagnosis for IgH sequencing. We observed a reduced efficiency of IgH sequencing starting from gDNA. The large amount of IgH transcripts is probably responsible for the improved results obtained with RNA. Indeed, we think that this aspect might be more critical in IgH sequencing of MM samples mostly owing to the high rate of somatic hypermutation, which might induce significant loss of primer efficiency in these patients. Trizol is our favorite reagent, although most commercially available kits can provide good-quality RNA *(5)*.

3.1.3. cDNA Synthesis

IgH-specific cDNA is usually prepared using standard room temperature reactions using the C-γ or C-α primers (**Table 1**), depending on the myeloma histotype. cDNAs from light chain MM are prepared using either random hexamers or oligo-T primers *(5)*.

3.1.4. Samples for Follow-Up Analysis

gDNA or cDNA of follow-up samples are usually employed for qualitative PCR. For real-time PCR, we employ only gDNA, because we favor absolute quantification for this purpose *(5)*.

3.2. Amplification of IgH Rearrangement

3.2.1. Primer Families

The strategy used to obtain the tumor-specific IgH is shown in **Fig. 1** *(5,13)*. Two microliters of cDNA is amplified using three sets of consensus forward primers, two derived from the framework region 1 (FR1) *(14,15)* and one derived from the leader region *(15)* together with a JH region antisense consensus primer *(13)* (**Table 1**). Two families of primers contain degenerated primers (**Table 1**).

Table 1
Primers for cDNA Synthesis and IgH Sequencing

Primers	Name	Sequences	Ref
cDNA	Cα	5′ GACCTTGGGGCTGGTCGGGGATGC 3′	*19*
	Cγ	5′ GACCGATGGGCCCTTGGTGGAAGC 3′	*19*
	Random Hex.	NA	NA
	Oligo dT	NA	NA
VHFD	VH1FD	5′ CCTCAGTGAAGGTCTCCTGAAGG 3′	*14*
	VH2FD	5′ TCCTGCGCTGGTGAAAGCCACACA 3′	*14*
	VH3FD	5′ GGTCCCTGAGACTCTCCTGTGCA 3′	*14*
	VH4aFD	5′ TCGGAGACCCTGTCCCTCACCTGCA 3′	*14*
	VH4bFD	5′ CGCTGTCTCTGGTTACTCCATCAG 3′	*14*
	VH5FD	5′ GAAAAAGCCCGGGGAGTCTCTGAA 3′	*14*
	VH6FD	5′ CCTGTGCCATCTCCGGGGACAGTG 3′	*14*
VHFSdeg	VH1FS	5′ CAGGTGCAGCTGGTGCARYCTG 3′	*15*
	VH2FS	5′ GAGGTGCAGCTGGTGSAGTCYG 3′	*15*
	VH4aFS	5′ CAGSTGCAGCTGCAGGAGTCSG 3′	*15*
	VH4bFS	5′ CAG GTGCAGCTACARCAGTGGG 3′	*15*
	VH5FS	5′ GAGGTGCAGCTGKTGCAGTCTG 3′	*15*
	VH6FS	5′ CAGGTACAGCTGCAGCAGTCAG 3′	*15*
VHLS	VH1LS	5′ CTCACCATGGACTGGACCTGGAG 3′	*15*
	VH2LS	5′ ATGGACATACTTTGTTCCACGCTC 3′	*15*
	VH3LS	5′ CCATGGAGTTTGGGCTGAGCTGG 3′	*15*
	VH4LS	5′ ACATGAAACAYCTGTGGTTCTTCC 3′	*15*
	VH5LS	5′ ATGGGGTCAACCGCCATCCTCCG 3′	*15*
	VH6LS	5′ ATGTCTGTCTCCTTCCTCATCTTC 3′	*15*
JH	JH/D	5′ ACCTGAGGAGACGGTGACCAGGGT 3′	*13*

We usually start using the VHFD family followed by the VHFSdeg and VHLS. If one of the three reactions gives a satisfactory PCR product, we proceed with a scale-up reaction for sequencing. In case of lack of clonal amplification in all of the three reactions, we relinquish VDJ sequencing for this patient. Often a fuzzy band appears. We usually try to improve the quality of the product by increasing the annealing temperature of 2°C for each experiment up to 6°C. If this strategy is unsatisfactory, we clone the best band that we obtained.

*3.2.2. PCR Conditions (see **Note 2**)*

Standard conditions for our baseline IgH sequencing reaction are as follows: 30–33 cycles with denaturation at 94°C for 1 min, annealing at 62°C for 30 s, and extension at 72°C for 30 s with a final extension of 10 min at 72°C. Samples are amplified "hot start" using Ampliwax 100 beads (PE Applied

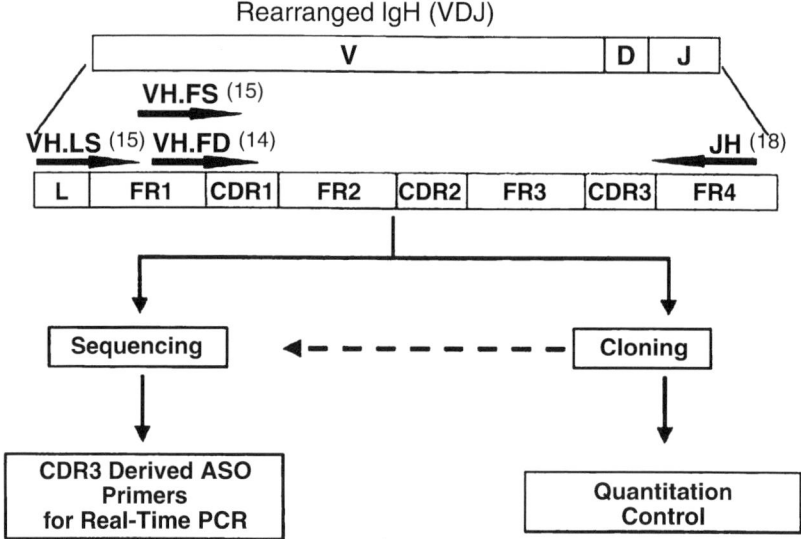

Fig. 1. Schematic representation of strategy used to amplify myeloma IgH sequences. The names and relative positions of the primers used for initial amplification are shown. V, variable region; D, diversity region; J, joining region; L, leader region; CDR, complementarity-determining region; FR, framework region.

Biosystems). PCR products are then analyzed by electrophoresis on 2% agarose gels. **Figure 2A** is a typical example of a IgH PCR that is expected to give a good sequence. **Figure 2B** shows a band that requires further improvement of PCR conditions. **Figure 2C** is a reaction that is unable to identify a clonal PCR product.

3.2.3. Scale-Up and Purification of the PCR Product

When an apparently clonal PCR product is observed, the sample of interest is reamplified in large scale for direct sequencing of the tumor IgH rearrangement. PCR products are run on low melting point agarose gels and are purified by gel excision using a QIAquick PCR purification kit (Qiagen, GmbH) and are directly sequenced from both strands usually using the same primers as in the amplification reaction. Sequencing analysis is performed in an external facility. The amount of PCR product required and sample preparation are highly variable, depending on the requirements of the sequencing facility. Usually a 200-μL reaction carried out in four separate tubes is enough. Sequencing is usually performed on both strands. Alignments for identification of hypervariable regions are performed using the GenBank data library as well as DNAPLOT (http://vbase.mrc-cpe.cam.ac.uk/index.php?module=pagemaster&PAGE_user_op=view_page&PAG

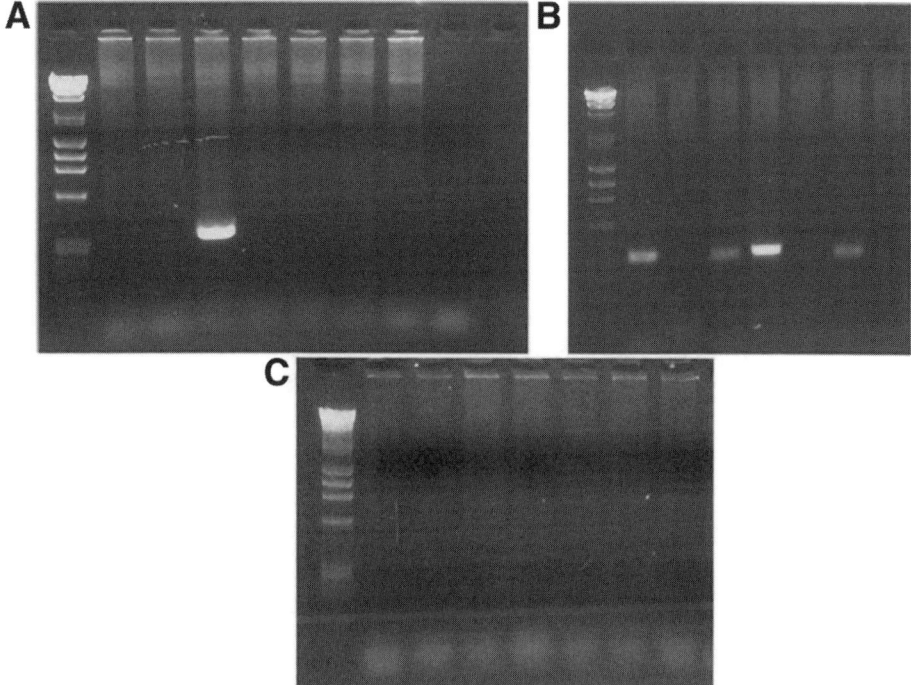

Fig. 2. Examples of PCR analysis of IgH genes. (**A**) Clear clonal product that can be sequenced without further tuning of reaction. (**B**) Multiple fuzzy bands. Such a reaction requires additional tuning of PCR conditions. (**C**) Total absence of clonal product. This indicates that no IgH sequencing is possible with this set of primers in that particular patient.

E_id=10&MMN_position=7:7) for comparison of the IgH rearranged variable region with the homologous germ-line sequences.

3.2.4. When Cloning Is Required to Sequence the IgH Rearrangement (see **Notes 3** and **4**)

When direct sequencing does not allow the reading of a clear sequence, cloning of PCR products can be beneficial. The procedure is identical to that described in the next section with the only difference that cloning and sequencing of 12–15 colonies is required. Given the good quality of plasmid clones, we usually sequence only one strand (usually the forward). Sequences repeated in at least three different clones are considered as pertaining to the tumor clone. If no repeated sequence is noticed following examination of 12 clones, sequencing of additional sequences is usually of no advantage.

3.3. Cloning of IgH Rearrangement to Prepare Quantitation Controls

Cloning is required to prepare quantitation standards. We usually employ the TOPO-TA Cloning kit (Invitrogen) according to the manufacturer's recommendations using blue-white colony selection. We have also employed the TA cloning kit from the same company with similar results (the kit provides all the required reagents). The procedure can be subdivided into four steps.

3.3.1. Ligation (see **Note 5**)

Briefly 1 µL of fresh (reaction performed the same day) PCR product is ligated using a mix containing SALT solution (1 µL), TOPO VECTOR (1 µL), and H_2O (3 µL). After mixing gently, the product is left for 30 min at room temperature. The ligation product can be stored at $-20°C$.

3.3.2. Chemical Transformation (see **Note 6**)

The ligation product is employed to transform competent cells according to the following procedure:

1. Gently thaw *E. coli*-competent cells in a vial on ice.
2. Add 2 to 3 µL of the ligation product to the vial of *E. coli*-competent cells and mix.
3. Incubate the cells and ligation product for 5–30 min on ice.
4. Heat-shock the cells for 30 s at 42°C without shaking and then incubate in ice for 2 min.

3.3.3. Recovery and Plating

1. Add 250 µL of room temperature SOC medium (available with the TOPO-TA Cloning Kit) to bacteria.
2. Cap all tubes and shake at 37°C for 1 h.
3. Spread 10–50 µL from each transformation product onto LB plates containing 5-bromo-4-chloro-3-indolyl-β-D-galactoside (X-gal) and ampicillin (*see* **Note 7**). Incubate overnight at 37°C. Reagents for plates are not available in the kit.

3.3.4. Analysis of Positive Clones

Approximately four white colonies are picked up and grown by overnight shaking in LB broth containing 50 µg/mL of ampicillin (*see* **Note 8**). Plasmid DNA is purified using Wizard Plus Minipreps resin and minicolumns (Promega). Plasmids are then sequenced in order to verify identity to the sequence obtained by direct sequencing. This step is required because, occasionally, a bacterial clone might not contain the sequence of interest. Plasmid aliquots can be stored indefinitely at $-70°C$ in 1X TE. Bacteria in liquid culture can be frozen at $-70°C$ by adding 30% glycerol.

3.3.5. Quantification and Dilution of Plasmids

Plasmids are quantified spectrophotometrically and diluted in order to obtain a concentration that is appropriate for real-time PCR. Since 10e6 copies in the first dilution tube are desired and usually 2.5 μL of test DNA is added to the PCR tube, the required final concentration is 400,000 plasmids/μL. Plasmid DNA is usually diluted into DNA from polyclonal peripheral blood at a concentration of 100 ng/μL.

3.3.6. Appropriate Controls

Several controls might be useful especially when the procedure still needs to be optimized, including a transformation positive control (a plasmid that is known to work), a plasmid-only control (in which the open plasmid is ligated without any insert), and a negative control (in which no plasmid is added). This might be helpful in understanding during which step of the procedure a problem has occurred.

3.4. How to Make Effective Clone-Specific Primers

Each nucleotide sequence is compared with other similar IgH sequences obtained from a database. Some softwares are commercially available, and others can be accessed through the Web (e.g., Primer 3). This step allows identification of conserved regions (FR) and variable regions (complementarity-determining region [CDR] of IgH. The most critical primer for PCR specificity is the CDR3-derived antisense primer. This primer should be chosen in the most hypervariable area of the patient sequence. The forward 5′ primer is less critical. If the reaction is used only for qualitative PCR, the most important criterion is obviously the variability of the region of interest. If the reaction is designed for real-time PCR, forward primers designed immediately upstream to the consensus probes usually allow having very robust real-time PCR reactions. Despite the fact that this area is rather conserved, we observed no significant specificity problems if the reverse primer was chosen correctly. We strongly discourage the use of the FR1 or leader primers employed for IgH sequencing as forward primers for real-time PCR, mainly for two reasons: (1) these primers produce amplicons that are too long, and (2) these primers are 100% homologous to the plasmid whereas they can be <100% homologous to the patient sequence. The lack of homology between patient and plasmid sequence can induce a right shift of unknown samples compared to standards that might induce an underestimation of the amount of clonal DNA up to 2 log (unpublished observation). A discussion of the use of the IgH-derived primers for standard qualitative PCR is beyond the scope of this chapter. However, additional indications on this methodology have been published (13).

3.5. Consensus or Patient-Specific Probes

Although several researchers employ patient-specific probes *(9,10)*, we prefer to use consensus probes, which allow a dramatic reduction in the cost of the procedure *(5,6,16)*. Consensus probes are not a fixed panel, and we are currently increasing the number of probes that we are using. Their use requires no additional experimental setup and is not associated with loss of sensitivity and specificity. **Table 2** provides consensus probes that allow amplification of a large proportion of MM sequences. Additional probes might be designed if required. All these probes were originally labeled with FAM and TAMRA. These probes can easily tolerate one and often two mismatches, provided that the first 5′ base is homologous. Historically, probes were preferentially chosen from the reverse strand, but now both sense and antisense probes are used as required. **Table 2** also provides probes that can amplify a high proportion of patients employing VH1, VH2, VH3, and VH4 families. These probes have been repeatedly and successfully employed at our institution. We suggest beginning experiments using one of these probes, possibly assessing patients with one or no mismatches. Once the methodology is working fine, it would be possible to move toward samples with two mismatches or design additional probes. We are currently testing minor groove binder (MGB) probes that seem to show even greater effectiveness and require shorter areas of homology, thus allowing them to work in a larger number of patients. When designing new probes, the common recommendations originally suggested by Applied Biosystems (especially those regarding the preference for G-poor sequences, particularly avoiding four G stretches and a G as first base) should be followed, if this is possible, based on the homologous areas of the IgH sequences of interest *(17)*.

3.6. Real-Time PCR Conditions: The "Appropriate" Standard Curve

Standard IgH real-time PCR conditions are as follows: 500–600 ng of target DNA in a 25-μL volume using the TaqMan PCR Core Reagent Kit reagents (PE Applied Biosystems). The following reagents are used: 1X PCR Core Reagent Kit Buffer, 25 mM MgCl$_2$, with the addition of 0.5 μL of dATP, dCTP, and dGTP (10 mM solution); 0.5 μL of dUTP (20 mM solution); 10 pmol of each primer; 5 pmol of reporting probe; 0.25 μL of AmpErase Uracil-N-Glycosylase; and 0.13 μL of Taq Platinum DNA polymerase (Gibco-BRL). After incubating for 2 min at 50°C for optimal activity of AmpErase Uracil-N-Glycosylase, and incubating for 10 min at 95°C to activate Taq Platinum, the following reaction is run: 42 cycles of denaturation at 95°C for 15 s and annealing at 60–62°C for 1 min. Reactions are performed in an ABI Prism 7700 or 7900 sequence detector system (PE Applied Biosystems). Note that we do not employ the Universal Master Mix because some tuning,

Table 2
Probe for Real-Time Polymerase Chain Reaction

Probe	Sequences	Report/Quencer	Ref
LVH1	CTGCTCAGCTCCATGTAGGCTGTGC	FAM/TAMRA	5
MVH1	CTGCCCTGGAACTTCTGTGCGTAG	FAM/TAMRA	5
MVH2	ACCACCTGGTTTTTGGAGGTGTCCTT	FAM/TAMRA	5
LVH3	CCGTGTCCTCGGCTCTCAGGC	FAM/TAMRA	5
MVH3TER	CTCTGGAGATGGTGAATCGCCC	FAM/TAMRA	6
MVH4	CGTGTCTGCGGCGGTCACAGA	FAM/TAMRA	5
MVH4TER	TGTCCGCGGCGGTCACAGA	FAM/TAMRA	unpublished
VH2TOR	TCAGCCCCCAGGAAC	FAM/MGB	unpublished

particularly of $MgCl_2$ concentrations, might be required that we add no more than 600 ng of DNA because larger amounts often induce significant inhibition of the reaction.

There are no objective criteria to define whether a standard curve can be used or not for sample quantitation. Indeed, this might change considerably depending on the target and the required level of sensitivity. However, we have defined some empirical criteria defining a standard curve that can be safely employed even in the case of extremely low copy numbers such as MRD for evaluation. Our classic test experiment employs 10-fold dilutions of plasmids starting from 10^6 up to 10 genomes. A no-template DNA is also included. Real-time PCR of a given patient rearrangement is considered effective if the reaction can fulfill the following criteria:

1. The amplification should show a clear positive signal in the dilution to which 10 plasmid copies were added.
2. No nonspecific PCR product should be observed when a DNA from healthy donor peripheral blood lymphocytes (PBL) is PCR amplified.
3. The correlation should be >0.98.
4. The Y-intercept should be <40 cycles.
5. The slope should be between −3.7 and −3.1.

Based on our experience >70% of the reactions fulfill these criteria using the standard approach; some tuning is required for the remaining 30% of samples. **Figure 3A** presents a typical curve that we obtain for IgH real-time PCR sequencing. **Figure 3B–D** shows some typical problems that might frequently occur (amplification of the no-template DNA **[Fig. 3B]**, no amplification of 10^2 and 10^1 copy samples **[Fig. 3C]**, reaction failure **[Fig. 3D]**). *See* **Notes 9–16** for tips on dealing with these common problems.

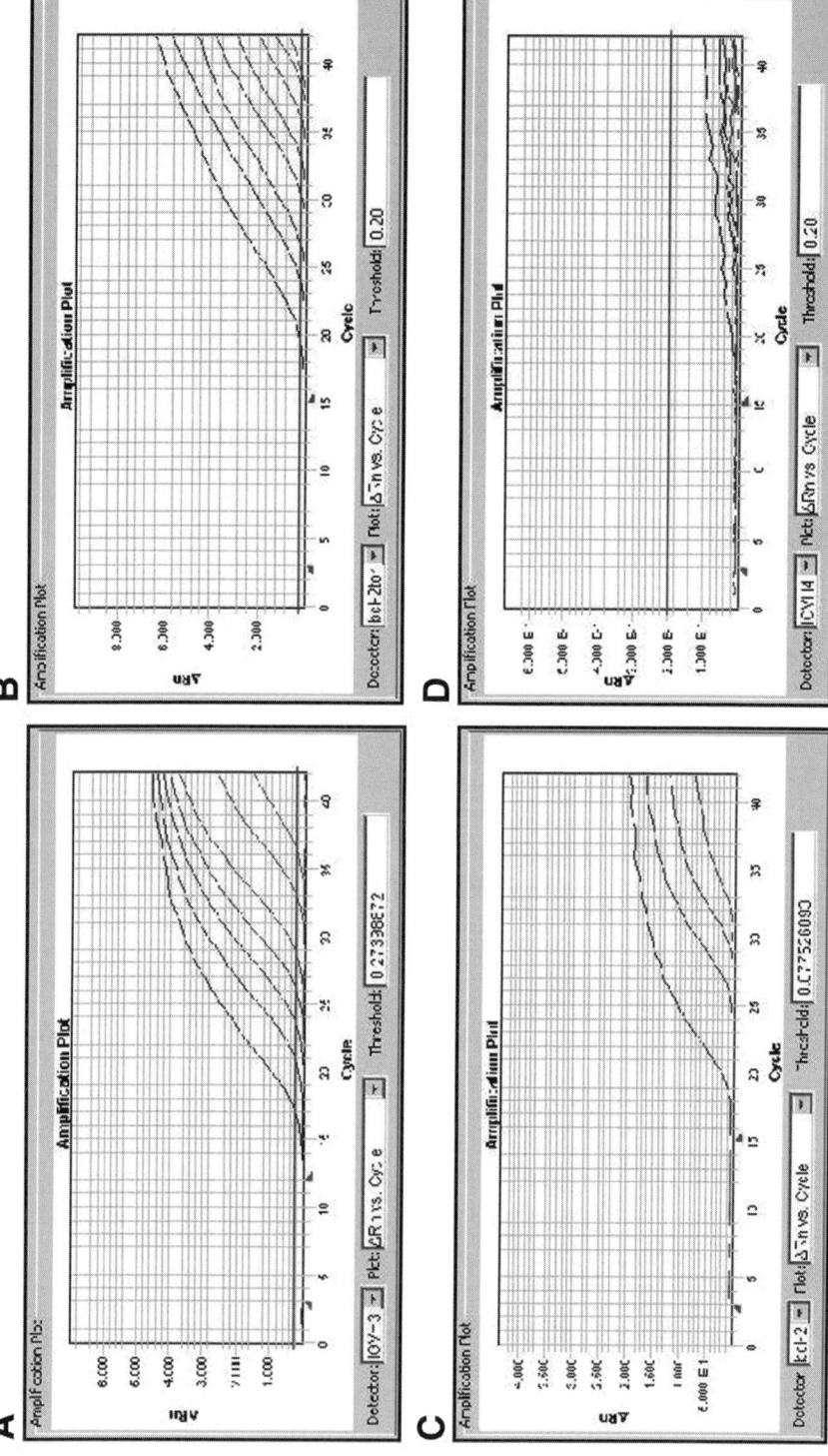

3.7. DNA Normalization (see Note 17)

Several genes have been employed for sample normalization of real-time quantitative PCR results. The basic characteristics for a gene to be employed for DNA normalization are the following: to be present in one single copy in each aploid genome; to be located on autosomic chromosomes; to lack polymorphisms, particularly within primer and probe sequences. We originally employed the GAPDH gene, as already described *(6,16)*. We have recently switched to the RNase P gene whose primers and probe are produced by Applied Biosystems (www.appliedbiosystems.com). This gene is highly recommended by the company and is commercially available. Real-time PCR conditions are as follows: 500–600 ng of target DNA in a 25-µL volume using the TaqMan PCR Core Reagent Kit reagents (PE Applied Biosystems) (we always use the same concentration and amount as in the IgH quantification experiment). The following reagents are used: 1X PCR Core Reagent Kit Buffer, 12.5 µL of 2X Universal Master Mix, 1.25 µL of 20X probe and primer mix, 0.5 U of AmpErase Uracil-*N*-Glycosylase. After incubating for 2 min at 50°C for optimal activity of AmpErase Uracil-*N*-Glycosylase, and incubating for 10 min at 95°C to activate Taq Gold, the following reaction is run: 42 cycles of denaturation at 95°C for 15 s and annealing at 60–62°C for 1 min. Reactions are performed in an ABI Prism 7700 or 7900 sequence detector system (PE Applied Biosystems). Obviously, the standard curve is made by diluting the plasmid in water instead of human DNA. If the results obtained with another target are satisfactory, there is no reason to switch to those described here when performing IgH real-time PCR.

Currently, we perform separate reactions for IgH and RNaseP real-time PCR. We tried multiplex PCR approaches in the past, but the reaction setup proved to be excessively complex, mostly because the IgH primers and probe were different in each patient, and conditions working for one patient gave unacceptable results in others.

Fig. 3. *(see opposite page)* Examples of real-time PCR standard amplification plots obtained using ABI Prism 7900 analytical thermal cycler. **(A)** Amplification plot that satisfies all criteria described in **Subheading 3.6**. **(B)** Amplification plot in which the no-template control is positive, indicating nonspecific amplification. **(C)** Amplification plot in which samples containing 10e2 and 10e1 target copies are not amplified, indicating poor efficiency. Note that also in this case the correlation coefficient and *Y*-intercept derived from these standards are not satisfactory. **(D)** Total failure of reaction. In these cases, refer to the flowchart in **Fig. 4**.

3.8. Analysis and Interpretation of Data

A full description of how to analyze and interpret real-time PCR results is beyond the scope of this chapter. Here we discuss three practical aspects that might be important for the most appropriate use of quantitative data.

3.8.1. When Results Should Not Be Considered

We prefer not to consider samples in which DNA copies of the normalization gene are $<1^4$ or $>1^6$ *(6)* for the following reasons: First, a low value often means that DNA is of very low quality especially if the amount appears much higher by spectrophotometry. If this is the case one might consider procedures to improve DNA quality. Second, when the amount of DNA is very high, we have noticed a significant loss of efficiency in the amplification, which might allow considerable underestimation of the amount of target. We thus prefer to dilute the DNA and test it again.

3.8.2. How to Express Data From Real-Time Quantitative PCR

We usually express our results in terms of IgH copies/1 million of diploid genomes. Several experiments on cell lines have shown that the approach provides values that are very close to absolute quantification *(5)*. Indeed, one might see some degree of difference between expected and calculated values, because a given number of cells is added that actually might be diploid or tetraploid according to the phase of the cell cycle. For this reason, we express the value in terms of rearrangements vs diploid genomes and not as cancer cells vs total cells. Obviously, some biases might result in selected cases owing to the presence of insertions and deletions of chromosomal portions containing the reference gene. If this is a concern in a specific investigational setting, the best option is to use multiple genes for DNA normalization.

3.8.3. How to Compare Qualitative and Quantitative PCR Results

If well performed, both nested PCR and real-time PCR should amplify up to a single copy of DNA. However, real-time PCR is usually performed with a smaller amount of DNA per tube and is thus slightly less sensitive. When we have a sample that is positive by nested PCR and negative by real time PCR, we score it as containing between 1 and 10 rearrangements/1 million diploid genomes. Indeed, real-time PCR is performed on an amount of DNA representative of 100,000 cells. Thus, you can detect the signal of 1 single cell in 1 million only by testing the sample on multiple tubes. This phenomenon has been verified experimentally.

4. Notes

1. This step is critical. Verify RNA extraction procedures (use of gloves, RNase-free reagents, and disposables). A good test for cDNA quality is to perform a PCR using a common housekeeping gene. We usually employ β_2-microglobulin on total cDNA *(18)*. Reassessment of cDNA quality should be performed if the sample is used again following more than 30 d from the first quality check. It is also possible to verify RNA quality by electrophoresis as already described *(19)*. This procedure is rarely required.

2. If PCR contamination is observed, verify the quality of reagents, cleanliness of the pre-PCR room, and manual skill of the operators. The most common source of contaminating DNA is PCR products and plasmids containing IgH inserts. Both should never remain in pre-PCR areas.

3. The most common causes of lack of clonal product are as follows:
   a. Lack of tumor cells in the sample: verify this point with the clinician.
   b. Amplification problems: check a positive control (PC). If the PC works, the problem is with cDNA quality. If the PC fails, review all the procedures and change all reagents.

4. If low-quality sequences (i.e., the presence of too many N) are observed, first note carefully the feedback from the sequencing facility. It might provide some important suggestions. Sequencing of a non-IgH template might be an important control. If the control sequence is good and IgH sequences are poor, the product is probably too rich in polyclonal IgH transcripts. One can try to improve the DNA by increasing the annealing temperature or reducing $MgCl_2$ concentrations. Alternatively, one might choose to clone the PCR product as previously described. One might also wish to try amplifying less heavily mutated IgH rearrangements such as those observed in chronic lymphocytic leukemias or mantle-cell lymphomas and then switch to MM.

5. IF ligation problems are encountered, remember that the TOPO-TA cloning requires fresh PCR products. If one is sure of the PCR product, try changing the enzyme tube.

6. If the transformation is not working, the following reasons can explain the problem:
   a. Competent cells are very sensitive to temperature: Check with another kit that no deterioration occurred.
   b. Heat-shock is performed at the wrong temperature: Try using another thermomixer.
   c. Growth in SOC medium is poor: Allow more time for growing to verify that SOC medium has not been supplemented with antibiotics.

7. If colonies are too dense or too sparse, tune the amount of colonies by spreading more or less medium on the plate. Plates with too many colonies are not good because there is the risk of picking up two colonies instead of one.

8. If there are too many white colonies with no insert, check that X-gal and iso-propyl-β-D-thiogalactopyranoside (IPTG) are spread correctly, check that the PCR

product is fresh and there is no excess plasmid, and, importantly, distinguish white and light blue colonies (put the plates over a blank sheet). The best option is to choose white colonies located quite near deep blue colonies. This will ensure that the colony is growing in an area that contains an appropriate amount of IPTG and X-gal.

9. If the no-template sample is positive (with a negative no-DNA sample) **(Fig. 3B)**, this means nonspecific amplification of clonal IgH sequences. Try annealing at 62°C and 64°C. If this fails, consider designing another CDR3-specific reverse primer.

10. If the 10^1 copy sample (or even the 10^2) is negative **(Fig. 3C)**, this means that the reaction is poorly efficient. Try to improve the reaction by adding more $MgCl_2$ or change the primers. This is common when amplicons are too long. The use of MGB probes can also help. Another potential problem unrelated to the PCR is a wrong dilution of the plasmid.

11. If no standard curve shows up or the curve looks very bad **(Fig. 3D)**, the most important thing to do is run the reaction on an agarose gel. This allows verification of the presence of amplicons. If no amplicons are noticed, the problem is either with the primers or with the amplification reaction. If the amplicons are good, the problem is related to the probe. We recommend following the simple flowchart detailed in **Fig. 4.**

12. If the no-DNA sample is positive, this means contamination. Follow the same rules as for IgH amplification by qualitative PCR.

13. If the correlation coefficient is poor, increasing the manual skill of the operator can usually solve this problem. In addition, try to fix the threshold for cycle threshold calculation. Running multiple standard curves can also be beneficial.

14. If the correlation coefficient is good and the Y-intercept is >40 cycles, one should expect not to see the 10e1 or to see it very late.

15. If the standard curve is too flat (slope >–0.30), this indicates that the accumulation of PCR product is far from exponential. Usually, if the curve is very flat, one probably will not notice amplification of sample containing low amounts of DNA.

16. If the standard curve is too steep (slope <–0.34): note that perfect exponential accumulation of PCR product results in a slope of –3.3. By definition, greater values thus cannot be reached. Usually, this feature is associated with a wrong dilution (dilutions are not 10-fold or some additional nonspecific IgH DNA is amplified).

17. With DNA normalization, one usually notices the same problems observed when performing IgH amplifications.

Acknowledgments

We are grateful to all the organizations that supported or are presently supporting our MM projects, including Associazione Italiana Ricerca sul Cancro (AIRC), Milan, Italy; Compagnia di San Paolo, Torino, Italy; Consiglio Nazionale delle Ricerche (CNR) and Ministero dell' Università e della Ricerca (MIUR); International Myeloma Foundation (IMF); and Associazione per lo Studio e la Cura delle Malattie del Sangue.

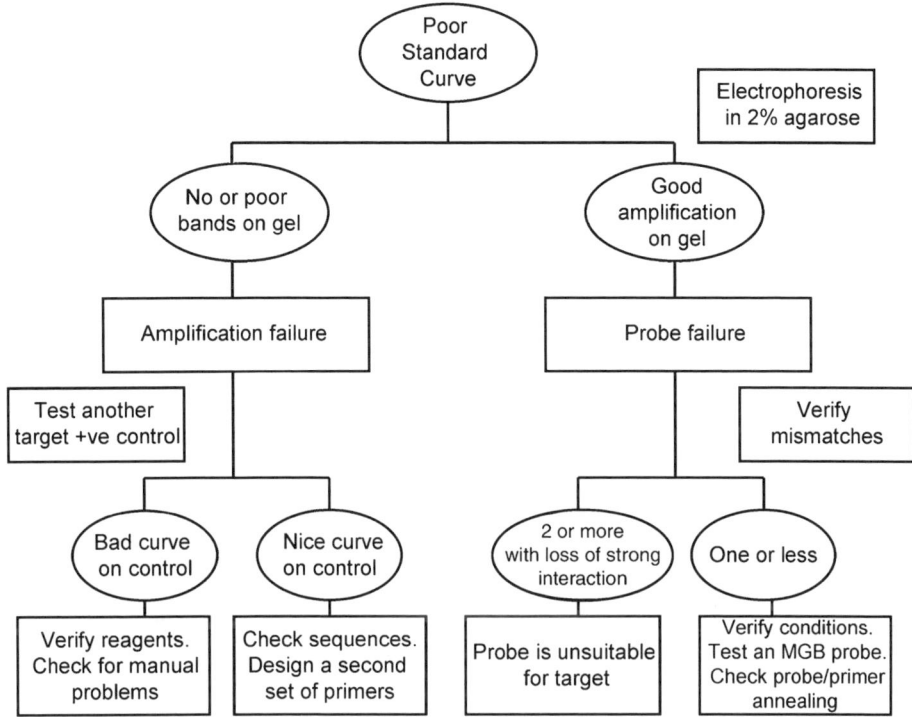

Fig. 4. Flowchart describing how it is possible to operate in case of reaction failure. Note that the basic step is always running the failed reaction on an agarose gel.

References

1. Van Dongen, J. J., Langerak, A. W., Bruggemann, M., et al. (2003) Design and standardization of PCR primers and protocols for detection of clonal immunoglobulin and T-cell receptor gene recombinations in suspect lymphoproliferations: report of the BIOMED-2 Concerted Action BMH4-CT98-3936. *Leukemia* **17,** 2257–2317.
2. Corradini, P., Cavo, M., Lokhorst, H., et al. Chronic Leukemia Working Party of the European Group for Blood and Marrow Transplantation (EBMT). (2003) Molecular remission after myeloablative allogeneic stem cell transplantation predicts a better relapse-free survival in patients with multiple myeloma. *Blood* **102,** 927–1929.
3. Corradini, P., Voena, C., Tarella, C., et al. (1999) Molecular and clinical remissions in multiple myeloma: role of autologous and allogeneic transplantation of hematopoietic cells. *J. Clin. Oncol.* **17,** 208–215.
4. Martinelli, G., Terragna, C., Zamagni, E., et al. (2000) Polymerase chain reaction-based detection of minimal residual disease in multiple myeloma patients receiving allogeneic stem cell transplantation. *Haematologica* **85,** 930–934.

5. Ladetto, M., Donovan, J. W., Harig, S., et al. (2000) Real-time polymerase chain reaction of immunoglobulin rearrangements for quantitative evaluation of minimal residual disease in multiple myeloma. *Biol. Blood Marrow Transplant.* **6,** 241–253.

6. Ladetto, M., Omede, P., Sametti, S., et al. (2002) Real-time polymerase chain reaction in multiple myeloma: quantitative analysis of tumor contamination of stem cell harvests. *Exp. Hematol.* **30,** 529–536.

7. Rasmussen, T., Poulsen, T. S., Honore, L., and Johnsen, H. E. (2000) Quantitation of minimal residual disease in multiple myeloma using an allele-specific real-time PCR assay. *Exp. Hematol.* **28,** 1039–1045.

8. Willems, P., Verhagen, O., Segeren, C., et al. (2000) Consensus strategy to quantitate malignant cells in myeloma patients is validated in a multicenter study. Belgium-Dutch Hematology-Oncology Group. *Blood* **96,** 63–70.

9. Gerard, C. J., Olsson, K., Ramanathan, R., Reading, C., and Hanania, E. G. (1998) Improved quantitation of minimal residual disease in multiple myeloma using real-time polymerase chain reaction and plasmid-DNA complementarity determining region III standards. *Cancer Res.* **58,** 3957–3964.

10. Voena, C., Locatelli, G., Castellino, C., et al. (2002) Qualitative and quantitative polymerase chain reaction detection of the residual myeloma cell contamination after positive selection of CD34+ cells with small- and large-scale Miltenyi cell sorting system. *Br. J. Haematol.* **117,** 642–645.

11. Cremer, F. W., Kiel, K., Wallmeier, M., Haas, R., Goldschmidt, H., and Moos, M. (1998) Leukapheresis products in multiple myeloma: lower tumor load after mobilization with cyclophosphamide plus granulocyte colony-stimulating factor (G-CSF) compared with G-CSF alone. *Exp. Hematol.* **26,** 969–975.

12. Gonzalez, D., Gonzalez, M., Alonso, M. E., et al. (2003) Incomplete DJH rearrangements as a novel tumor target for minimal residual disease quantitation in multiple myeloma using real-time PCR. *Leukemia* **17,** 1051–1057.

13. Voena, C., Ladetto, M., Astolfi, M., et al. (1997) A novel nested-PCR strategy for the detection of rearranged immunoglobulin heavy-chain genes in B cell tumors. *Leukemia* **11,** 1793–1798.

14. Deane, M. and Norton, J. D. (1991) Immunoglobulin gene 'fingerprinting': an approach to analysis of B lymphoid clonality in lymphoproliferative disorders. *Br. J. Haematol.* **77,** 274–281.

15. Sahota, S. S., Leo, R., Hamblin, T. J., and Stevenson, F. K. (1996) Ig VH gene mutational patterns indicate different tumor cell status in human myeloma and monoclonal gammopathy of undetermined significance. *Blood* **87,** 746–755.

16. Donovan, J. W., Ladetto, M., Zou, G., et al. (2000) Immunoglobulin heavy-chain consensus probes for real-time PCR quantification of residual disease in acute lymphoblastic leukemia. *Blood* **95,** 2651–2658.

17. Corradini, P., Voena, C., Astolfi M., et al. (1995) High-dose sequential chemo-radiotherapy in multiple myeloma: residual tumor cells are detectable in bone marrow and peripheral blood cell harvests and after autografting. *Blood* **85,** 1596–1602.

18. Suggs, S. V., Wallace, R. B., Hirose, T., Kawashima, E. H., and Itakura, K. (1981) Use of synthetic oligonucleotides as hybridization probes: isolation of cloned cDNA sequences for human beta 2-microglobulin. *Proc. Natl. Acad. Sci. USA* **78,** 6613–6617.
19. Sambrook, J., Fritsch, E. F., and Maniatis, T. (1989) Extraction, purification, and analysis of messenger RNA from eucaryotic cells, in *Molecular Cloning: A Laboratory Manual*, 2nd ed., Cold Spring Harbor Laboratory Press, Cold Spring Harbor, NY: pp. 7.28–7.52.

12

Incomplete DJH Rearrangements

David González and Ramón Garcia-Sanz

Summary

Analysis of Ig genes in B-cell malignancies has become an essential method in molecular diagnosis, and polymerase chain reaction (PCR) amplification of Ig heavy chain gene (IgH) rearrangements is now widely used for detection of clonality and minimal residual disease (MRD). Although several different sensitive protocols are now available for PCR analysis of IgH genes, they are frequently hampered owing to the high rate of somatic hypermutation present in multiple myeloma (MM). We recently described a new approach using incomplete DJH rearrangements as an alternative target. About 60% of MM samples contain an incomplete DJH rearrangement, 90% of them lacking on somatic mutations. This approach allows resolution of problems derived from primer mismatches, making DJH rearrangement a reliable and sensitive target for detection of clonality and MRD investigation in MM.

Key Words

Multiple myeloma; polymerase chain reaction; IGH rearrangements; DJH rearrangements; somatic hypermutation.

1. Introduction

Analysis of immunoglobulin (Ig) rearrangements is a very useful tool for the diagnosis of clonality, characterization, and detection of minimal residual disease (MRD) in multiple myeloma (MM). Polymerase chain reaction (PCR) amplification of the variable region of Ig heavy chains (IgH) is now widely performed as a rapid method for diagnosis of clonality in many B-cell lymphoid malignancies, including MM *(1–5)*. Assessment of clonality is usually based on the detection of a single PCR "clonal" band in an agarose or polyacrylamide gel, as opposed to the characteristic smear, containing bands of different sizes, obtained from polyclonal samples.

During early B-cell development, the process of V-D-J recombination takes place in the bone marrow. First, one diversity (D) segment is juxtaposed to a

From: *Methods in Molecular Medicine, Vol. 113: Multiple Myeloma: Methods and Protocols*
Edited by: R. D. Brown and P. J. Ho © Humana Press Inc., Totowa, NJ

joining (J) segment to form an incomplete DJH rearrangement. Then, one of the many variable (V) gene segments will recombine to the DJH complex leading to the completion of a VDJH rearrangement *(6)* **(Fig. 1)**. These processes occur in either one or both alleles at the same time. However, once a functional VDJH rearrangement is obtained, further recombination in the other allele is excluded, and the cell subsequently undergoes downstream processes of B-cell maturation *(7–9)*. Thus, according to the regulatory model of allelic exclusion, there are three possible *IGH* gene configurations in a given mature Ig(+)B-cell. First, both *IGH* alleles have undergone complete VDJH rearrangement, one productive and one nonproductive; second, there is one productive VDJH allele and one incomplete DJH rearrangement; and, third, there is one productive VDJH rearrangement and the second allele in germ-line configuration. Theoretically, the frequency of incomplete DJH rearrangements in normal mature B-cells is supposed to be 60% *(6)*. Recently, it has been shown that this frequency also occurs in malignant mature B-cells such as MM *(1)* and B-cell chronic lymphocytic leukemia (unpublished results). The enormous variability obtained by the random combination of different V, D, and J gene segments is further accomplished by the insertion and deletion of nucleotides at both V-D and D-J junctions by an enzyme known as terminal deoxynucleotidyl transferase (TdT) *(10)*. Thus, IgH rearrangements can be regarded as the fingerprint of a given B-cell, which makes them a perfect target for molecular diagnosis of clonality. Furthermore, mature B-cells entering the germinal centers may undergo further diversification by insertion of point mutations in Ig variable genes during the process of somatic hypermutation *(11–13)*.

PCR analysis of VDJH rearrangements leads to the detection of clonality in the majority of samples (see previous chapters). However, in the case of malignancies derived from mature postgerminal center B-cells, the high rate of somatic hypermutation in VDJH rearrangement may prevent PCR amplification in a considerable number of patients. This is particularly true for MM in which the malignant repertoire derives from the most mature B-cells, i.e., plasma cells *(5,12,14)*. Because incomplete DJH rearrangements are normally unmutated, they have become a reliable alternative target for diagnosis of clonality in mature B-cell malignancies such as MM *(1)*. Furthermore, somatic hypermutation in VDJH rearrangements also makes it difficult to establish a consensus strategy for MRD follow-up by real-time quantitative PCR in many patients with MM. On the contrary, analysis of unmutated DJH rearrangements overcomes these technical problems *(15)*.

In this chapter, we describe the protocols for PCR detection and molecular characterization of clonal incomplete DJH rearrangements as tumor targets.

IGH germinal configuration

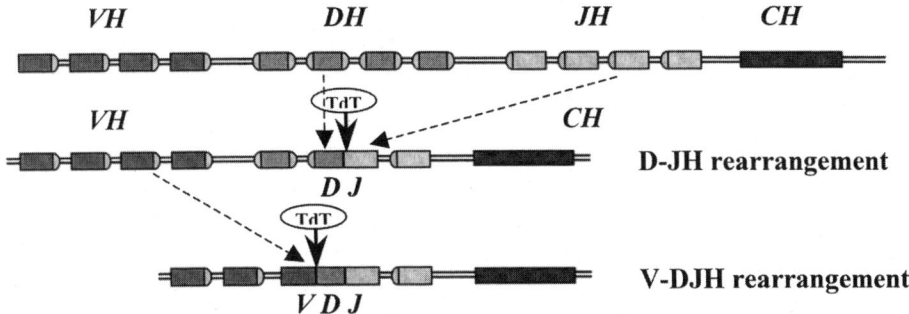

Fig. 1. Recombination of *IGH* genes. TdT is involved in both DJH and VDJH rearrangements, increasing the diversity in the joining regions.

2. Materials

1. DH and JH primers (JH-Fam-labeled primer for Genescan analysis) (BIOMED-2 primers *[16]*). These primers are now commercially available from InVivoScribe (Carlsbad, CA).
2. AmpliTaq Gold, PCR buffer, and $MgCl_2$ (Applied Biosystems, Foster City, CA).
3. dNTPs (Amersham Pharmacia Biotech, Roosendaal, The Netherlands).
4. Polyacrylamide (19:1), 40% for heteroduplex analysis (Amresco, Venlo, The Netherlands).
5. Deionized formamide (Sigma-Aldrich, St. Louis, MO).
6. Ammonium persulfate (APS) (Invitrogen, Life Technologies, Paisley, UK).
7. TEMED (Applied Biosystems).
8. Long Range™ gel solution, 50% stock solution for Genescan analysis (Cambrex Bioscience Rockland, Solon, OH).
9. Molecular weight marker for heteroduplex analysis: 1-kb ladder (Invitrogen).
10. Molecular weight marker for Genescan analysis: 500 ROX™ Size Standard (Applied Biosystems).
11. 2X and 1X TAE buffer.
12. 10X and 1X TBE buffer.
13. Ethidium bromide (EtBr) (Amresco).
14. ABI PRISM Big-Dye terminators sequencing kit and 5X sequencing buffer (Applied Biosystems).
15. ABI PRISM 377 DNA sequencer (Applied Biosystems) or equivalent.

3. Methods

3.1. DJH PCR

The human DH locus has evolved by duplication of a minor population of DH segments. Thus, although they all share some similarities, DH segments have been grouped in seven different families containing DH segments sharing

>80% homology in both coding and noncoding sequences. During the BIOMED-2 Concerted Action, seven different family-specific DH primers were designed, each covering every single member of a given DH family *(16)* (**Fig. 2**). Two different sets of PCR are needed for amplification of DJH rearrangements (*see* **Note 1**).

1. Prepare the master mix containing 1X PCR buffer, 1.5 m*M* MgCl$_2$, 200 µ*M* dNTPs, 10 pmol of each primer (DH1 to DH6 plus JH consensus primer for tube A or DH7 plus JH primer for tube B) (*see* **Fig. 2** and **Note 1**), 1 U of AmpliTaq Gold, and ultrapure water up to 49 µL/sample.
2. Add 1 µL (equivalent of 100 ng) of DNA sample.
3. Use the following thermal cycler conditions: denaturation and AmpliTaq Gold activation at 95°C for 10 min, followed by 35 cycles of 94°C for 30 s, 60°C for 30 s, and 72°C for 30 s, and an additional 10-min final extension at 72°C.

3.2. Heteroduplex Analysis

This simple analysis allows discrimination between PCR products derived from clonal and polyclonal samples using polyacrylamide gel electrophoresis (PAGE).

1. Prepare 6% polyacrylamide gel in 1X TAE (*see* **Note 2**). For 30 mL of gel mixture, 4.5 mL of 40% polyacrylamide, 15 mL of 2X TAE, 210 µL of 10% APS, 45 µL of TEMED, and 10.25 mL of water are needed.
2. Pour the gel and let stand for at least 30 min (1 h recommended).
3. After performing the PCR, heat the tubes at 95°C for 10 min in the same thermal cycler to denature the PCR products, and immediately cool down to 4°C for 60 min. This allows the single strands to hybridize with their respective homologous population (homoduplex) or between the heterogeneous population (heteroduplex) in the case of clonal and polyclonal PCR products, respectively.
4. Immediately after formation of heteroduplex, load 30 µL of PCR product and proceed to PAGE. Electrophoresis can be run overnight at low voltage (25–30 V) or, alternatively, at high voltage (200 V) for 2 h (*see* **Note 3**).
5. Take the gel out of the plates and place in a tray containing 50 µL of EtBr solution in 250 mL of water (*see* **Note 4**) and gently shake/rock for 30 min. Discard the staining solution in a proper decontamination tank (*see* **Note 4**), and wash with 250 mL of water by shaking it for 15 min. Repeat the washing step once more.
6. Remove the gel from the plate, place it under ultraviolet light, and take a picture. Single bands falling into the proper size range are considered clonal bands (*see* **Notes 5** and **6**). Polyclonal samples, by contrast, will produce a smear of heteroduplexes.

3.3. Genescan Analysis

Alternatively, DJH PCR products can be analyzed by Genescan using an automated DNA sequencer. This type of analysis easily discriminates clonal

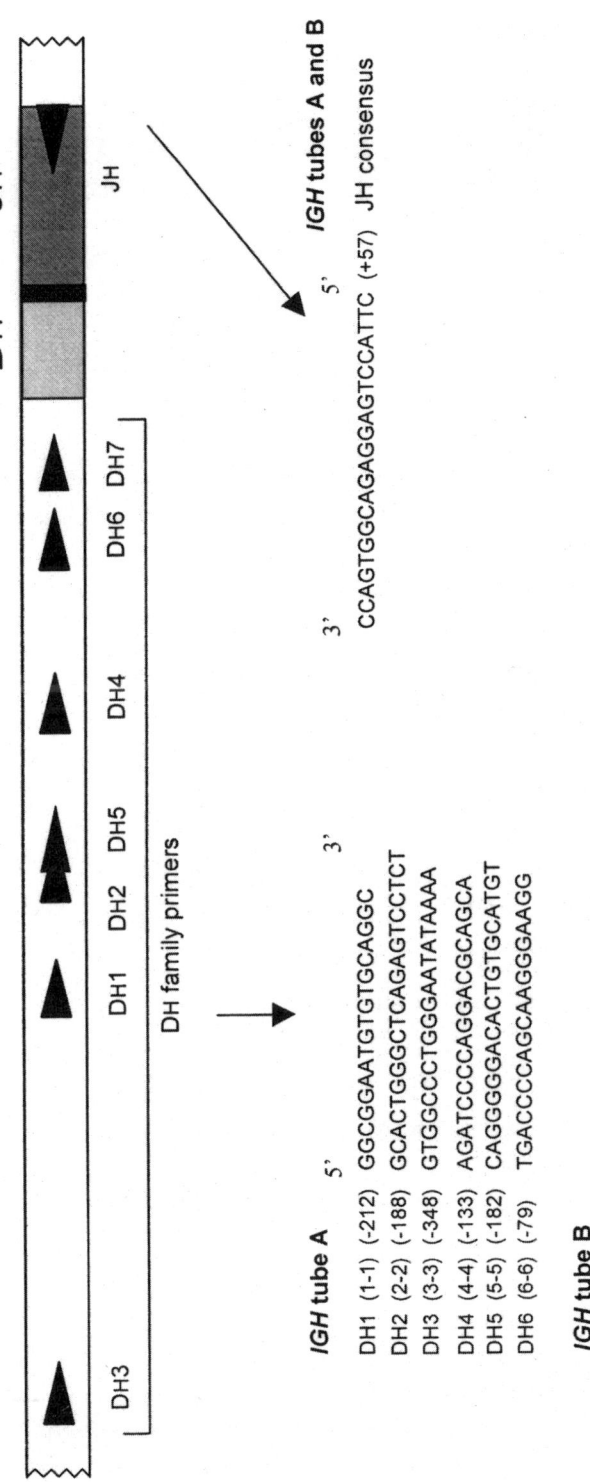

Fig. 2. PCR analysis of DJH rearrangements. Schematic diagram of DH-JH PCR with seven DH family primers and one JH consensus primer, divided over two tubes (A and B). The DH7 primer was separated from the other six DH primers, because the DH7 and JH consensus primers will give a germ-line PCR product of 211 bp. The relative position of the DH and JH primers is given according to their most 5' nucleotide upstream (−) or downstream (+) of the involved recombination signal sequences (RSS). The DH gene segment used as a representative DH family member for primer design is indicated in parentheses. (Taken with permission from **ref. 16**.)

from polyclonal samples, because they appear as a single fluorescent peak or a Gaussian distribution of different sized peaks, respectively (*see* **Note 7**).

1. Prepare and pour a Genescan gel following the manufacturer's instructions (Applied Biosystems).
2. Prepare the loading buffer solution by mixing deionized formamide, loading buffer, and Genescan molecular weight marker in a 5:1:0.5 ratio.
3. Add 0.5 µL of the PCR product to 5 µL of loading buffer solution.
4. Denature this PCR solution at 95°C for 10 min and let it cool down on ice.
5. Load 1.5–2 µL of this solution into the gel.
6. Run for approx 3 h or until the 500-bp band of the molecular weight marker appears in the gel.
7. Analyze with the GeneScan™ software (Applied Biosystems).

3.4. Sequencing and Analysis of DJH Rearrangements

3.4.1. Sequencing Reaction

1. Cut the band(s) of interest out of the gel with a razor blade and place in a 0.6-mL microfuge tube.
2. Add the appropriate amount of ultrapure water (*see* **Note 8**) and leave overnight (*see* **Note 9**).
3. Prepare the reaction mix for a total reaction volume of 10 µL by adding 2 µL of Sequencing Mastermix, 2 µL of 5X Sequencing buffer, and 3.2 pmol of JH primer (0.3 µL of a 10-µ*M* aliquot) per sample (make enough mix for the number of samples plus 10%).
4. Add 4.3 µL of reaction mix and 5.7 µL of DNA solution (*see* **Note 8**) to a PCR tube, and perform the sequencing reaction in a thermal cycler.

3.4.2. Purification of Sequencing Products

1. To a 0.6-mL microfuge tube add 10 µL of water; 2 µL of 3 *M* sodium acetate, pH 4.6; 50 µL of 96% ethanol; and 10 µL of the sequencing reaction.
2. Vortex briefly and leave on ice for 15–20 min.
3. Centrifuge at full speed for 20 min.
4. Carefully remove as much supernatant as possible with a 200 µL micropipet without disturbing the DNA pellet.
5. Add 180 µL of 70% ethanol and centrifuge for 3 min at full speed.
6. Again, remove the supernatant and dry in a thermal cycler for 1 min at 94°C.
7. Resuspend each sample in 5 µL of loading buffer solution (formamide:loading buffer in a 5:1 ratio), denature at 94°C for 4 min, and leave on ice.
8. Load 2 to 3 µL of sample into the automated DNA sequencer.

3.4.3. Analysis of DJH Rearrangements

The analysis of complete VDJH rearrangements is now facilitated by Web-assisted tools such as DNAPLOT (http://www.mrc-cpe.cam.ac.uk/

DNAPLOT.php, MRC Centre for Protein Engineering) *(17)*. However, these databases do not offer the possibility of analyzing incomplete DJH rearrangements. For analysis of DJH sequences, we recommend a BLAST search (http://www.ncbi.nih.gov/) by entering accession no. X97051, which contains the complete sequence for the DH and JH loci (*see* **Note 10**). Once the DH and JH segments involved in a rearrangement are identified, it is easy to characterize the N-region present in the DH to JH joint.

4. Notes

1. Owing to the proximity of the DH7-27 gene segment to the JH locus, amplification of germ-line DH7-JH transcripts is usually obtained from nonrearranged normal cells. To facilitate the interpretation of results, two different sets of PCR were designed, one containing the JH consensus primer together with DH1 to DH primers, and the second containing the JH consensus primer and the DH7 primer *(16)*. DH7-JH PCR will amplify products of 211 bp from nonrearranged alleles (i.e., DH7-JH1 and also 419, 1031, 1404, 1804, and 2420 bp in the case of primer annealing to downstream JH gene segments) and will be detected as a ladder of germ-line bands in virtually every sample with good-quality DNA.

2. It is very important to use 1X TAE buffer instead of 0.5X TBE buffer in case further analyses such as direct sequencing or cloning are needed. First, unlike TAE buffer, TBE buffer interferes with subsequent reactions, including cycle sequencing and cloning. Second, 1X TAE buffer allows higher yields of DNA recovery from PCR bands in polyacrylamide gels than 0.5X TAE buffer (see DNA extraction from polyacrylamide gels in **Subheading 3.4.1.**).

3. Usually, better results are obtained when running PAGE overnight. However, it is also possible to run the electrophoresis at higher voltage (200–250 V) for 2 h if time is limiting. The latter option allows having results in 1 d, and the bands of interest can be sequenced the next day, if necessary.

4. The staining and washing steps are easily accomplished if only one plate is carefully removed, leaving the gel on the remaining one. EtBr is highly toxic and a suspected teratogen. *Do not* allow EtBr-containing solutions to contact the skin. To discard solution, partially fill an appropriate tank with decontaminating solution containing 5% bleach and 3% nonionic detergent and pour all EtBr solutions into it. In addition, use decontamination solution to wash the trays used for staining the gels.

5. The size range for DJH PCR products depends on the DH family primer used: DH1, 260–290 bp; DH2, 230–260 bp; DH3, 390–420 bp; DH4, 175–205 bp; DH5, 225–255 bp; DH6, 110–150 bp; and DH7, 100–130 bp. A nonspecific band of 348 bp is amplified in virtually all samples. The sequence corresponds to the germ-line JH4 that is amplified with the JH consensus primer and the DH2 primer annealing upstream the JH4 segment. This nonspecific band does not interfere with the interpretation of clonality results because it is out of the range of all rearranged DJH fragments. Furthermore, it can be used as a good control for DNA quality of the MM samples.

6. Sometimes, the bands corresponding to DH3 rearrangements (400 bp on average) are difficult to amplify. This is particularly true when using bad-quality DNA (i.e., extracted from paraffin-embedded tissue) or when the number of clonal cells is very low. Thus, in those difficult cases in which a very faint band is suspected within the DH3-PCR products size range, we recommend further confirmation by amplifying the sample(s) with DH3 and JH primers alone, because it increases the sensitivity up to 1%.

7. Note that for Genescan analysis the JH primer must be fluorescent labeled. Always use compatible fluorochromes for JH primer and molecular weight markers (i.e., Fam-labeled JH primer and Rox-labeled molecular weight markers). Once the fluorochromes are chosen, use the appropriate Matrix file on the Genescan run.

8. The amount of water added to the polyacrylamide slice varies according to the intensity of the band. The minimum recommended amount is 8 μL for the faintest bands and can go up to 25–30 μL for brighter bands (we recommend performing initial experiments with bands of different intensity to establish a protocol in the laboratory). It is useful for subsequent steps in the sequencing reaction to have the same DNA concentration on average in every sample, so that the volume of DNA solution added for sequencing remains the same. The yield of recovered DNA increases if the polyacrylamide slice is virtually dry before adding the water because the process is based on osmotic force driving the DNA from a saline solution (1X TAE in the polyacrylamide gel) to deionized pure water. In our experience, using 1X TAE buffer allows better recovery from the polyacrylamide gels than 0.5X TAE, probably because the higher the saline concentration, the higher osmotic force. However, higher concentration of TAE buffer also means a higher amperage during electrophoresis, so we do not recommend using TAE buffers at a concentration higher than 1X owing to overheating during PAGE.

9. Alternatively, if the intensity of the clonal band is high, the polyacrylamide slice can be left in ultrapure water for only 2 h before proceeding with the sequencing reaction. Normally, enough DNA is eluted out from the gel to the water in this short time if the amount of PCR product is adequate, making it very useful when time is limiting.

10. The following guidelines for identification and analyses of junctional regions may be helpful: Check IgH junctional regions manually (i.e., comparing with the germ-line DH exon sequences) for the presence of more than one DH segment in the CDR3 region, particularly in cases with more than 10 "unknown" inserted nucleotides.

References

1. Gonzalez, D., Balanzategui, A., Garcia-Sanz, R., et al. (2003) Incomplete DJH rearrangements of the IgH gene are frequent in multiple myeloma patients: immuno-biological characteristics and clinical implications. *Leukemia* **17,** 1398–1403.

2. Gonzalez, M., Gonzalez, D., Lopez-Perez, R., et al. (1999) Heteroduplex analysis of VDJ amplified segments from rearranged IgH genes for clonality assessments in

B-cell non-Hodgkin's lymphoma: a comparison between different strategies. *Haematologica* **84,** 779–784.

3. Diss, T. C. and Pan, L. (1997) Polymerase chain reaction in the assessment of lymphomas. *Cancer Surv.* **30,** 21–44.
4. Linke, B., Bolz, I., Fayyazi, A., et al. (1997) Automated high resolution PCR fragment analysis for identification of clonally rearranged immunoglobulin heavy chain genes. *Leukemia* **11,** 1055–1062.
5. Garcia-Sanz, R., Lopez-Perez, R., Langerak, A. W., et al. (1999) Heteroduplex PCR analysis of rearranged immunoglobulin genes for clonality assessment in multiple myeloma. *Haematologica* **84,** 328–335.
6. Alt, F. W., Yancopoulos, G. D., Blackwell, T. K., et al. (1984) Ordered rearrangement of immunoglobulin heavy chain variable region segments. *EMBO J.* **3,** 1209–1219.
7. Tarlinton, D. (1998) Germinal centers: form and function. *Curr. Opin. Immunol.* **10,** 245–251.
8. Han, S., Dillon, S. R., Zheng, B., Shimoda, M., Schlissel, M. S., and Kelsoe, G. (1997) V(D)J recombinase activity in a subset of germinal center B lymphocytes. *Science* **278,** 301–305.
9. Pierre, D. M., Goldman, D., Bar, Y., and Perelson, A. S. (1997) Somatic evolution in the immune system: the need for germinal centers for efficient affinity maturation. *J. Theor. Biol.* **186,** 159–171.
10. Komori, T., Okada, A., Stewart, V., and Alt, F. W. (1993) Lack of N regions in antigen receptor variable region genes of TdT-deficient lymphocytes. *Science* **261,** 1171–1175.
11. Klein, U., Goossens, T., Fischer, M., et al. (1998) Somatic hypermutation in normal and transformed human B cells. *Immunol. Rev.* **162,** 261–280.
12. Kosmas, C., Stamatopoulos, K., Papadaki, T., et al. (1998) Somatic hypermutation of immunoglobulin variable region genes: focus on follicular lymphoma and multiple myeloma. *Immunol. Rev.* **162,** 281–292.
13. Neuberger, M. S. and Milstein, C. (1995) Somatic hypermutation. *Curr. Opin. Immunol.* **7,** 248–254.
14. Kosmas, C., Stamatopoulos, K., Stavroyianni, N., et al. (2000) Origin and diversification of the clonogenic cell in multiple myeloma: lessons from the immunoglobulin repertoire. *Leukemia* **14,** 1718–1726.
15. Gonzalez, D., Gonzalez, M., Alonso, M.E., et al. (2003) Incomplete DJH rearrangements as a novel tumor target for minimal residual disease quantitation in multiple myeloma using real-time PCR. *Leukemia* **17,** 1051–1057.
16. van Dongen, J. J., Langerak, A. W., Bruggemann, M., et al. (2003) Design and standardization of PCR primers and protocols for detection of clonal immunoglobulin and T-cell receptor gene recombinations in suspect lymphoproliferations: report of the BIOMED-2 Concerted Action BMH4-CT98-3936. *Leukemia* **17,** 2257–2317.
17. Cook, G. P. and Tomlinson, I. M. (1995) The human immunoglobulin VH repertoire. *Immunol. Today* **16,** 237–242.

13

Identification of Malignant Plasma Cells by mRNA *In Situ* Hybridization

Ross D. Brown and P. Joy Ho

Summary

Patients with multiple myeloma have a clonal proliferation of malignant plasma cells, each with an identical rearrangement of immunogloblin heavy and light chain genes. When these unique sequences are determined, a valuable molecular tool is available that can been used to detect the presence of the malignant population. Previous methods have employed oligonucleotides derived from these sequences and allele-specific polymeraes chain reaction to detect clonality. The method described in this chapter uses mRNA *in situ* hybridization (ISH) to demonstrate the presence of individual malignant cells. Single-cell analysis using mRNA ISH provides opportunities that when combined with immunophenotyping offer a valuable new investigative tool.

Key Words

Multiple myeloma; *in situ* hybridization; plasma cells; probes; oligonucleotides.

1. Introduction

Multiple myeloma (MM) is a hematological malignancy characterized by an increased number of bone marrow plasma cells (PCs) and the presence of high levels of a serum monoclonal immunoglobulin (Ig) that is coded by a unique genetic sequence in the variable region of the Ig heavy chain gene. Morphological examination of bone marrow biopsy samples prior to therapy and serum immunofixation studies of the monoclonal Ig are usually sufficient to clearly diagnose this disease. However after therapy, when the number of malignant cells is reduced, it is not possible to differentiate between the small number of malignant and normal (polyclonal) PCs using traditional microscopic staining methods. In addition, although the malignant cells are generally found predominantly in the bone marrow, in many patients with progressive disease the malignant cells may spill over into the peripheral blood.

From: *Methods in Molecular Medicine, Vol. 113: Multiple Myeloma: Methods and Protocols*
Edited by: R. D. Brown and P. J. Ho © Humana Press Inc., Totowa, NJ

Flow cytometry has provided a tool to demonstrate the presence of PCs with light chain restriction, which infers clonality. Studies of peripheral blood stem cell harvests have shown that the contaminating PCs are predominantly poly-clonal and thus not malignant *(1)*. However the true identity of the malignant cells can only be demonstrated when gene probes are used that correspond to the unique genetic sequence that is generated by recombination of the variable region and somatic hypermutation. This tumor-specific genetic signature does not change throughout the course of MM *(2)*. Many laboratories have now per-formed polymerase chain reaction (PCR) with allele-specific oligonucleotides to identify the presence of the malignant clone in blood and bone marrow sam-ples from patients with myeloma. One clinical application of this technique has been to demonstrate the presence of minimal residual disease after intensive therapy *(3,4)*. However, the PCR method detects the presence of cell popula-tions without distinguishing malignancy at the level of a single cell.

The technique of mRNA *in situ* hybridization (ISH) *(5–8)* was developed using patient and tumor-specific probes to identify individual cells belonging to the malignant clone and to characterize other features of the malignant PCs at the single-cell level *(9,10)*. Thus, it has been shown that

1. The malignant cells are present in the blood of all patients at concentrations of about 0.1–25% of the mononuclear cell fraction.
2. There is a direct correlation between disease activity and the number of malignant cells in blood.
3. Only a small proportion of the B-cells (CD19[+]) belong to the malignant clone.
4. Malignant CD34[+] cells either do not exist or are below the level of sensitivity of the assay *(9,10)*.

The mRNA ISH method that we describe has been used with a number of different oligonucleotide and cDNA probes. The mRNA ISH technique is highly sensitive owing to the high level of heavy and light chain mRNA present in the cytoplasm of PCs. Thus, mRNA ISH using heavy or light chain probes has a good chance of overcoming any sensitivity problems, and strong staining of patient and tumor-specific IgH chain mRNA can be achieved (*see* **Fig. 1**). The sensitivity of detection can be further increased by ISH-PCR, but this should not be necessary. The technique consists of two major steps. In the first step, the CDR3 region of the Ig heavy chain gene of the malignant cell popu-lation is sequenced, from which the non-germ-line sequences are determined and biotinylated antisense oligonucleotide probes to these unique sequences are prepared *(2,4,8–10)*. The protocol we outline describes the second step, which involves the ISH staining procedure for cytospin preparations of blood and bone marrow cells. The steps in this staining procedure are fixation and permeabilization, hybridization, detection, and visualization.

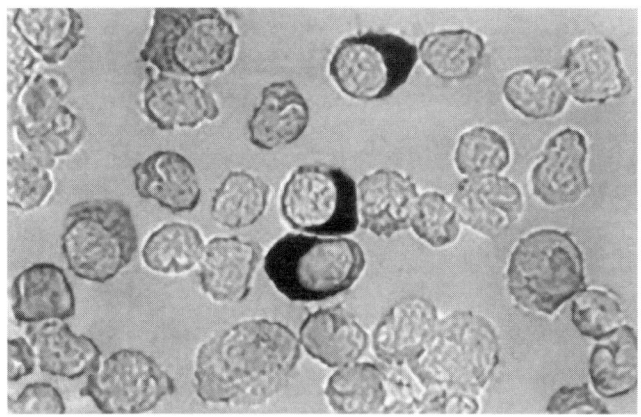

Fig. 1. ISH of bone marrow cells from a patient with MM. The Ig heavy chain mRNA in the cytoplasm of PCs is stained with probes that are patient and tumor specific.

2. Materials

1. TBS buffer 1: 0.1 M Tris-HCl; 1.0 M NaCl; 5 mM MgCl$_2$, pH 7.6. For l L: 12.1 g of Tris, 59.4 g of NaCl, 1 g of MgCl$_2$. Autoclave and store at room temperature.
2. TBS buffer 2: 0.1 M Tris-HCl; 0.1 M NaCl; 10 M MgCl$_2$, pH 9.2. For 1 L: 12.1 g of Tris, 5.84 g of NaCl, 2.0 g of MgCl$_2$. Autoclave and store at room temperature.
3. Developing reagent A: 1 mL of TBS buffer 2, 10 μL of nitro blue tetrazolium (NBT), 10 μL of 5-bromo-4-chloro-3-indolyl phosphate (BCIP). Add NBT (Sigma) to buffer 2, mix well, and then add BCIP (Sigma, St. Louis, MO) and mix. Prepare immediately before use. Store NBT and BCIP in the dark at –20°C.
4. Developing reagent B: 1 mL of TBS buffer 2, 10 μL of naphthol AS-MX phosphate (Sigma), 10 μL of Fast Red TR salt (Sigma), 10 μL of 0.5 M levamisole (Sigma). Dissolve 20 mg of naphthol AS-MX phosphate in 1 mL of dimethylformamide in a glass tube, and dissolve 20 mg of Fast Red TR salt in 1 mL of distilled water. Add 10 μL of each solution to 1 mL of buffer 2 and mix well. Add 10 μL of levamisole and mix. Prepare immediately before use. Store naphthol AS-MX, Fast Red solutions, and levamisole at –20°C in the dark.
5. Hybridization buffer (for 10 mL): 1 g of dextran sulfate (mol wt = 500,000) (Sigma), 5 mL of formamide (Aldrich), 2.5 mL of 20X saline sodium citrate (SCC). Add herring sperm DNA and water, and then add formamide and mix well. Store at –20°C until required.
6. Phosphate-buffered saline (PBS): For 1 L of 10X stock solution: 2 g of KCl, 80 g of NaCl, 11.5 g of Na$_2$HPO$_4$, 2 g of KH$_2$PO$_4$.
7. SSC: For 1 L of 10X stock: 87.7 g of NaCl, 44.1 g of trisodium citrate.

3. Methods

This protocol does not describe the methods concerning extraction of DNA from the malignant PCs, amplification of the variable region of the

IgH genes, DNA sequencing, probe design, and construction of biotinylated probes. Details of these techniques have been published previously
(2,4,9,10).

3.1. Fixation and Permeabilization

3.1.1. Preparation of Slides

1. Wash slides in ethanol and then place in poly-L-lysine hydrobromide (0.005%)
   for 5 min. Air-dry the slides for 10 min and then at 37°C overnight. These slides
   may be used for up to 2 mo.
2. Prepare cytospin preparations of cells from a primary sample or from cell cultures on the treated slides.

3.1.2. Fixation With Ethanol and Acetic Acid

Several different fixation methods may be used. It is recommended that fixation with ethanol and acetic acid be attempted first. However, owing to the
variability of the probes, one of the other methods (*see* **Notes 1** and **2**) should
be trialed if results are not as good as expected.

1. Fix the air-dried slides of cells in a 3:1 ethanol:acetic acid mixture for 30 min.
2. Place the slides in 100% ethanol for 5 min.
3. Immerse the slides in acetone for 5 min to extract lipids and perforate the cell
   membrane.
4. Air-dry the slides in an incubator at 37°C and store in a dust-free place.

3.2. Hybridization With Oligonucleotide Probes

1. Add 20–50 µL of biotin-labeled oligonucleotide probe (20–100 ng) to the slides
   (*see* **Notes 3–7**).
2. Cover with cover slips.
3. Incubate at 42°C for 12 h or overnight, but place in a moist chamber.

3.3. Posthybridization and Detection

1. Remove the cover slips and rinse the slides in two changes of 2X SSC, 0.1%
   sodium dodecyl sulfate (SDS) at 42°C.
2. Incubate the slides for 15 min in 2X SSC, 0.1% SDS at 42°C.
3. Incubate for 15 min in 0.4X SSC, 0.1% SDS at 42°C.
4. Incubate the slides for a further 15 min in 2X SSC, 0.1% SDS at 42°C.
5. Incubate for 15 min in 0.4X SSC, 0.1% SDS at 42°C.
6. Rinse the slides in two changes of 0.4X SSC at room temperature.
7. Rinse the slides in two changes of PBS.
8. Place the slides in two changes of TBS buffer for 1–5 min each.
9. Drain the slides and apply streptavidin (1:100 dilution in buffer 1 of a Dako ISH
   Detection kit K0600) to the slides for 10–20 min with occasional rocking.
10. Rinse the slides in TBS buffer 1 and again drain.

11. Apply biotinylated alkaline phosphatase (1:100 dilution in buffer 1 of Dako ISH Detection kit) to the slides for 10 min with occasional rocking.
12. Rinse the slides in TBS buffer 1.
13. Drain the slides and apply streptavidin (1:500 dilution in buffer 1 of Dako ISH Detection kit) to the slides for 10–20 min with occasional rocking.
14. Rinse the slides in TBS buffer 1 and again drain.
15. Apply biotinylated alkaline phosphatase (1:500 dilution in buffer 1 of Dako ISH Detection kit) to the slides for 10 min with occasional rocking.
16. Rinse the slides in TBS buffer 1.
17. Incubate the slides with two changes of TBS buffer for 5 min.

3.4. Visualization

1. Drain the slides rapidly and add excess developing reagent A or B (i.e., more than 50 µL). At the same time, place a cover slip over the slide to avoid bubbles. Blot off the excess developing agent, and store the slides in a cool, dark place.
2. View the slides quickly under a microscope at 30-min intervals until the intensity of staining is satisfactory. The mRNA staining should be most intense in the cytoplasm.
3. Wash the slides several times with distilled water, and counterstain (*see* **Note 8**) with Nuclear Fast Red (Sigma) for 5 min, wash with water, then metanil yellow for 3 to 4 min, and wash with distilled water again.
4. Mount the slides while wet using an aqueous mounting medium such as glycerol-gelatin.

4. Notes

1. All glassware should be baked at 180°C for 2 h, and all solutions should be made in autoclaved water and treated with 0.2% diethylpyrocarbonate. Salts should be RNase free. Wear gloves and use sterile disposable plastic ware. See a technical manual, such as *Molecular Cloning (11)*, for additional details of basic molecular techniques.
2. There are other fixation methods that can be trialed as alternatives if poor results are obtained:
   a. Fixation with paraformaldehyde:
      i.   Fix cells on slides in 4% paraformaldehyde dissolved in PBS for 30 min.
      ii. Rinse the slides with two changes of PBS for 5 min each.
      iii. Wash the slides with two changes of 0.25% Triton X-100 (Sigma) and 0.25% Nonidet P40 (Sigma) in PBS for 5 min each to extract lipids and perforate the cell membrane.
      iv. Rinse the slides with two changes of PBS for 5 min each.
      v.   Dip the slides in 20% acetic acid (in water) for 5 min.
      vi. Rinse the slides in two changes of distilled water for 5 min each.
      vii. Place in 100% ethanol for 5 min.
      viii. Air-dry at 37°C in a dust-free place.

   b. Fixation with Histochoice Fixative-Astral (HTCF):
     i.   Fix slides in 1X HTCF (20X HTCF;alcohol;water = 1;4;15) for 30–40 min.
     ii. Place the slides in 100% ethanol for 5 min, then acetone for 5 min to extract lipids and perforate the cell membrane.
     iii. Air-dry the slides and store in a dust-free place.
     Cells must not be allowed to dry. This is likely to cause elevated levels of non-specific binding, indicated by an overall blue background. BCIP/NBT positivity has a purple hue.

3. The oligonucleotides that we have successfully used were 18mer to 24mer. The optimum conditions may vary for different probes owing to size and GC content. It is advisable to end-label with biotin during the construction of the probe. Longer probes will need higher temperatures for hybridization. Whenever there are several nongerminal sequences, a cocktail of two or more different probes can be used to enhance detection.

4. cDNA probes do not have as good penetration as oligonucleotide probes and require a longer incubation. One hundred microliters of photobiotin-labeled probe (5 µg) and 20 µL of 10X SSC are placed in a sterile Eppendorf tube and heated at 90°C for 15 min to dissociate double-stranded DNA into single strands and immediately chilled on ice to prevent reannealing. Cold hybridization buffer (900 µL) is then added and mixed well. The preparation is stored at –20°C until required. To the prepared slides is added the appropriate DNA probe in hybridization buffer (20–40 µL), and then the slides are completely covered with a cover slip. The slides are placed in a closed chamber containing absorbent paper moistened with water and incubated for 22–28 h at 42°C.

5. Gene sequences should be checked for uniqueness using an appropriate sequence database such as GenBank.

6. Control slides of cells from different patients hybridized with the same oligonucleotide probe should be used. A probe of irrelevant specificity may also be used as a negative control. Non-PCs act as an internal negative control. Sense probes may be weakly positive.

7. Some cells have high levels of endogenous biotin to which streptavidin will bind nonspecifically. This may be overcome by using a different label. Digoxigenin-labeled probes have been effective *(12,13)*.

8. Counterstaining with nuclear stains may make interpretation difficult. This is especially true for hematoxylin. A light counterstain with Nuclear Fast Red is recommended. Alternatively, Methyl Green (Sigma) for 1 min can be used to counterstain the slides. The slides are then washed with water or Mayer's hematoxylin for about 10 min, rinsed with water and placed in a weak solution of ammonia solution for 1 min, and then rinsed with two changes of water.

Acknowledgments

We gratefully acknowledge the technical assistance of Xiao-Feng Luo and the financial support of the Anthony Rothe Memorial Trust, Foundation IV, and Multiple Myeloma Research Foundation.

References

1. Pope, B., Brown, R., Gibson, J., and Joshua, D. (1997) Plasma cells in peripheral blood stem cell harvests from patients with multiple myeloma are predominantly polyclonal. *Bone Marrow Transplant.* **20,** 205–210.
2. Ralph, Q. M., Brisco, M. J., Joshua, D. E, Brown, R., Gibson, J., and Morley, A. (1993) Advancement of multiple myeloma from diagnosis through plateau phase to progression does not involve a new B cell clone: evidence from the Ig heavy chain gene. *Blood* **82,** 202–206.
3. Swedin, A., Lenhoff, S., Olofsson, T., Thuresson, B., and Westin, J. (1988) Clinical utility of immunoglobulin heavy chain gene rearrangement identification for tumour cell detection in multiple myeloma. *Br. J. Haematol.* **103,** 1145–1151.
4. Brisco, M. J., Tan, L. W., Osborn, A. M., and Morley, A. A. (1990) Development of a highly sensitive assay based on the polymerase chain reaction for rare B-lymphocyte clones in a polyclonal population. *Br. J. Haematol.* **75,** 163–167.
5. Lawrence, J. B. and Singer, R. H. (1985) Quantitative analysis of *in situ* hybridization methods for the detection of actin gene expression. *Nucleic Acids Res.* **13,** 1777–1799.
6. Gee, C. E. and Roberts, J. L. (1983) *In situ* hybridisation histochemistry: a technique for the study of gene expression in single cells. *DNA* **2,** 157–171.
7. Pringle, J. H., Primose, L., Kind, C. N., Talbot, I. C., and Lauder, I. (1989) *In situ* hybridization demonstration of poly-adenylated RNA sequences in formalin-fixed paraffin sections using a biotinylated oligonucleotide poly d(T) probe. *J. Pathol.* **158,** 279–286.
8. Markovic, B., Kwan, Y.-L., Nicholls, E. M., Walsh, C., and Crouch, R. L. (1992) A sensitive method for the detection of poly-A tails of mRNA using a biotin labelled heteropolymer of dT:rA. *J. Pathol.* **167,** 369–373.
9. Brown, R. D., Luo, X.-F., Gibson, J., et al. (1995) Idiotypic oligonucleotide probes to detect myeloma cells by mRNA in situ hybridization. *Br. J. Haematol.* **90,** 113–118.
10. Joshua, D. E., Brown, R. D., Luo, X.-F., and Gibson, J. (1996) Circulating clonal lymphocytes in myeloma determined by mRNA in situ hybridization. *Blood* **88,** 1125.
11. Sambrook, J., Fritsch, E. F., and Maniatas, T. (1989) *Molecular Cloning: A Laboratory Manual*, 2nd ed., Cold Spring Harbor Laboratory Press, Cold Spring Harbor, NY.
12. Kessler, C. (1990) The digoxigenin system: principle and applications of the novel nonradioactive DNA labelling and detection system. *BioTechnol. Int.* **1990,** 183–194.
13. Hotlke, H. J. and Kessler, C. (1990) Non-radioactive labelling of RNA transcripts in vitro with the hapten digoxigenin (DIG): hybridization and ELISA-based detection. *Nucleic Acids Res.* **18,** 5843–5851.

14

The SCID-hu Myeloma Model

Joshua Epstein and Shmuel Yaccoby

Summary

The severe combined immune deficient human (SCID-hu) myeloma model is the only available model in which primary myeloma cells grow in vivo in a human bone marrow microenvironment. A SCID mouse receives an implanted human fetal bone into which myeloma cells are directly injected. Through interaction with the human bone marrow microenvironment, the myeloma cells induce typical myeloma manifestations in the SCID host, such as the appearance of M protein in the serum, and changes in the implanted human bone, which often result in osteolysis of the human bone. The model provides the only platform for in vivo investigation of the biology and therapy of primary human myeloma in a human microenvironment. This chapter describes in detail all the steps necessary to establish this model and evaluate its success.

Key Words

SCID-hu; myeloma; model; human bone microenvironment; growth; bone marrow; identification chip.

1. Introduction

Myeloma cells do not grow or survive in culture, which presents a major hurdle to the study of myeloma biology. The clinical characteristics of myeloma—myeloma cell dissemination is restricted to the bone marrow, myeloma is frequently associated with lytic bone disease, and the conversion of monoclonal gammopathy of undetermined significance to overt myeloma is preceded by changes in the cellular composition of the bone marrow (activation of osteoclasts, inhibition of osteoblastogenesis, and stimulation of angiogenesis)—all indicate that in order to grow primary myeloma cells, one must provide a supportive bone marrow microenvironment.

An animal model that provides a human bone marrow microenvironment is a valuable tool for growing and studying myeloma cells. Not only does such a

From: *Methods in Molecular Medicine, Vol. 113: Multiple Myeloma: Methods and Protocols*
Edited by: R. D. Brown and P. J. Ho © Humana Press Inc., Totowa, NJ

model provide the necessary support for sustaining the survival and growth of myeloma cells, but it also approximates the human disease by providing an in vivo system in which primary myeloma cells grow in a human bone marrow microenvironment. This model also facilitates research on the bone manifestations of myeloma and the effects of treatment on the myeloma cells, their microenvironment, and the host organism.

The mouse model developed for primary myeloma was successfully adapted from that used for the study of human hematopoiesis, lymphopoiesis, and leukemia *(1)*. Construction of the severe combined immune-deficient human (SCID-hu) myeloma model consists of three major steps: constructing the SCID-hu mouse, preparing the myeloma cells, and establishing and monitoring myeloma in the SCID-hu mouse. Human fetal bone fragments are implanted into SCID mice, resulting in SCID-hu mice. After allowing 6 wk for vascularization, the fetal bones are directly injected with myeloma cells freshly obtained from patients with myeloma. The development of myeloma in the SCID-hu mouse occurs as effectively when using purified myeloma plasma cells (PCs) as with whole bone marrow from patients. The SCID-hu host is monitored for development of myeloma and changes in tumor burden. This is determined by a rise in the host's serum level of human immunoglobulin (hIg) of the M protein isotype. Changes in bone calcification can be detected by X-radiography. Typically, myeloma is established in the human bone, and bone manifestations can be observed within a few weeks from injection of myeloma cells *(2–5)*. Because the process of establishing a myelomatous SCID-hu mouse is laborious, lengthy, and expensive, electronic identification chips are recommended in order to minimize the likelihood of misidentifying mice.

2. Materials

2.1. Construction of SCID-hu Mice

1. Human fetal femurs and tibias from physical extractions obtained at 17–22 gestational weeks (*see* **Note 1**).
2. Culture medium (e.g., RPMI-1640 from Mediatech, Herndon, VA) with antibiotics.
3. Six- to 8-wk-old homozygous CB-17/Icr scid/scid mice (e.g., from Harlan, Indianapolis, IN) (*see* **Note 2**).
4. Sterile phosphate-buffered saline (PBS) (e.g., from Mediatech).
5. Syringe (1 mL) and anesthetic cocktail of ketamine hydrochloride and xylazine: To a glass vial containing 5.6 mL of PBS, add 2 mL of ketamine (100 mg/mL) and 0.4 mL of xylazine (20 mg/mL). The final 8-mL solution contains 25 mg/mL of ketamine and 1 mg/mL of xylazine.
6. 70% Ethanol.
7. Sterile gauze, surgical scissors, forceps, stapler, and staple remover.
8. Implantable identification chips and reader (e.g., IMI-1000 from BioMedic Data Systems, Seaford, DE).

2.2. Preparation of Myeloma Cells

1. Heparinized bone marrow aspirates, blood, biopsies of soft-tissue lesions, and fine-needle aspirates from myeloma patients' focal lesions (*see* **Note 3**).
2. Ficoll-paque.
3. Conjugated monoclonal antibodies (MAbs):
   a. Phycoerythrin (PE)-conjugated anti-CD38 or -CD138.
   b. Fluorescein isothiocyanate (FITC)-conjugated anti-CD45. Conjugated antibodies (e.g., CD38 PE, CD138 PE, CD45 FITC; Becton-Dickinson, San Jose, CA) are light sensitive and should be stored in dark bottles at 4°C.
4. Sterile PBS.
5. Immunomagnetic beads and magnet for purification of plasma cells (e.g., Mini-Macs or AutoMACs automated separation system from Miltenyi Biotec, Auburn, CA); store immunomagnetic beads at 4°C.
6. Pyrogen-free 0.9% saline, for injection.

2.3. Establishment and Monitoring of Myeloma in SCID-hu Mice

1. Syringe (mL) and anesthetic cocktail of ketamine hydrochloride and xylazine (*see* **Subheading 2.1., item 5**).
2. 70% Ethanol.
3. Sterile gauze.
4. Syringe (0.5–1 mL) (to inject myeloma cells).
5. Enzyme-linked immunosorbent assay (ELISA) kits to measure hIg levels (e.g., Human Ig Quantitation Kit from Bethyl, Montgomery, TX).
6. ELISA plate reader.

3. Methods

3.1. Construction of SCID-hu Mice

1. To prepare bones for implantation, clean away the surrounding muscle tissue. Cut the femur and tibia into halves crosswise (approx $5 \times 5 \times 10$ mm each). Keep in culture medium containing antibiotics on ice until ready to implant into mice.
2. Anesthetize a mouse using an intramuscular injection of ketamine/xylazine cocktail (0.00335 mL/g of mouse weight, i.e., 0.067 mL for a mouse weighing 20 g). The mouse should be anesthetized and ready for implantation within 10 min of injection (*see* **Note 4**).
3. Clean the site of implantation with 70% ethanol and dry with sterile gauze.
4. Make a small incision in the skin on one side of the mouse, toward the mouse's front legs.
5. Insert one bone fragment into the incision, open end first. Once inserted, the closed end of the bone should be closest to the incision.
6. Staple the incision closed.

7. On the other flank of the mouse, insert an identification chip using the same technique as for inserting the bone. Read the chip and record the mouse number and type of bone implanted (e.g., sample identity, femur or tibia) (*see* **Note 5**).

8. Return the mouse to its cage. Keep watch until it regains consciousness, usually within 20–30 min of administration of anesthesia. Myeloma cells can be injected into the human bone 6–10 wk after the bone is implanted.

3.2. Preparation of Myeloma Cells

Separate cells over a Ficoll-paque density gradient. If desired, purify myeloma cells using immunomagnetic beads according to the manufacturer's protocols. Determine the percentage of PCs in the preparation. Prepare myeloma PCs as follows:

1. Place 5×10^5 cells into a 1.5-mL microcentrifuge tube (*see* **Note 6**).
2. Spin for 3–5 s in a microcentrifuge at 1500*g* to pellet the cells and decant.
3. Resuspend the cell pellet in 5 µL (or according to the manufacturer's protocol) each of CD38 PE– (or CD138 PE) and CD45 FITC-conjugated MAbs.
4. Let stand on ice for 20 min.
5. Add 1 mL of PBS, mix by pipetting up and down several times, spin as in **step 2** to pellet the cells, and decant.
6. Repeat the 1-mL PBS wash and decant.
7. Resuspend the cell pellet in 0.5 mL of PBS.
8. Analyze the cells on a flow cytometer to determine the proportion of cells with high levels of CD38 (or CD138) and low-intermediate levels of CD45 (*see* **Note 7**).
9. Prepare the cells for injection by diluting to 1×10^7 cells/50 µL in pyrogen-free saline or PBS.

3.3. Establishment and Monitoring of Myeloma in SCID-hu Mice

1. Anesthetize a mouse with ketamine/xylazine cocktail (*see* **Subheading 3.1., step 2**).
2. Take an X-ray image of the human bone prior to injection.
3. Bleed the mouse (*see* **Note 8**) to use as a control for determining background hIg levels. Separate serum and store at –80°C for future analysis.
4. Sterilize the site of injection using 70% ethanol. Dry the area with sterile gauze.
5. Inject the cells (50 µL/bone) into the open end of the human bone.
6. Read the identification chip to confirm the mouse's identity. In the corresponding record, document all relevant information connected with the injected myeloma cells.
7. Return the mouse to its cage and observe until fully recovered (about 20 min from administration of anesthesia).
8. Starting 2 wk after injection and continuing every 2 wk, bleed the mouse from the tail vein. At this stage it is possible to store the murine serum frozen at –80°C.
9. Four weeks after injection and every 2 wk thereafter, perform ELISA to measure the levels of hIg of the M protein isotype (heavy and light chains).

10. Two weeks after hIgs are first detected in the serum, bleed the mouse again and perform ELISA for all hIg isotypes, heavy and light chains, to ascertain the clonality of the cells.

Once the isotype of the hIg is confirmed as that of the M protein, and once hIg concentrations increase in two sequential measurements, myeloma is established in the human bone, and the SCID-hu mouse is ready for further experimentation. It is important to store aliquots of the serum at –80°C until the end of the experiment so that a final ELISA can be performed with all samples on the same plate or in the same assay. To confirm myeloma growth, take an X-ray image of the human bone to examine changes in bone calcification. It is advisable to determine the clonality of the myeloma cells in the human bone by *in situ* hybridization for CDR3 and to confirm the lack of Epstein-Barr virus (EBV) infection in the tumor by PCR or other method. EBV lymphomas are not usually a problem but should be checked nevertheless.

4. Notes

1. Tissues should be derived from physical extraction procedures not involving administration of prostaglandins or related drugs. Only human immunodeficiency virus- and hepatitis-free tissues should be used. Universal Precaution Procedures for the use of human tissues should be implemented, signed informed consent forms should be obtained and kept on file, and all patient confidentiality regulations should be followed.
   Note that if the bones are too large (e.g., the femur from a large fetus implanted into a small mouse), they may protrude through the skin of the mouse within a few weeks of implantation. Use judgment as to the proper size of bone to implant.
2. All experimental protocols using laboratory animals must be approved by the local Animal Care and Use Committee. Because SCID mice are immune deficient, they must be housed in isolation cages in a protective environment and receive sterile food and water. All procedures (surgical, imaging, and so on) must be carried out under sterile conditions. Use a laminar flow hood as much as possible.
3. In all experiments involving human tissues, approved informed consent forms must be signed by the patient/donor prior to any procedure and kept on file. All regulations and rules, including those governing patient confidentiality and safe procedures for handling human tissues, should be strictly adhered to.
   a. Use only preservative-free heparin to prevent damage to the cells.
   b. Process and use myeloma cells as soon after aspiration as possible.
   c. Remember that myeloma cells do not survive freezing, and cells thawed from frozen storage do not grow in this model.
4. Anesthetizing mice using inhalation of isoflurane or other inhalants is not recommended because the depth of anesthesia and duration of unconsciousness are difficult to control, frequently resulting in death of the animals. The use of a cocktail

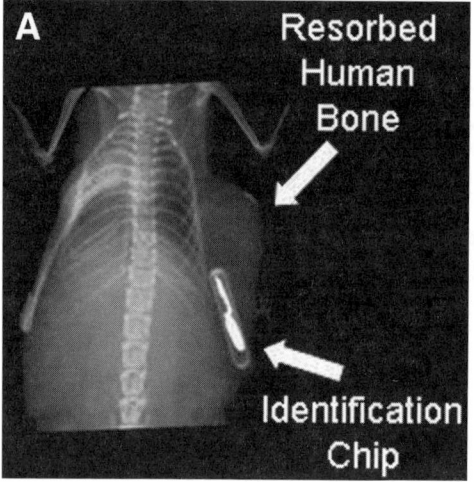
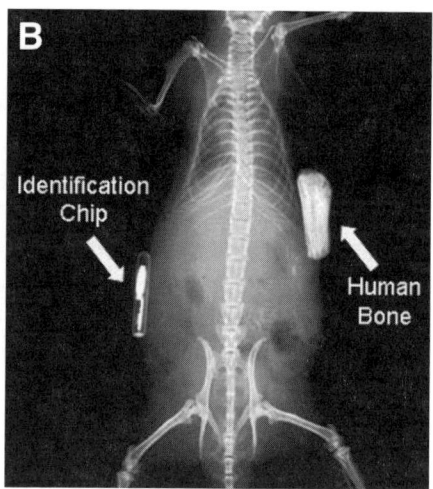

Fig. 1. X-radiographs of SCID-hu mice after implantation of human fetal bone and identification chip. (**A**) The human bone and the identification chip were implanted through the same incision. Although the chip was pushed away from the bone during insertion, it later migrated to the same area as the bone. (**B**) The human bone and the identification chip were implanted through separate incisions contralaterally and remained in place. Note the low contrast of human bone injected with myeloma cells (A) compared with the control bone (B). This indicates complete resorption of the human bone owing to myeloma.

that combines ketamine and xylazine yields safe, predictable effects. The mice are usually ready for surgical implantation within 10 min of injection.

It is important to prevent hypothermia of anesthetized mice. Place a mouse on a sterile pad so that it is not in contact with the metal surface of the hood. Use ethanol sterilization only on the necessary areas of the animal's body, and dry with sterile gauze. The use of a heat lamp is very helpful in preventing death owing to hypothermia.

5. It is possible to insert the identification chip and human bone through the same incision; however, often the chip moves within close proximity to the human bone. On X-ray, part of the bone is then obscured by the identification chip (**Fig. 1A**). Therefore, it is recommended that the chip be inserted contralateral to the bone (**Fig. 1B**). In the event that two bones are implanted into the same mouse, they should be implanted contralaterally through two separate incisions, and the chip should be inserted through its own incision at the back of the neck.

6. To achieve a high success rate, use samples with ≥15% myeloma PCs when injecting unseparated cells, and ≥1 × 10^6 cells when injecting purified myeloma cells.

7. The percentage of PCs in bone marrow aspirates after Ficoll separation and the purification product can be determined histologically or immunohistochemically

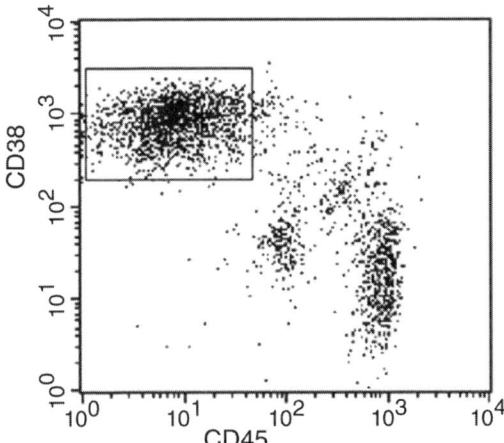

Fig. 2. Flow cytometry profile of myeloma cells. Bone marrow cells were separated on a Ficoll gradient. Light-density cells were reacted with conjugated MAbs (CD38 PE and CD45 FITC) and analyzed on a FacScan flow cytometer. The boxed area indicates myeloma PCs (high levels of CD38, low-intermediate levels of CD45) that can be enumerated or purified, as desired.

(e.g., staining for cytoplasmic Igs); however, flow cytometry is the preferred method for this task. Using flow cytometry, one can interrogate a large pool of cells (e.g., 10^4–10^6 cells), thus achieving much higher sensitivity for identifying myeloma cells and detecting contaminating cells in purified specimens than by any microscopic procedure (**Fig. 2**).

8. Because the mice in these experiments are bled repeatedly, it is best to bleed through the tail vein. To make this procedure easier, use Mouse Tail Illuminator (Braintree Scientific, Braintree, MA). This device efficiently illuminates and warms the mouse tail for easy bleeding (and injection).

References

1. Kyoizumi, S., Baum, C. M., Kaneshima, H., McCune, J. M., Yee, E. J., and Namikawa, R. (1992) Implantation and maintenance of functional human bone marrow in SCID-hu mice. *Blood* **79,** 1704–1711.
2. Yaccoby, S., Pearse, R. N., Johnson, C. L., Barlogie, B., Choi, Y., and Epstein, J. (2002) Myeloma interacts with the bone marrow microenvironment to induce osteoclastogenesis and is dependent on osteoclast activity. *Br. J. Haematol.* **116,** 278–290.
3. Pearse, R. N., Sordillo, E. M., Yaccoby, S., et al. (2001) Multiple myeloma disrupts the TRANCE/osteoprotegerin cytokine axis to trigger bone destruction and promote tumor progression. *Proc. Natl. Acad. Sci. USA* **98,** 11,581–11,586.

4. Yaccoby, S. and Epstein, J. (1999) The proliferative potential of myeloma plasma cells manifest in the SCID-hu host. *Blood* **94,** 3576–3582.
5. Yaccoby, S., Barlogie, B., and Epstein, J. (1998) Primary myeloma cells growing in SCID-hu mice—a model for studying the biology and treatment of myeloma and its manifestations. *Blood* **92,** 2908–2913.

15

The 5T2MM Murine Model of Multiple Myeloma

Maintenance and Analysis

Karin Vanderkerken, Kewal Asosingh, Angelo Willems,
Hendrik De Raeve, Pedro Couck, Frans Gorus,
Peter Croucher, and Ben Van Camp

Summary

Multiple myeloma is a B-cell neoplasm characterized by the monoclonal proliferation of plasma cells in the bone marrow, the development of osteolytic lesions, and the induction of angiogenesis. These different processes require three-dimensional interactions, with both humoral and cellular contacts. The 5TMM models are suitable to study these interactions. These are murine models that originate from spontaneously developed myeloma in elderly mice. They are propagated by in vivo transfer of the myeloma cells into young syngeneic mice. We report methods involving the maintenance of the 5T2MM model and the quantification of tumor burden (by determining serum paraprotein concentration and plasmacytosis), assessment of bone lesions, and quantification of angiogenesis. The combination of these different techniques in these models not only helps in unraveling basic biological processes but also in the testing of potentially new therapeutic targets.

Key Words

Multiple myeloma; animal model; angiogenesis; osteolytic lesions.

1. Introduction

The 5TMM models belong to the *de novo* models of myeloma (*1*) and originate from spontaneously developed multiple myeoloma (MM) in elderly mice of the C57BlKaLwRij strain (*2*). The models are initiated and are continued by transplantation of the diseased bone marrow into young syngeneic recipients. Several 5TMM models exist, each with its own characteristics; the 5T2MM and 5T33MM are the best characterized and the most commonly used (*3*). The

From: *Methods in Molecular Medicine, Vol. 113: Multiple Myeloma: Methods and Protocols*
Edited by: R. D. Brown and P. J. Ho © Humana Press Inc., Totowa, NJ

clinical characteristics of the 5T2MM model, including the selective localization of the MM cells in the bone marrow, the presence of serum M-component, the induction of osteolytic bone disease, and an increased angiogenesis in the bone marrow, are similar to the human disease *(2,4–8)*. These cells grow exclusively in vivo and can only be maintained in vitro for a short period of coculture with bone marrow stromal cells.

2. Materials

2.1. Isolation of 5TMM Cells

1. Dulbecco's modified essential medium supplemented with penicillin-streptomycin, L-glutamine, nonessential amino acids, and Na pyruvate (Gibco), called "supplemented medium." Cold medium is used during the whole procedure.
2. Trypan blue.
3. Lympholyte M (Cedarlane, Hornby, Ontario, Canada).
4. Petri dishes (60×15 mm), 50- and 15-mL Falcon tubes, nylon filter (70-μm mesh diameter), 1-mL syringes with needle (26-gage $\times$ 1/2 in., 0.45×12 mm), and 5-mL syringes.
5. Forceps and dissection scissors.

2.2. Enzyme-Linked Immunosorbent Assay

1. Phosphate-buffered saline (PBS) containing 0.05% NaN_3.
2. Blocking buffer RPMI-1640 culture medium with 10% fetal clone I (FCI).
3. Multichannel pipets and disposable pipet tips.
4. Microtiter plates, Sterilin plates 611F96 from Seriwell.
5. Spectrophotometer with 405-nm filter.
6. Washing buffer (18 g of NaCl + 1 mL of Igepal CA-630 [Sigma, St. Louis, MO]/ 1 L of water).
7. 2-2′-azino-di-(3-ethylbenzthiazoline sulfonic acid), diammonium salt (ABTS) solution: 10 mL of 0.1 *M* citrate, pH 4.0 + 100 μL of ABTS (Roche) (150 mg/ 10 mL of water) + 3.3 μL of 30% H_2O_2.
8. Goat anti-mouse IgG and goat anti-mouse IgG_1 (Oxford Biotechnology).

2.3. Electrophoresis

1. Pipets.
2. Disposable tips.
3. Paragon CZE™ 2000 (Beckman).

2.4. Fluorescent-Activated Cell Sorter Analysis

1. Fluorescent-activated cell sorter (FACS) tubes (Becton Dickinson).
2. FACSflow (Becton Dickinson).
3. Flow cytometer.
4. Centrifuge.
5. Solution A: Make a stock solution of 36% formaldehyde and 45% acetone in FACSflow. Dilute (1/1) in FACSflow before using.

   6. Solution B: 0.01% saponin and 1% bovine serum albumin in FACSflow.

   7. Rat anti-mouse IgG_1-PE (Pharmingen).

2.5. Morphology

   1. 10% FCI medium.
   2. Trypan blue buffered solution.
   3. Degreased 76 × 26 mm microscope slides.
   4. Glass cover slips.
   5. Mounting DPX resin/xylene.
   6. Shandon Cytospin 2 centrifuge.
   7. May-Grünwald Giemsa staining solution (May-Grünwald & Giemsa).
   8. Buffered water.
   9. Solution C (9.1 g/L of KH_2PO_4), solution D (11.9 g/L of $Na_2HPO_4 \cdot 2H_2O$): Mix 73 mL of solution C and 27 mL of solution D until a pH of 6.4 is reached. Add 50 mL of this mixed solution to 950 mL of millQ water.

2.6. Assessment of Bone Lesions

   1. 4% Formol.
   2. EDTA.
   3. Hematoxylin, eosin.
   4. Naphthol AS-BI-phosphate.
   5. Dimethylformamide (DMF).
   6. Tartrate.
   7. Sodium acetate trihydrate.
   8. Pararosaniline.
   9. 4% Sodium nitrite.
 10. Paraffin tissue processor.
 11. Paraffin microtome.
 12. Faxitron X-ray system (Hewlett Packard, McMinnville, OR).
 13. UMAX PowerLook 1100 scanner (UMAX UK, Gomshall, UK).
 14. Adobe™ Photoshop (Adobe Systems).
 15. Leica QWin image analysis system (Leica Microscope Systems, Milton Keynes, UK).
 16. PIXImus scanner (Lunar, Madison, WI).
 17. Leica TP1020 carousel tissue processor.

2.7. Quantification of Angiogenesis

   1. Zinc fixative: 1000 mL of 0.1 M Tris buffer, pH 7.4 (before adding additives), 0.5 g of calcium acetate, 5.0 g of zinc acetate, and 5.0 g of zinc chloride.
   2. Decalcification solution: 100 g of EDTA, 12 g of NaOH, 50 mL of 4% formalin, 950 mL of demineralized water.
   3. Paraffin.
   4. Toluol.
   5. Isopropyl alcohol.
   6. Superfrost Plus Slides (8613967; International Medical n.v., Marche en Famenne, Belgium).

7. Modular Vacuum Processor Renaissance (Ventana Medical Systems, Tucson, AZ).
8. Rotation microtome HM 335E (Microm GmbH, Walldorf, Germany).
9. TNT wash buffer: 0.1 M Tris-HCl, pH 7.5; 0.15 M NaCl; 0.05% Tween-20.
10. Methanol.
11. Hydrogen peroxide (H_2O_2).
12. Working solution of trypsin: dissolve 0.07 g of trypsin (Trypsin 0109819; Roche, Mannheim, Germany) at 37°C in 70 mL of demineralized water containing 0.07 g of $CaCl_2$.
13. TNB Blocking Buffer: 0.1 M Tris-HCl, pH 7.5; 0.15 M NaCl; 0.5% Blocking Reagent. Blocking Reagent is supplied in a Tyramide Signal Amplification kit (NEL700A; NEN, Boston, MA).
14. Normal goat serum solution: 4/5 TNB Blocking Buffer and 1/5 normal goat serum.
15. Normal mouse serum.
16. Monoclonal antibody (MAb) rat antimouse CD31 (platelet endothelial cell adhesion molecule-1) (MEC 13.3; Becton Dickinson, Pharmingen, LA).
17. Goat anti-rat Specific Polyclonal Immunoglobulin (559286; Becton Dickinson).
18. Streptavidin-horseradish peroxidase (HRP), supplied in a Tyramide Signal Amplification kit (NEL700A; NEN).
19. Biotinyl tyramide (amplification reagent supplied in a Tyramide Signal Amplification kit, NEL700A).
20. Biotinyl tyramide stock solution: add 0.3 mL of dimethyl sulfoxide (8.02912.1000; Merck, Darmstadt, Germany) to biotinyl tyramide. Aliquot the biotinyl tyramide stock solution and store at 4°C.
21. Biotinyl tyramide working solution: dilute the biotinyl tyramide stock solution 1/50 with Amplification Diluent (supplied in a Tyramide Signal Amplification kit, NEL700A).
22. 3,3′-Diaminobenzidine (DAB) (Dako Liquid DAB+, K3468; DakoCytomation, CA).
23. Hematoxylin.
24. Mounting medium (Coverquick; Labonord, Templemars, France).
25. Light microscope.
26. Eyepiece graticule.

3. Methods

3.1. Isolation of 5TMM Cells

1. Sacrifice terminally diseased 5T2MM-bearing mice by cervical dislocation or CO_2 asphyxiation.
2. Dissect the hind legs and the vertebrae. Remove all tissues around the bones and put them in a Petri dish with 5 mL of supplemented medium. Cut the hind legs through the knee. Cut open both ends of the tibiae and femora. Aspirate medium in a 1-mL syringe with a needle, and flush the contents of the bones into a Petri dish with 5 mL of medium (final volume). Aspirate and flush the medium several times to disperse the bone marrow cells.

3. Crush the vertebrae with the back side of a 5-mL syringe in 5-mL of medium.
4. Filtrate the cell suspensions through a nylon filter (70-μm mesh diameter) into a 50-mL tube.
5. Pipet 5 mL of Lympholyte M into a 15-mL tube, and overlay carefully with 5 mL of cell suspension. Use one tube/mouse.
6. Centrifuge for 20 min at 1000g and remove the cells at the interface of the Lympholyte M and medium.
7. Wash the mononuclear cells two times in 5 mL of medium, and count the viable cells following trypan blue exclusion.
8. Adjust the cell concentration to 10×10^6/mL for 5T2MM.

3.2. Injection of 5TMM Cells

Two hundred microliters of the cell suspension is injected into one of the lateral tail veins of naive 6- to 8-wk-old recipients (C57BlKaLwRijHsd; Harlan CPB, Horst, The Netherlands) with a 29-gage syringe. The development of the disease is monitored by the quantification of the serum paraprotein concentration. When a concentration of >10 mg/mL is reached, the mice are sacrificed and used for the maintenance of the model. No more than five generations are used (*see* **Note 1**); at that time, frozen early generations of cells are thawed and injected.

3.3. Quantification of Tumor Load

3.3.1. Serum Paraprotein Concentration

The serum should be physically separated (centrifuged) from contact with cells within 2 h from the time of collection. Whole blood is incubated for 30 min at 37°C, followed by 1 h of incubation at 4°C and centrifugation. If serum samples are not assayed within 8 h from the time of collection, they should be stored at 2–8°C. Serum samples stored at –20°C are stable for a maximum of 40 d. Frozen samples should be thawed only once. Hemolyzed, lipemic samples are not recommended for analysis.

3.3.2. Enzyme-Linked Immunosorbent Assay

1. Disperse 50 μL of goat anti-mouse IgG solution at 5 μg/mL (*3*) PBS containing 0.05% NaN$_3$ into each well of the plate. Tap or shake the plate to ensure that the solution is evenly distributed over the bottom of the plate. Seal the plate and incubate for 2 h at room temperature and overnight at 4°C or for 2 h at 37°C.
2. Rinse the coated plate with washing buffer three times, each time flicking the washing buffer into the sink.
3. Fill each well with 50 μL of blocking buffer and incubate for at least 30 min at room temperature.
4. Rinse the plate three times in washing buffer. After the last rinse, remove residual liquid by gently flicking the plate face down onto tissue on the benchtop.

5. Add 100 µL of serum samples (diluted 1:2) to each sample well of the first row of wells, and dilute 1:2 for the following wells of each column, obtaining 50 µL of solution in each well.
6. Add purified 5T2MM protein to control wells starting at 5 µg/mL and diluting 1:2 with blocking buffer to obtain a standard curve.
7. Incubate for 1 h at room temperature.
8. Wash three times with washing buffer.
9. Add anti-5T2 idiotype antibodies (*6*) at 5 µg/mL and incubate for 1 h.
10. Wash three times with washing buffer.
11. Add goat anti-mouse IgG$_1$ antibodies at a 1/10,000 dilution in blocking buffer (50 µL/well) and incubate for 1 h.
12. Wash three times with washing buffer.
13. Add 100 µL of ABTS to each well and incubate in the dark.
14. Read on an enzyme-linked immunosorbent assay (ELISA) reader at 405 nm when optical density values of the first control wells reach about 900.
15. Calculate the serum paraprotein concentration by interpolation from the standard curve.

3.3.3. Electrophoresis

The Paragon CZE 2000 is a dedicated automated system for the routine analysis of human serum proteins by capillary zone electrophoresis. Proteins are measured by direct absorption at 214 nm through a small optical window in the capillary. Instrument settings for serum protein electrophoresis are as follows: 1-min conditioning, 1-s injection, 0.5-min wash, 0.5-min rinse, 9000 V, and 24°C. The Paragon CZE 2000 automatically selects pattern fractions, using an involved software package. The instrument attempts to find valleys to delimit the different fractions. Manual editing of the delimitation is possible and often necessary owing to inadequate separation of the fractions. Delimitation of monoclonal spikes has to be done manually by visual interpretation of the electrophoretic patterns (**Fig. 1**). The absolute concentration of the detected monoclonal spikes is calculated automatically by the obtained relative amount of the monoclonal component (percent) and the protein concentration (g/dL) in the sample.

The procedure is linear for protein concentrations between 3.5 and 12 g/dL. Samples with a protein content >12 g/dL have to be diluted with saline (0.9% NaCl solution).

3.3.4. Plasmacytosis

3.3.4.1. FACS ANALYSIS (*SEE* **NOTE 2**)

1. Wash 1 × 10^6 cells two times with FACSflow. Decant the supernatant after the last washing step, and resuspend the pellet in the remaining volume of FACSflow.
2. Add 75 µL of solution A and incubate for 10 min in the dark at room temperature.
3. Wash with 2.5 mL of FACSflow and aspirate the supernatant.

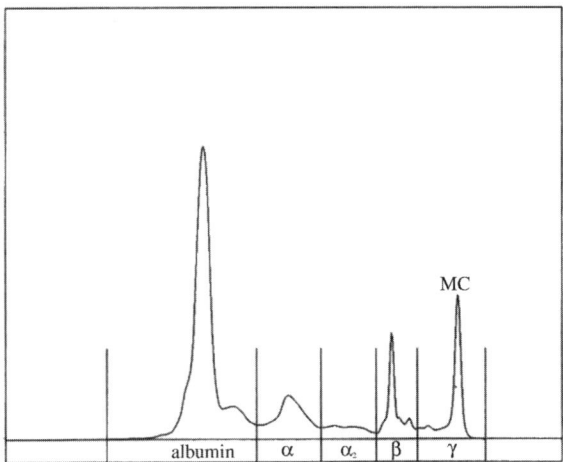

Fig. 1. Electrophoretic pattern obtained with Paragon CZE 2000 in a murine serum sample, showing different fractions and presence of a monoclonal component (MC) in γ fraction. The delimitation of this MC protein resulted in a concentration of 0.82 g/dL, with a total protein concentration of 7.84 g/dL.

4. Add 75 µL of solution B and 75 µL of anti-5T2MM supernatant (mouse IgG₁) *(6)*. Incubate for 15 min in the dark at room temperature. Use a mouse IgG₁ as the control antibody.

5. Wash with 2.5 mL of FACSflow, decant the supernatant after the last washing step, and resuspend the pellet in the remaining volume of FACSflow.

6. Add 75 µL of solution A and incubate for 10 min in the dark at room temperature.

7. Wash with 2.5 mL of FACSflow and aspirate the supernatant.

8. Add 75 µL of Rat-anti-mouse IgG₁-PE (Pharmingen) diluted in solution B. Incubate for 15 min in the dark at room temperature.

9. Wash with 2.5 mL of FACSflow and aspirate the supernatant.

10. Resuspend the pellet in 300 µL of FACSflow.

11. Acquire 10,000 events with a flow cytometer.

12. Gate the cells on a forward scatter/side scatter dot plot (R1).

13. Display events falling into R1 on an FL1/FL2 dot plot and put quadrant markers on the control sample (**Fig. 2**).

14. Analyze the anti-idiotype-stained sample with the same gate and quadrants (**Fig. 2**).

3.3.4.2. MORPHOLOGY

1. Dilute total viable cell concentration, determined by trypan blue exclusion, to a concentration of 4×10^5/mL in medium with 10% FCI.

2. Add 200 µL (8×10^4) of this suspension to a sample chamber assembly, and centrifuge (Shandon Cytospin 2) for 7 min at 900 rpm (~72G).

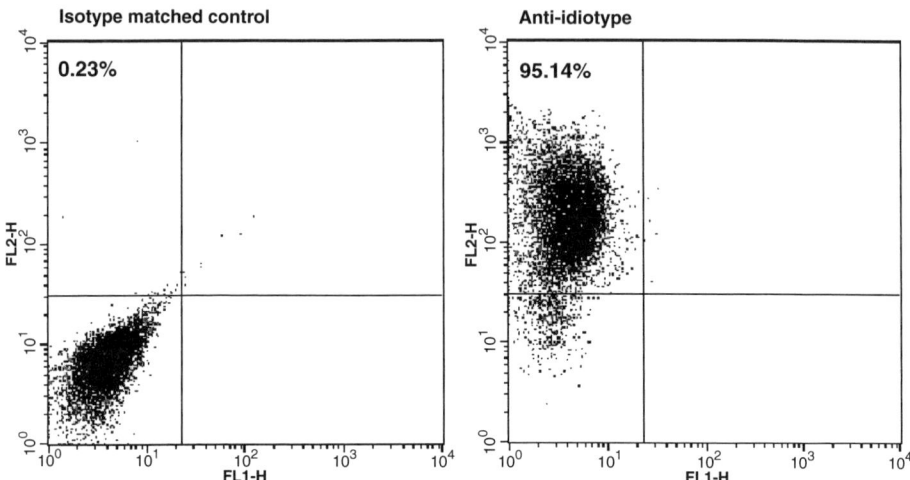

Fig. 2. FACS analysis illustrating 95.14% 5T2MM idiotype-positive cells.

3. After air-drying, stain the cells using the May-Grünwald Giemsa staining protocol as follows:
   a. Bath 1 = May-Grünwald undiluted: 5 min.
   b. Bath 2 = May-Grünwald/buffered water (1/1): Immerse two to three times.
   c. Bath 3 = Giemsa/buffered water (1/9): 20 min.
   d. Bath 4 = buffered water: Immerse.
   e. Bath 5 = buffered water: immerse.
   f. Bath 6 = buffered water: 1 min.
4. After air-drying the microscope slides, mount a cover slip using DPX resin. Then
   determine tumor burden using a microscope (×1000) (**Fig. 3**).

3.4. Assessment of Bone Lesions

A combination of radiographic and histomorphometric techniques are used.
MicroCT approaches are now also available although access to equipment is
limited; therefore, these approaches are not discussed.

3.4.1. Radiographic and Bone Densitometric Analysis

Following sacrifice the femur, tibia, and lumbar vertebrae are dissected free
of soft tissue and fixed in either 4% formol or 4% paraformaldehyde (*see*
Subheading 3.4.4.).

3.4.2. Radiographic Analysis

The femur, tibia, and lumbar vertebrae are placed on plastic film and retained
in position using 3M tape. To ensure comparability all tibiae, femora, and vertebrae from individual experiments are placed on one film. Bones are X-rayed

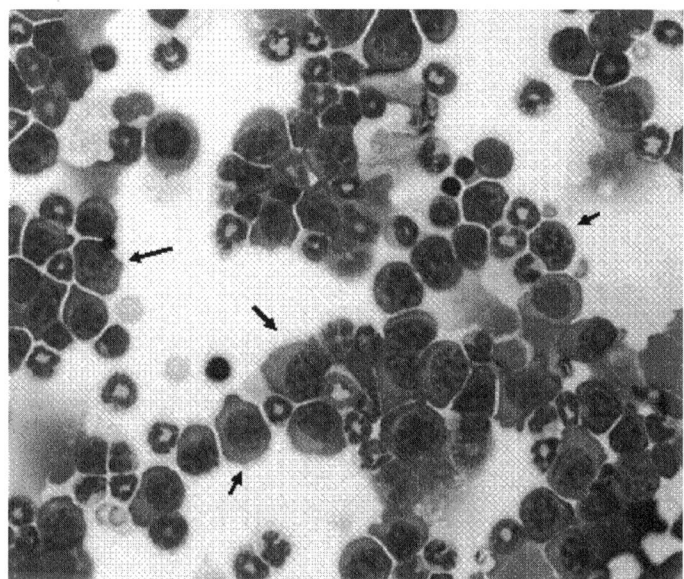

Fig. 3. Morphology on cytosmears. Arrows indicate 5T2MM cells.

on a Faxitron X-ray system with an exposure time of 10 s (35 kV). X-ray film is developed using an automatic film processor. X-rays are scanned on a UMAX PowerLook 1100 scanner into Adobe Photoshop. The images are enlarged and the numbers of osteolytic bone lesions in the tibia and femur are counted manually. The area of osteolytic bone lesions is determined by importing images into the Leica QWin image analysis system. Lytic bone lesions are traced manually and the area of lesion is expressed in square millimeters (**Fig. 4**).

3.4.3. Analysis of Total Bone Mineral Density (BMD)

Individual tibiae and femora and lumbar vertebrae 1–4 are scanned using a PIXImus scanner. Total bone mineral density (BMD) of scanned bones is determined using the dedicated small animal software. The coefficient of variation for femoral BMD was obtained after scanning 30 femurs five times each, following repositioning between scans, and was found to be 2.7%. BMD is expressed as milligrams/square centimeters *(7)*.

3.4.4. Histological and Histochemical Analysis

Tibiae and femora are fixed and decalcified in one of two ways:

1. Formalin fixation: Following dissection immerse the bones in 4% formol for a minimum of 4 d. Then transfer the bones to 0.5 *M* EDTA for decalcification and maintain at room temperature. Change the EDTA solution each week.

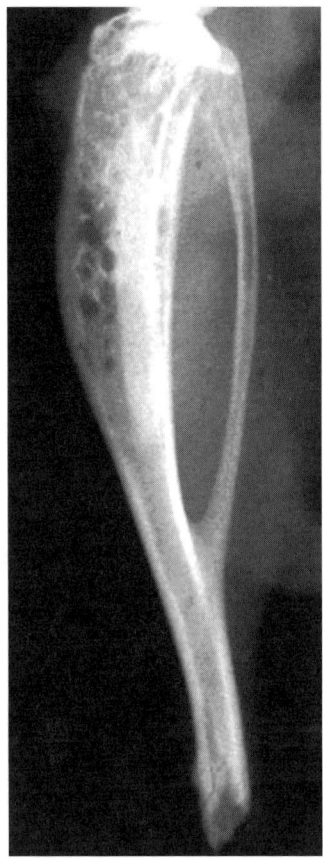

Fig. 4. Radiographic analysis demonstrating lytic bone lesions in a 5T2MM-invaded bone marrow.

   Decalcification is complete within 4 wk. Confirm decalcification by X-ray analysis as detailed in **Subheading 3.4.2.**
2. Paraformaldehyde fixation: Following dissection immerse the bones in 4% paraformaldehyde (in PBS, pH 7.4, prepared on the day of fixation) at 4°C for a minimum of 24 h. Then transfer the bones to decalcification solution (0.5 *M* EDTA/0.5% paraformaldehyde in PBS, pH 8.0) and incubate at 4°C for 1 to 2 wk. Change the decalcification solution two to three times per week. Confirm decalcification by X-ray analysis as detailed in **Subheading 3.4.2.**

   Paraformaldehyde fixation and the associated decalcification approach are used when sections are to be used for immunohistochemical studies. Following decalcification, bones are washed in distilled H_2O to remove EDTA and processed in paraffin using a Leica TP1020 carousel tissue processor and standard processing protocol (3 × 70% ethanol, 2 × 95% ethanol, 2 × 100% ethanol, 2 × xylene, and 2 × paraffin wax [56°C congealing point], each for 2 h). Samples are then embedded in paraffin and 3-µm sections cut on a Leica RM2135 microtome using disposable steel blades. Sections are cut at a minimum of three levels separated by 100 µm. Sections from each level are stained with hematoxylin and eosin (H&E) or reacted for tartrate-resistant acid phosphatase (TRAP) activity to identify osteoclasts using the following methods:

1. For H&E, dewax the sections and take to H_2O. Immerse in Gill's hematoxylin for 90 s, wash in tap water, and counterstain in 1% aqueous eosin for 3 min. Dehydrate in graded ethanol, clear in xylene, and mount.
2. For tartrate-resistant acid phosphatase, prepare the following solutions:
   a. Naphthol AS-BI-Phosphate (20 mg/mL), prepared in DMF.
   b. 0.2 *M* Acetate buffer containing sodium tartrate (100 m*M*), pH 5.2: dissolve 2.72 g of sodium acetate trihydrate in 100 mL of dH_2O, adjust the pH to 5.2 with 1.2% acetic acid, and add 2.3 g of sodium tartrate/100 mL on the day of use.
   c. Pararosaniline: dissolve 1 g of pararosaniline in 20 mL of distilled H_2O with heating, add 5 mL of concentrated HCl, cool, and filter.
   d. 4% Sodium nitrite: dissolve 80 mg of sodium nitrite in 2 mL of dH_2O.
3. Warm acetate buffer to 37°C. Dewax the sections in xylene, rehydrate through ethanol to distilled H_2O, and then immerse in acetate buffer.
4. Prepare solution A: into a glass jar add 1 mL of naphthol-AS-Bi phosphate to 50 mL of acetate buffer. Incubate the sections for 30 min at 37°C.
5. Prepare solution B: Hexazotize the pararosaniline by mixing 2 mL of pararosaniline stock with 2 mL of sodium nitrite solution. Add 2.5–50 mL of acetate buffer, and incubate the sections for 15 min at 37°C. Rinse in tap water, counterstain with hamatoxylin, dehydrate in graded ethanol, clear in xylene, and mount.

After staining, the following assessment is undertaken using the Leica QWin image analysis system:

1. Cancellous bone area: Determine the cancellous bone area as a proportion of the total area (Cn.Ar/T.Ar, %) in the distal femoral metaphysis and proximal tibial metaphysis, in an area of 0.64 mm^2 and 0.25 mm from the growth plate. Examine H&E-stained sections on a Leica DMRB microscope using an objective magnification of ×4. Capture images on the Leica QWin system, trace cancellous bone manually, and express as a proportion of the total area (percent). Examine a minimum of two sections from two separate levels from each bone.
2. Osteoclast number and osteoclast surface: In 5T2MM-bearing animals, cancellous bone area is significantly decreased and there is little bone surface on which to examine osteoclast numbers. Therefore, count the number of osteoclasts present on 3 mm of each cortical-endosteal surface, beginning 0.5 mm from the growth plate. Examine the sections reacted for TRAP activity at an

objective magnification of ×10. Store the images on the QWin imaging system. Trace the corticoendosteal surface manually, and count the number of TRAP-positive osteoclasts lining the bone surface. Express the number of osteoclasts per millimeter of corticoendosteal bone surface. The surface covered by osteoclasts can also be traced manually and expressed as a percentage of total surfaces.

3.5. Quantification of Angiogenesis

3.5.1. Preparation, Fixation, Embedding, and Cutting of Sections

1. Dissect the hind leg of a mouse.
2. Remove all tissue around the bone. Make two holes at the extremities of the bone through the cortex into the bone marrow cavity with a needle (29-gage) in order to allow penetration of the fixative into the medullary cavity.
3. Fix the long bone by immersion for 48 h in zinc fixative.
4. Immerse the samples for 48 h in a decalcification solution.
5. Put the bones into cassettes.
6. Dehydrate and impregnate the bones in paraffin with a Modular Vacuum Processor Renaissance.
7. Embed in paraffin.
8. Cut 5-μm sections of the paraffin blocks with a rotation microtome.

3.5.2. CD31-Immunohistochemical Staining for the Visualization of Microvessels in Bone Marrow (see **Note 3**)

1. Deparaffinate the sections by immersing the slides, respectively, twice for 15 min in toluol and once for 1 min in each of 100% isopropyl alcohol, 95% isopropyl alcohol, 75% isopropyl alcohol, and demineralized water.
2. Wash the slides three times for 5 min each time in TNT wash buffer at room temperature with agitation.
3. Immerse the slides in a solution of 50 mL of methanol and 0.5 mL of H_2O_2 (30%) for 30 min (quenching of the endogenous peroxidase).
4. Wash the slides twice for 5 min each time in TNT wash buffer at room temperature with agitation.
5. Immerse the slides for 5 min in demineralized water at 37°C.
6. Immerse the slides in a working solution of trypsin for 20 min at 37°C (antigen retrieval).
7. Stop the trypsinization by immersing the slides in demineralized water for 4 min at 4°C.
8. Wash the slides three times for 5 min each time in TNT wash buffer at room temperature with agitation.
9. Preincubate the slides with normal goat serum solution for 30 min.
10. Pipet 200 μL/slide of the primary MAb rat anti-mouse CD31 diluted 1/10 in TNB Blocking Buffer containing 10% mouse serum, and incubate overnight at 4°C.

11. Wash the slides three times for 5 min each time in TNT wash buffer at room temperature with agitation.
12. Pipet 200 μL/slide of a biotin-conjugated goat anti-rat specific polyclonal immunoglobulin diluted 1/70 in TNB Blocking Buffer containing 10% mouse serum, and incubate for 1 h at room temperature.
13. Wash the slides three times for 5 min each time in TNT wash buffer at room temperature with agitation.
14. Pipet 200 μL/slide of streptavidin-HRP diluted 1/100 in TNB Blocking Buffer, and incubate for 30 min at room temperature.
15. Wash the slides three times for 5 min each time in TNT wash buffer at room temperature with agitation.
16. Pipet 200 μL/slide of biotinyl tyramide working solution, and incubate for 10 min at room temperature.
17. Wash the slides three times for 5 min each time in TNT wash buffer at room temperature with agitation.
18. Pipet 200 μL/slide of streptavidin-HRP diluted 1/100 in TNB Blocking Buffer, and incubate for 30 min at room temperature.
19. Wash the slides three times for 5 min each time in TNT wash buffer at room temperature with agitation.
20. Immerse the slides in a DAB solution in the dark for 10 min.
21. Wash the slides for 4 min in demineralized water.
22. Counterstain with hematoxylin for 15 s.
23. Dehydrate the sections by immersing the slides, respectively, for 1 min in 75% isopropyl alcohol, 1 min in 95% isopropyl alcohol, twice for 1 min each time in 100% isopropyl alcohol, and three times for 1 min each time in toluol.
24. Mount the slides with mounting medium.

3.5.3. Determination of Microvessel Density

Consider only CD31-positive cells as being endothelial cells. The presence of a lumen with or without red blood cells is not considered an exclusive criterion for identifying a vessel.

1. On the CD31-immunostained sections, select the areas with the highest density of microvessels (hot spots) with a light microscope at low magnification (×10 ocular and ×10 objective).
2. In these areas, count the number of cross-sections of the microvessels within an area defined by an eyepiece graticule at a magnification of ×200 (×10 ocular and ×20 objective) (**Fig. 5**).

4. Notes

1. To preserve the characteristics described for the 5TMM lines, it is important to limit the number of in vivo generations and to limit the route of tumor inoculation to intravenous injection.

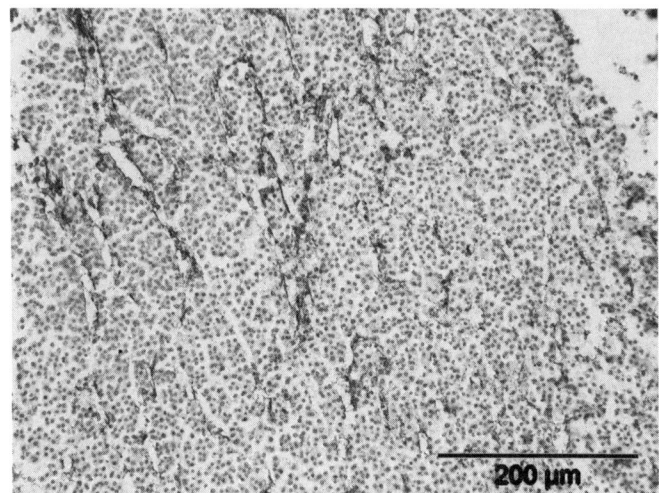

Fig. 5. CD31 staining on 5T2MM-invaded bone marrow.

2. For FACS analysis, a solution A and B are described to permeabilize and to fix the
   cells. Commercial kits (Fix and Perm) are also available.
3. To obtain a strong CD31 staining on the bone marrow sections, it is important to
   limit the time of fixation and decalcification, as described in the protocol.

Acknowledgments

This work was supported by the Fund for Scientific Research-Flanders
(FWO-Vlaanderen). K.V. and K.A. are postdoctoral fellows and H.R. has a
clinical doctoral grant from the FWO-Vlaanderen. P.C. is funded by the
Leukemia Research Fund. The development of a core facility for the 5TMM
model was supported by the Multiple Myeloma Research Foundation (senior
grants for K.V. and P.C.).

References

1. Radl, J. (1990) Age-related monoclonal gammapathies: clinical lessons from the
   aging C57BL mouse. *Immunol. Today* **11,** 234–236.
2. Radl, J., De Glopper, E. D., Schuit, H. R., and Zurcher, C. (1979) Idiopathic para-
   proteinemia. II. Transplantation of the paraprotein-producing clone from old to
   young C57BL/KaLwRij mice. *J. Immunol.* **122,** 609–613.
3. Vanderkerken, K., Asosingh, K., Croucher, P., and Van Camp, B. (2003) Multiple
   myeloma biology: lessons from the 5TMM models. *Immunol. Rev.* **194,** 196–206.
4. Asosingh, K., Radl, J., Van Riet, I., Van Camp, B., and Vanderkerken, K. (2000)
   The 5TMM series: a useful in vivo mouse model of human multiple myeloma.
   Hematol. J. **1,** 351–356.

5. Vanderkerken, K., Goes, E., De Raeve, H., Radl, J., and Van Camp, B. (1996) Follow-up of bone lesions in an experimental multiple myeloma mouse model: description using X-ray dedicated for mammography. *Br. J. Cancer* **73,** 1463–1465.

6. Vanderkerken, K., De Raeve, H., Goes, E., et al. (1997) Organ involvement and phenotypic adhesion profile of 5T2 and 5T33 myeloma cells in the C57BL/KaLwRij mouse. *Br. J. Cancer* **76,** 451–460.

7. Croucher, P. I., Shipman, C., Lippitt, J., et al. (2001) Osteoprotegerin inhibits the development of osteolytic bone disease in multiple myeloma. *Blood* **98,** 3534–3540.

8. Van Valckenborgh, E., De Raeve, H., Devy, L., et al. (2002) Murine 5T multiple myeloma cells induce angiogenesis in vitro and in vivo. *Br. J. Cancer* **86,** 796–802.

16

Determination of Telomerase Activity and Telomere Length

Kai-da Wu and Malcolm A. S. Moore

Summary

Telomerase is an enzyme that has been attracting much attention in recent years because its activities are so central to the processes of malignant transformation. It is a reverse transcriptase enzyme that can synthesize telomeric DNA using its own RNA component as a template. Without telomerase, telomeres will shorten until, at a critical length, cells enter senescence and die. The low level or absence of telomerase activity in most nonneoplastic tissues and somatic cells, and its presence in almost all malignant tumors is thus of great interest for potential diagnostic, prognostic, and therapeutic applications in the management of human cancer. It has been documented that high telomerase activity and short telomere length correlate with poor prognosis in patients with multiple myeloma, and antitelomerase therapy has become a novel therapeutic approach for the disease. Thus, determination of telomerase activity and telomere length is essential in the study of cancer. In this chapter, we provide a standard telomeric repeat amplification protocol for telomerase activity assay and a Southern blot terminal restriction fragment protocol for telomere length assay. We also discuss comparison with related assay methods.

Key Words

Multiple myeloma; telomerase; telomere activity; telomere length; telomeric repeat amplification protocol; Southern blot analysis.

1. Introduction

Telomeres are specialized DNA-protein structures located at each chromosome terminus where noncoding sequences are arranged in tandemly repeated units of the hexanucleotide $(TTAGGG)_n$ with an estimated length ranging between 5 and 15 kb in human cells. The length of the repeated telomere region is highly variable among the chromosomes of a single cell and among different cells within a population *(1)*. It has been suggested that telomeres protect chromosome ends against degradation, rearrangement, and fusion with

From: *Methods in Molecular Medicine, Vol. 113: Multiple Myeloma: Methods and Protocols*
Edited by: R. D. Brown and P. J. Ho © Humana Press Inc., Totowa, NJ

other chromosomes *(2)*. In addition to maintaining chromosome stability, telomeres play multiple roles in spatial organization of the cell nucleus and in chromosomal separation during cell division *(3)*. They can also regulate gene expression and cellular senescence *(2)*. In somatic cells, telomere length (TL) is progressively shortened with each cell division both in vivo and in vitro, owing to the inability of the DNA polymerase complex to replicate the very end of the lagging strand *(4)*. Stabilization of telomeric DNA via telomerase upregulation or activation of alternative mechanisms of telomere maintenance is essential if cells are to avoid senescence and proliferate extensively *(5)*. Telomerase is a specialized reverse transcriptase enzyme that can synthesize telomere strands *de novo* by using its own template to compensate for the loss of telomere repeats. Telomerase activity (TA) has been detected in up to 85–90% of human cancers but is absent in the majority of normal tissues, supporting the notion that immortalization is associated with the upregulation of telomerase. Although telomerase is not an oncogene *(6)*, transfection of hTERT into normal epithelial or endothelial cells transformed with simian virus 40 large T antigen and N-ras oncogene allows cells to bypass crisis and ultimately achieve malignant phenotype, confirming the role of telomerase in cellular immortalization and tumorigenesis *(7)*.

There are limited telomerase and telomere studies in multiple myeloma (MM) biology *(8–10)*. In one study, telomerase level was not elevated in plasma cells (PCs) from five patients with monoclonal gammopathy of undetermined significance, but it was elevated in 21 of 27 patients with MM and in all 4 patients with PC leukemia *(9)*. In another study of 25 patients with MM, elevated TA level correlated with high β_2-microglobulin levels, clinical stage III disease, and shorter survival *(10)*.

We have demonstrated in a large group of patients with MM that there is considerable heterogeneity in tumor TA and TL *(8)* (**Fig. 1**). Increased TA correlated positively with age and negatively with TL. Strong correlations were determined between various prognostic features (β_2-microglobulin and interleukin-6 levels, platelet counts at diagnosis) and TA, TL, or both. Various cytogenetic abnormalities, including poor prognosis abnormalities involving chromosome 13, strongly correlated with TA and, in many instances, with short TL. High TA significantly correlated with 2-yr survival among patients, pointing to the prognostic value of TA evaluation in the survival of MM *(8)*. Based on these findings, antitelomerase therapy has become a novel therapeutic approach for MM *(11,12)*.

In this chapter, we describe a sensitive and efficient polymerase chain reaction (PCR)-based telomerase activity detection method, telomeric repeat amplification protocol (TRAP) assay *(13,14)*, and a modified Southern blot analysis

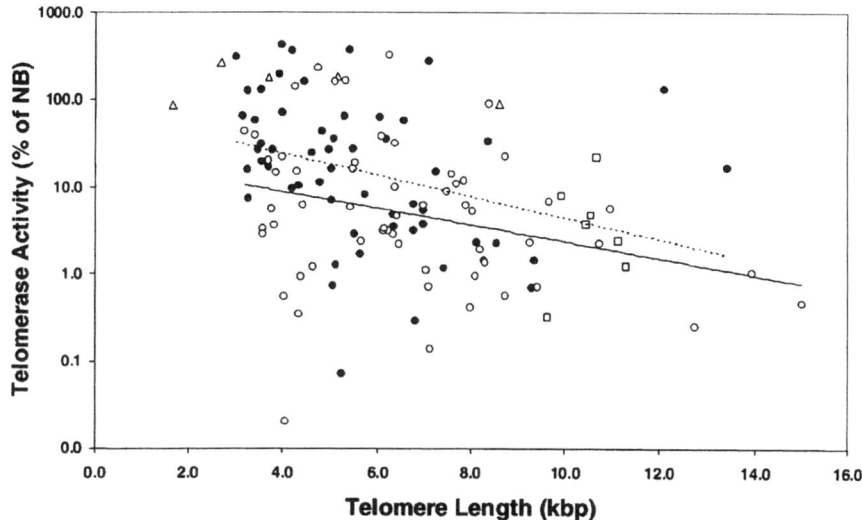

Fig. 1. Correlations between telomerase activity and telomere length in myeloma and normal PCs. The results showed that there was a strong negative correlation between TA and TL in the myeloma samples from treated (●) and untreated (○) patients. The dotted line indicates treated patients with MM, and the solid line indicates untreated patients with MM. MM cell lines (△) had high TA and short TL, and seven healthy donors (□) had low TA and relatively long TL. Seven patients with MM exhibited unusually long TL (longer than 10.8 kbp) with TA <5.8% of neuroblastoma (NB) control in five patients.

of terminal restriction fragment to determine telomere length in MM in our laboratory *(8,11)*.

2. Materials

2.1. Determination of Telomerase Activity by TRAP Assay

1. Protein assay kit (cat. no. 500-0006; Bio-Rad, Hercules, CA).
2. 3-[(3-Cholamidopropyl)dimethylammonio]-1-propanesulfonate (CHAPS) (cat. no. 28300; Pierce, Rockford, IL) lysis buffer (10 mM Tris-HCl, pH 7.5; 1 mM MgCl$_2$; 1 mM EGTA; 0.1 mM phenylmethylsulfonyl fluoride; 5 mM β-mercaptoethanol; 0.5% [w/v] CHAPS; and 10% [v/v] glycerol).
3. RNase inhibitor (cat. no. 3335399; Roche, Indianapolis, IN).
4. AmpliTaq DNA polymerase (5 U/μL) (Applied Biosystems, Foster City, CA).
5. Phosphate-buffered saline (PBS) (Mg^{++} and Ca^{++} free).
6. 40% Polyacrylamide/bisacrylamide stock solution (19:1) (cat. no. 161-0145; Bio-Rad).
7. TEMED (cat. no. 161-0801; Bio-Rad).

8. Ammonium persulfate (cat. no. BP179-100; Fisher, Fairview, NJ).
9. 10X Tris–boric acid–EDTA buffer (108 g of Tris base; 55 g of boric acid; 40 mL of 0.5 M EDTA, pH 8.0).
10. 3MM chromatography paper (cat. no. 3030917; Whatman).
11. γ^{32}P-ATP (3000 Ci/mmol, 10 mCi/mL) (cat. no. NEG002A; New England Nuclear).
12. T4 polynucleotide kinase and 10X buffer (cat. no. 174645; Applied Biosystems).
13. Bovine serum albumin (BSA) (cat. no. A-3059; Sigma, St. Louis, MO).
14. Telomerase-positive control cells (SK-N-SH neuroblastoma; a cell line was established by the Memorial Sloan-Kettering Cancer Center [MSKCC]).
15. Primers:
    a. Telomerase substrate (TS) primer (5′-AATCCGTCGAGCAGAGTT-3′, high-performance liquid chromatography (HPLC) purified, 1 μg/μL).
    b. Reverse primer (RP) (5′-GCGCGG[CTTACC]₃CTAACC-3′, HPLC purified, 0.1 μg/μL).
    c. Internal control (NT) primer (5′-ATCGCTTCTCGGCCTTTT-3′, HPLC purified, 0.1 μg/μL).
    d. Telomerase substrate internal control (TSNT) primer (5′-AATCCGTCGAGC AGAGTTAAAAGGCCGAGAAGCGAT-3′, HPLC purified, 0.01 amol/μL).
16. R8 quantitation standard (5′-AATCCGTCGAGCAGAGTTAG[GGTTAG]₇-3′, HPLC purified, 0.1 amol/μL).
17. Acrylic Work Station (cat. no. 3045-5000; USA Scientific).
18. Brem Shield (cat. nos. BR-202 and BR-008; Research Products).
19. T3 thermocycler (Biometra).
20. Adjustable water bath (VWR).
21. Polyacrylamide vertical gel electrophoresis apparatus (Protean II XiCell; Bio-Rad).
22. Power supply (Buchler 3-1500).
23. Tubes (0.5 mL) for PCR amplification (part no. N801-0180; Applied Biosystems).
24. Aerosol-resistant pipet tips (RNase free).
25. Gel dryer (Bio-Rad model 583).
26. Fuji Imaging Plate (Fujifilm, Type BAS-IIIs).
27. PhosphorImager (Fujifilm Bio-Imager analyzer, model BAS-2500).
28. Spectrophotometer (Thermo Spectronic, Genesys 5).

2.2. Determination of Telomere Length by Southern Blot Analysis

1. Telo TAGGG Telomere Length Assay Kit (cat. no. 2209136; Roche).
2. 50X TAE buffer (cat. no. BP1332-1; Fisher).
3. DNase-free RNase (cat. no. 1119915; Roche).
4. 10% Sodium dodecyl sulfate (SDS): Dissolve 100 g of electrophoresis-grade SDS (cat. no. 5525-017; Invitrogen) in 900 mL of H_2O. Heat to 68°C to assist dissolution. Adjust the pH to 7.2 by adding a few drops of concentrated HCl. Adjust the volume to 1 L with H_2O. Dispense into aliquots. Wear a mask when weighing SDS.

5. 20X Saline sodium citrate (SSC): Dissolve 175.3 g of NaCl and 88.2 g of sodium citrate in 800 mL of H_2O. Adjust the pH to 7.0, and then adjust the volume to 1 L with H_2O. After dispensing into aliquots, sterilize by autoclaving.

6. 3 M NaCl: Dissolve 175.32 g of NaCl in 800 mL of H_2O. Adjust the volume to 1 L with H_2O. Dispense into aliquots and sterilize by autoclaving.

7. 10 M NaOH: Dissolve 400.1 g of NaOH in 800 mL of H_2O. Adjust the volume to 1 L with H_2O. Dispense into aliquots.

8. 1 M Tris, pH 7.5: Dissolve 121.1 g of Tris base in 800 mL of H_2O and add about 60 mL of concentrated HCl. Allow the solution to cool to room temperature before adjusting the final pH to 7.5. Adjust the volume of solution to 1 L with H_2O. Dispense into aliquots and sterilize by autoclaving.

9. Denaturing solution: Mix 500 mL of 3 M NaCl and 50 mL of 10 M NaOH. Adjust the volume of the solution to 1 L with H_2O.

10. Neutralization solution: Mix 500 mL of 3 M NaCl and 500 mL of 1 M Tris. Adjust the volume of the solution to 1 L with H_2O.

11. 2X SSC, 0.1% SDS solution: Mix 100 mL of 20X SSC and 10 mL of 10% SDS. Adjust the volume of the solution to 1 L with H_2O.

12. 0.2X SSC, 0.1% SDS solution: Mix 10 mL of 20X SSC and 10 mL of 10% SDS. Adjust the volume of the solution to 1 L with H_2O.

13. Agarose (cat. no. 5510-027; Invitrogen).

14. Nylon membrane, positively charged (cat. no. 1417240; Roche).

15. Autography film (cat. no. XAR ALF 2025; Lab Scientific).

16. Hybridization bag (item no. 502; Kapak).

17. Microcentrifuge (Costar model 10).

18. Electrophoresis power supply (Bio-Rad model 250/2.5).

19. Ultraviolet (UV) crosslinker (UV Stratalinker 2400; Stratagene).

20. Orbital shaker (Lab-Line model no. 4626).

21. Hybridization oven (Robbins model 400).

22. Hybridization bottle (cat. no. 308-8; Lab-Line).

23. Hybridization mesh (cat. no. J2-2017; Marsh Bio Products).

24. Film scanner (Linotype-Hell, Ultra).

25. Medical film processor (Konica Medical model SRX-101).

26. Data analysis software, such as MacBase V2.5 (Fuji, Stamford, CT) or Lumi-Analyst (Roche).

3. Methods

3.1. Determination of Telomerase Activity by TRAP Assay (see Note 1)

3.1.1. Preparation of Protein Extract

1. Harvest and wash the cells with PBS (Ca^{++}, Mg^{++} free) twice. Pellet the cells at 850g for 6 min and aspirate all PBS carefully. When frozen material is thawed for extraction, the cells or tissue should be resuspended immediately in 1X CHAPS lysis buffer.

2. Resuspend the cell pellet in 200 μL of 1X CHAPS lysis buffer per 10^5–10^6 cells by vortexing briefly. If using tumor tissue, RNase inhibitor should be added to lysis buffer for a final concentration of 100–200 U/mL.
3. Incubate the suspension on ice for 30 min.
4. Spin the extract in a microcentrifuge at 12,000g for 20 min at 4°C.
5. Transfer about 160 μL of the supernatant into a fresh tube (or aliquot the supernatant into a small volume of tubes). Use one sample to determine the protein concentration.
6. Quick freeze the cell extract and store at –80°C. Do not freeze and thaw the extract more than three times. Under these conditions, the telomerase activity of the extract will be stable for at least 12 mo (*see* **Notes 2** and **3**).
7. Evaluate the samples by Western blot and Coomassie blue staining to exclude the degradation of protein.

3.1.2. Determination of Protein Concentration

1. Dilute Bio-Rad protein assay solution 1:5 with distilled water.
2. Prepare five dilutions of BSA, 0.2–1 mg/mL in CHAPS lysis buffer for a standard curve.
3. Add 2 μL of standard or extract to a disposable cuvet containing 1 mL of the diluted protein assay solution and mix by vortexing briefly. The sample volume can be scaled up using a ratio of 1:500, sample:diluted protein assay solution.
4. Prepare a sample blank by adding 2 μL of CHAPS lysis buffer to 1 mL of diluted protein assay solution.
5. Measure the absorbance of standards and extracts on a spectrophotometer at a wavelength of 595 nm and from a standard curve determine the protein concentration of the extracts. If the protein concentration of any sample is >1 mg/mL (outside the liner range of standard BSA), dilute the extract 1:5 with CHAPS lysis buffer and remeasure the protein concentration. The typical protein range for cell extracts is 10–750 ng/mL.
6. Dilute the samples down to 0.5 μg/μL with CHAPS lysis buffer.
7. Store at –80°C until assayed.

3.1.3. End Labeling of TS Primer With γ^{32}P-ATP (see **Note 4**)

For this protocol, be sure to work behind a beta shield.

1. Take standard precautions when working with ^{32}P. Mix the following reagents (for 22 assays) in a 1.5-mL centrifuge tube: 5.5 μL of γ^{32}P-ATP (3000 Ci/mmol, 10 μci/μL)
2. 2.2 μL of TS primer (1 μg/μL), 2.2 μL of 10X polynucleotide kinase buffer, 1.1 μL of T4 polynucleotide kinase (10 U/μL), and 11 μL of diethylpyrocarbonate (DEPC)-treated water for a total of 22 μL.
3. Incubate in a water bath at 37°C for 30 min in lead pig.

Table 1
Reagants for Master Mix

Reagent	1 Reaction (μL)	22 Reactions (μL)
10X TRAP buffer	5.0	110
RP primer (0.1 μg/μL)	1.0	22
NT primer (0.1 μg/μL)	1.0	22
TSU2 primer (0.05 μg/μL)	1.0	22
^{32}P-TS primer	1.0	22
2.5 mM dNTPs	1.0	22
DEPC-treated water	37.6	827.2
Taq Polymerase	0.4	8.8
Total	48	1056

4. Heat inactivate the polynucleotide kinase at 85°C for 5 min.
5. Store at –20°C in an acrylic box.

3.1.4. PCR Reaction

For this protocol, be sure to work behind a beta shield.

1. Thaw the reagents in **Table 1** and store on ice to prepare a "master mix."
2. Determine the number of assays to be run by adding the number of samples to the three controls (*see* **step 4**), and multiply each reagent in **Table 1** by that amount to determine the total volume of "master mix" for the run.
3. Aliquot 1 μg of protein of each sample (2 μL of 0.5 μg/μL protein) into a fresh 0.5-mL PCR tube. Add no more than 2 μL of protein extract (*see* **Note 5**).
4. Prepare the following controls (*see* **Note 6**):
    a. CHAPS negative control: 2 μL of CHAPS.
    b. Heat-inactivated control: 2 μL of sample extract (heated at 85°C for 10 min).
    c. R8 quantitation control: 2 μL of 0.5 amol/μL.
5. Mix the master mix thoroughly with a pipettor and aliquot 48 μL to each sample and the controls.
6. Quick spin the PCR tubes in a microcentrifuge to get the reaction mix to the bottom of the tube and to remove any bubbles.
7. Place the tubes in a thermocycler and run the following program: 1 cycle at 30°C for 30 min; 1 cycle at 94°C for 2 min; 30 cycles at 94°C for 30 s, 60°C for 30 s, and 72°C for 30 s; 1 cycle at 72°C for 5 min; and hold at 4°C. Add one drop of mineral oil if not using a thermocycler with a heated lid.

3.1.5. Polyacrylamide Gel Electrophoresis

3.1.5.1. 12.5% POLYACRYLAMIDE GEL

1. Assemble the electrophoresis casting chamber and prepare the following mix: 17.8 mL of sterile H_2O, 1.8 mL of 10X TBE, 10 mL of 30% Polyacrylamide-Bis

Solution (Bio-Rad), 400 μL of 10% ammonium persulfate (prepare weekly), and 45 μL TEMED for a total of 30 mL.
2. Mix well and quickly add to the casting chamber, taking care to prevent any bubbles.
3. Place a 20-well comb, again dispersing any bubbles, and let the gel polymerize for approx 1 h.
4. Remove the comb from the gel and wash with 0.5X TBE running buffer using a syringe with needle.

3.1.5.2. LOADING POLYACRYLAMIDE GEL

For this protocol, be sure to work behind a beta shield.

1. Add 7.5 μL of 6X loading dye to each amplified PCR reaction tube. Mix a few times and carefully load 25 μL of dye plus sample to the gel. Take every precaution not to carry over samples between adjacent wells because this can result in false positive bands. Load the R8 quantitation control in the last lanes of the gel.
2. Run the gel at 100 V for 20 min, and then at 150 V until the purple bromophenol blue band just runs off the gel. The blue xylene cyanol band should be about two-thirds of the way down the gel. At this point, the internal control band (36 bp) usually runs just above the xylene cyanol, and the smallest telomerase product is 50 bp.

3.1.5.3. DRYING POLYACRYLAMIDE GEL

For this protocol, be sure to work behind a beta shield.

1. Cut a piece of Whatman 3MM filter paper approximately the same size of the gel and wet with distilled water.
2. Disassemble the electrophoresis apparatus, remove one glass plate and spacers from the gel, and place filter paper onto the exposed face of the gel. Flip the gel over and lift off the second glass plate.
3. Place the gel filter paper side down on a gel dryer and cover with plastic wrap. Dry at 80°C for approx 1 h.
4. After shutting off the vacuum, very slowly lift the cover seal to break the vacuum so that the gel does not shatter.
5. Remove the gel with filter paper and plastic wrap, and place in an autoradiography cassette with the gel side up.

3.1.6. Gel Exposure

For this protocol, be sure to work behind a beta shield.

1. Place a Fuji Imaging Plate with the white exposure side facing down over the dried gel.
2. Expose the plate an adequate time (*see* **Note 7**).

3.1.7. Imaging

1. Remove the exposed plate and immediately place in a protective sleeve. Both moisture and light can affect the quality of the exposure.
2. Scan the plate in a Phosphor-Imager. A dynamic range of L5–4000 is sufficient.

3.1.8. Quantification of Telomerase Activity

1. Use MacBAS v2.5 or IQMAC V1.2 software for both quantification and labeling of samples.
2. Determine the signal from the internal standard 36-bp band by drawing a rectangle around the band and duplicating the box for each internal standard band for all samples and controls. Do the same for the telomerase product ladder beginning at 50 bp and increasing in size 6 bp apart.
3. Define the total product generated (TPG) as follows:

$$TPG = \frac{\text{(sample telomerase product} - \text{CHAPS control)} / \text{(sample internal control)}}{\text{(R8 standard product} - \text{CHAPS control)} / \text{(R8 internal control)}} \times 100$$

3.2. Measurement of Telomere Length by Terminal Restriction Fragment Assay

3.2.1. Extraction of High Molecular Genomic DNA (see **Note 13**)

3.2.2. Analysis of Genomic DNA for Degradation (see **Note 14**)

1. Combine the following reagents: 0.5 µg of undigested DNA, 1 µL (5 U/µL) of DNase-free RNase, and water to 10 µL. Incubate in a 37°C water bath for 15 min to allow the RNase to digest, and then add 2 µL of load dye.
2. Set up premade 1X TAE 1% agarose gel containing 0.5 µg/mL of ethidium bromide (EtBr), place the gel in an electrophoresis chamber, cover with 1X TAE, and shake to dislodge any bubbles from the wells.
3. Load the total sample volume onto the gel, and include an *Hind*III DNA ladder in a separate well as the marker (usually add 1 µg/lane).
4. Run the gel at approx 75 V for 1 h.
5. View under a UV light to examine the DNA quality. Make a video print to document.

3.2.3. Digestion of Genomic DNA With RsaI and HinfI Enzymes

1. Calculate the appropriate amount of DNA (*see* **Note 15**) to digest for each sample (usually 2 µg). Then add each component (we used a high amount of enzyme to allow a short period of digestion as follows: 2 µL of 10X restriction enzyme buffer, 0.5 µL of 40 U/µL of *Hinf*I, 0.5 µL of 40 U/µL of *Rsa*I, 17 µL of DNA (2 µg) in H$_2$O to a total of 20 µL.
2. Add all the components and mix gently. Centrifuge briefly to collect all of the sample at the bottom of the tube and place in a 37°C water bath for 2.5 h.

3. To stop the reaction, add 4 µL of gel electrophoresis loading buffer (bottle 8 in the kit) and quick spin the vials.

3.2.4. TRF Length Gel and Southern Transfer

1. Make a 0.8% agarose gel in 1X TAE by adding 1.2 g of agarose to 150 mL of 1X TAE, and bring to a boil to dissolve the agarose.
2. Use a 12 × 14 cm gel frame so that the path length of DNA is 14 cm. Tighten both ends of the gel frame securely to ensure that there is no leakage of hot gel mix.
3. Cool the gel to 60–80°C, add 7.5 µL of 10 mg/mL EtBr to the gel mix, and pour into the prepared frame. The depth of the gel should be 0.5–1 cm. Put the appropriate comb in the gel (20 wells). When the gel is solid (after about 60 min), remove the gel tub and place the whole frame in the chamber. Cover with 1X TAE and remove the comb just before loading the samples.
4. Prepare a Dig-labeled molecular weight marker (MWM, bottle 7) mixture by adding 4 µL of Dig-MWM, 12 µL of DEPC-treated water, and 4 µL of loading dye; incubate for 10 min at 65°C; and quick spin the vial.
5. Load 2 µg/lane of digested DNA samples including control DNA high and control DNA low (make sure there are no bubbles in the sample), and load 10 µL of Dig-MWM mixture on either side of the respective samples.
6. Run the gel at 5 V/cm (*see* **Note 16**) in 1X TAE buffer until the bromophenol blue tracking dye is separated about 12 cm from the starting wells (total run time is about 5 to 6 h).
7. Take a picture of the gel under a UV light.
8. Submerge the gel in 0.25 *M* HCl for 5–10 min for acid depurination with gentle agitation at room temperature.
9. Rinse the gel two times with deionized H_2O.
10. Submerge the gel in denaturation solution (1.5 *M* NaCl; 0.5 *M* NaOH) two times for 15 min each at room temperature.
11. Wash off the gel two times with deionized H_2O.
12. Neutralize the gel with neutralization solution (1.5 *M* NaCl; 0.5 *M* Tris-HCl, pH 7.5) two times for 15 min each at room temperature.
13. Soak the gel in transfer buffer (10X SSC) for 10 min at room temperature with gentle agitation.
14. Conduct capillary transfer using buffer (10X SSC) overnight. Prior to transfer, float the membrane in deionized H_2O to wet thoroughly, and then soak in 10X SSC transfer buffer for 5 min.
15. Fix the transferred DNA on the membrane by UV crosslinking or by baking at 80°C for 1 h (*see* **Note 17**).
16. Wash the membrane with 2X SSC for 5 min to remove bits of gel or particles from the membrane. Then proceed to prehybridization or air-dry the membrane and store at 2–8°C.

3.2.5. Hybridization and Detection of Chemiluminescence

1. Aliquot hybridization solution (Dig Easy Hyb, bottle 7 in the kit) to 15-mL Falcon tubes (10 mL/each), and prewarm 10 mL of Dig Easy Hyb to 42°C in a water bath.
2. Prepare a middle-size hybridization glass bottle. Turn on the oven and set the temperature at 42°C.
3. Prewet a piece of mesh and nylon membrane in a buffer of 2X SSC in a tub.
4. Lay the membrane on a piece of mesh and roll up; then put it into the hybridization bottle.
5. Add 10–15 mL of prewarmed, Dig Easy Hyb solution (without adding telomere probe) to the prehybridization bottle.
6. Roll the bottle for 60 min of prehybridization.
7. Prepare the hybridization solution by adding 1 µL of telomere probe (bottle 10 in the kit)/5 mL of fresh, prewarmed Dig Easy Hyb solution and mix. We use 10–12 mL of solution for each hybridization (*see* **Notes 18** and **19**).
8. Discard the prehybridization solution completely, and immediately add hybridization solution to the bottle enclosed with the membrane.
9. Place the bottle back in the oven and rotate at 42°C for 3 h.
10. Discard the hybridization solution.
11. Wash the membrane two times with sufficient 2X SSC, 0.1% SDS solution for 5 min at room temperature with gentle agitation.
12. Wash the membrane two times with sufficient prewarmed 0.2X SSC, 0.1% SDS solution for 15 min at 50°C with gentle agitation.
13. Rinse the membrane in at least 100 mL of washing buffer (1X solution 10 in the kit) for 1–5 min at room temperature with gentle agitation.
14. Incubate the membrane in 20 mL of freshly prepared blocking solution (1X solution 11 in the kit) for 30 min at room temperature with gentle agitation.
15. Prepare Anti-Dig-AP working solution (centrifuge at 15,000g for 5 min before use) by adding 2 µL of Anti-Dig-AP antibody to 20 mL of freshly made blocking solution.
16. Discard the blocking solution, and incubate the membrane in 20 mL of Anti-Dig-AP working solution for 30 min at room temperature with gentle agitation.
17. Wash the membrane two times for 15 min with 200 mL of washing buffer (1X solution 10 in the kit) at room temperature with gentle agitation.
18. Incubate the membrane in 100 mL of detection buffer (1X solution 14 in the kit) for 2–5 min at room temperature with gentle agitation.
19. Discard the detection buffer and pour off excess liquid by placing the membrane DNA side up on a sheet of 3M paper. Do not let the membrane dry.
20. Immediately place the wet membrane with the DNA side facing up on an opened hybridization bag, and very quickly apply approx 20 drops of substrate solution to the membrane.
21. Immediately cover the membrane with the second sheet of the bag to spread the substrate solution homogeneously without air bubbles over the membrane.
22. Incubate the membrane for 5 min at room temperature.

23. Squeeze out excess substrate solution and seal the bag.
24. Put the blot in a cassette. Expose to X-ray film for 1–5 min in a dark room (*see* **Note 20**).
25. Develop the film.

3.2.6. Telomere Smear Analysis (see **Note 21**)

1. Scan the exposed X-ray film with a scanner.
2. Overlay each sample lane of the scanned image with a grid (we use MacBAS v2.5 software to do the analysis). The vertical size of the individual squares of the grid defines the resolution in determining the TRF length. Typically, ≥25 squares/lane is recommended.
3. For background subtraction, select several boxes in each lane in which no telomere-specific signal is found and that are representative of the background of the corresponding lane. Signals of these boxes should be averaged and substrated from each grid box.
4. For each square, determine the signal *(ODi)* and the corresponding length *(Li)*, in which *ODi* is the total signal intensity within the grid box and *Li* is the molecular weight at the midpoint of the corresponding box.
5. Calculate the mean TRF length using the formula TRF = $\sum(ODi)/\sum(ODi/Li)$.

4. Notes

1. The most important consideration for performing the telomerase activity assay is the environment where the initial reaction mixtures are set up. An area free of contaminating ribonucleases and amplified PCR DNA products is a must for the assay. The ideal setup utilizes separate rooms (or, at a minimum, separate areas) for the extraction, PCR setup, and PCR amplification. It is essential that no PCR products enter the area designated for extraction or for PCR setup. Gloves should be changed as often as possible to prevent carryover, especially after handling the R8 quantitation control.
2. The cell or tissue pellet should be stored at –80°C. The telomerase in frozen cells or tissues is stable for at least 1 yr.
3. The extracts for the TRAP assay should be quick frozen in liquid nitrogen or on dry ice after each use. Aliquots should not be freeze thawed more than three times, to avoid loss of telomerase activity. Additionally, aliquoting reduces the risk of contamination.
4. Standard precautions regarding radioisotope use should be strictly followed.
5. We usually use 1 µg of protein cell extract and 0.1 µg of protein tissue extract for the telomerase activity assay.
6. The controls for telomerase activity assay should include a heat-inactivated control for each sample run on the gel adjacent to the sample, a positive telomerase extract control (we used the neuroblastoma cell line SK-N-SH that was established at Memorial Sloan-Kettering Cancer Center [MSKCC]), PCR amplification control

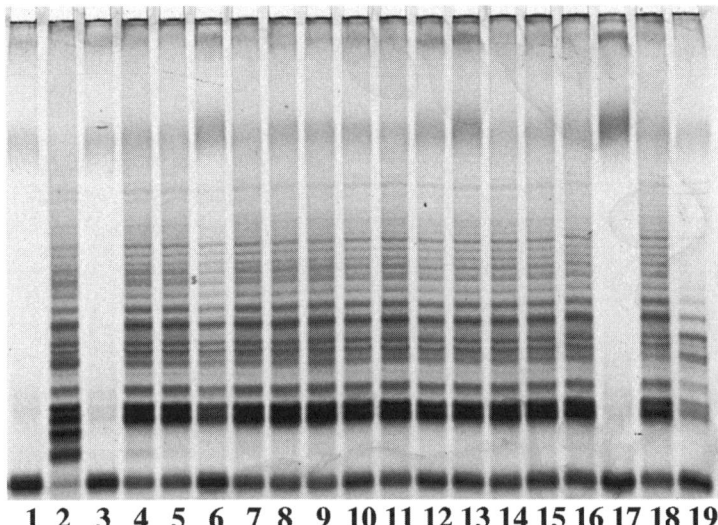

Fig. 2. Representative TRAP assay. Lane 1, PCR control (CHAPS buffer); lane 2, positive telomerase control (SK-N-SH neuroblastoma cells, 1 µg/lane); lane 3, heat inactivation control; lanes 4–17, experimental samples; lane 18, positive telomerase control (SK-N-SH neuroblastoma cells, 0.1 µg/lane); lane 19, telomerase quantitation control TSR8.

(36-bp internal standard), a primer-dimer/PCR contamination control (CHAPS buffer); and a telomerase quantitation control template-TSR8.

7. Exposure time depends on the age of the isotope. Generally, follow these guidelines: 1 wk (20–30 min), 2 wk (45 min), 3 to 4 wk (1+ h). These are only suggestions, but we have found that it is better to overexpose than underexpose.

8. For a valid TRAP assay, the following conditions should be met: For the primer/dimer/PCR contamination control lane, no product should be visible except the 36-bp internal control band; for the telomerase-positive control lane, no product should be visible except the 36-bp internal control band and a ladder of products at 6-bp increments starting at 50 bp (i.e., 50, 56, 62, 68, and so on); for the heat-treated sample extract lane, no product should be visible except the 36-bp internal control band (**Fig. 2**).

9. When the cell/tissue extract contains an inhibitor of *Taq* polymerase, few or no TRAP ladder bands are visible in the sample lanes, and the internal standard band (36 bp) in these lanes shows reduced intensity or disappearance. To solve the problem, dilute the extract 10-, 100-, and 1000-fold with 1X CHAPS lysis buffer and then reanalyze. In most cases, positive telomerase activity that cannot be detected in more concentrated extracts can be detected in the diluted extract.

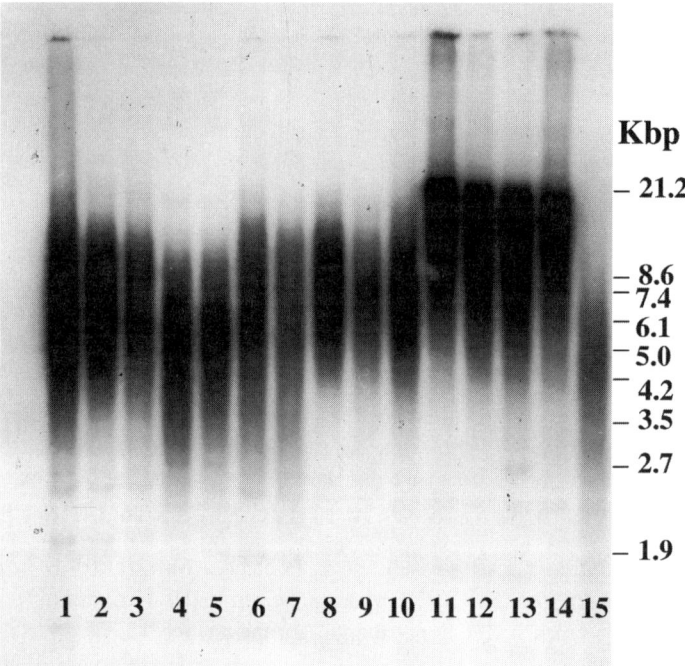

Fig. 3. Representative TRF assay on CD138⁺ PCs patients with MM and healthy donors. Telomere length was measured by Southern blot terminal restriction fragment analysis. Lanes 1–7, marrow myeloma cell from MM; lanes 8–10, peripheral blood granulocytes from MM; lanes 11–14, marrow PCs from healthy donors; lane 15, telomere standard; Kbp = kilobase pair DNA marker.

10. It is often observed that bands are present between the internal standard band (36 bp) and the first (50 bp) of the TRAP ladder bands. The potential problem is that telomerase activity in the sample extracts is too high. We either dilute the sample extracts (1:10) and reanalyze or ignore the extra band because it does not affect overall detection of telomerase activity.

11. There are two major methods for measuring the telomere length: terminal restriction fragment by Southern blot analysis and quantitative fluorescence *in situ* hybridization using either digital fluorescence microscopy (Q-FISH) or flow cytometry (flow-FISH). Southern blotting still serves as a "gold standard" for measurement of telomere length *(15–18)*, which, although relatively cumbersome, is accurate and reproducible. Compared with traditional TRF assay requiring a large amount of DNA (5 μg) and radioactive material and lasting 7 d, the modified protocol described previously does not use radioactive material, has a process time of about 2 d, and requires only a small amount of DNA (1 to 2 μg) to perform the assay (**Fig. 3**). Several other improvements to the Southern blot technique, such as pulse-field electrophoresis, slot blot, and centromere-to-telomere ratio measurement, have been

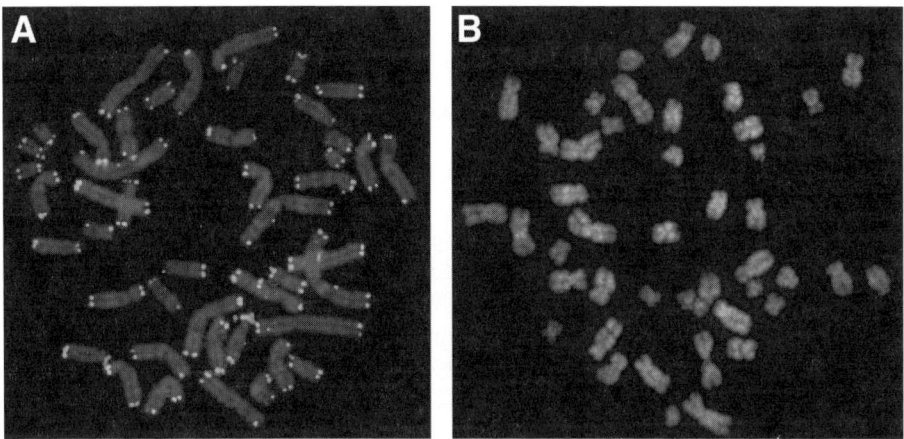

Fig. 4. Q-FISH assay. (**A**) Normal peripheral blood mononuclear cells and (**B**) SKO-007 myeloma cell telomeres were visualized using FITC-labeled peptide nucleic acid $(CCCTAA)_3$ telomere probe.

proposed *(19–21)*. However, each of these refinements to the Southern blot method increases rather than decreases the complexity of the assay. Q-FISH has specific limitations and is time-consuming (**Fig. 4**), whereas the flow-FISH technique using FISH with fluorescein isothiocyanate (FITC)–labeled peptide nucleic acid probes to measure the telomere length in interphase cells requires relatively few cells (10^5) and can be completed in a single day. A further advantage of the flow-FISH method is that data on the telomere length from individual cells and subsets of cells can be acquired from the same sample *(22)*. However, flow-FISH still has its disadvantages, such as large variation, poor reproducibility, and presence of T2AG3 repeat sequences in interstitial or centromeric sites, which limit its application *(23)*.

12. It is important to emphasize that the entire assay procedure must be performed under nuclease-free conditions: using only autoclaved, redistilled water; preparing appropriate aliquots of the kit solutions and keeping them separate from other reagents in the laboratory; using autoclaved or heat-sterilized labware as well as wearing gloves while performing the assay.

13. The method chosen for genomic DNA extraction and purification should give maximum recoveries of high molecular weight DNA with a low shearing protocol, such as by using a Nucleon DNA extraction and purification kit (cat. no. RPN 8502; Amersham).

14. Degradation of genomic DNA can significantly influence the TRF result. Therefore, it is important to run a DNA degradation gel assay for each sample to check the quality of DNA, especially when working on frozen samples with long-term cryopreserved specimens.

15. To obtain valid quantitative analysis of the telomere length, each sample should contain the same amount of DNA.

16. To guarantee a better resolution of the digested DNA, the voltage of electrophoresis must be <5 V/cm gel.
17. Fixing the transferred DNA on the wet blotting membrane by UV crosslinking is better than the baking method because the latter always gives a higher background.
18. Sufficient prehybridization and hybridization solution is necessary to keep a low blot background.
19. It is critical to control the amount of telomere probe and Anti-Dig-AP antibody so that they do not exceed the protocol's recommendation.
20. To obtain a reliable signal on the film, always acquire several films with different exposure times to obtain a satisfactory image.
21. The normal variation in this assay is approx 1% for identical samples within a single gel, and approx 2% between gels in the range of 3–14 kbp of telomere length.

Acknowledgments

We thank Sheik Baksh for critical reading and modification of the TRAP protocol, Gouri Nanjangud for providing excellent Q-FISH images, and Kate deBeer for helping in the preparation of the manuscript.

References

1. Lansdorp, P. M., Verwoerd, N. P., van de Rijke, F. M., et al. (1996) Heterogeneity in telomere length of human chromosomes. *Hum. Mol. Genet.* **5,** 685–691.
2. Sandell, L. L. and Zakian, V. A. (1993) Loss of a yeast telomere: arrest, recovery, and chromosome loss. *Cell* **75,** 729–739.
3. Kirk, K. E., Harmon, B. P., Reichardt, I. K., Sedat, J. W., and Blackburn, E. H. (1997) Block in anaphase chromosome separation caused by a telomerase template mutation. *Science* **275,** 1478–1481.
4. Watson, J. D. (1972) Origin of concatemeric T7 DNA. *Nat. N. Biol.* **239,** 197–201.
5. Collins, K. and Mitchell, J. R. (2002) Telomerase in the human organism. *Oncogene* **21,** 564–579.
6. Harley, C. B. (2002) Telomerase is not an oncogene. *Oncogene* **21,** 494–502.
7. MacKenzie, K. L., Franco, S., Naiyer, A. J., et al. (2002) Multiple stages of malignant transformation of human endothelial cells modelled by co-expression of telomerase reverse transcriptase, SV40 T antigen and oncogenic N-ras. *Oncogene* **21,** 4200–4211.
8. Wu, K. D., Orme, L. M., Shaughnessy, J., Jr., Jacobson, J., Barlogie, B., and Moore, M.A. (2003) Telomerase and telomere length in multiple myeloma: correlations with disease heterogeneity, cytogenetic status, and overall survival. *Blood* **101,** 4982–4989.
9. Xu, D., Zheng, C., Bergenbrant, S., et al. (2001) Telomerase activity in plasma cell dyscrasias. *Br. J. Cancer* **84,** 621–625.
10. Shiratsuchi, M., Muta, K., Abe, Y., et al. (2002) Clinical significance of telomerase activity in multiple myeloma. *Cancer* **94,** 2232–2238.

11. Wang, E. S., Wu, K., Chin, A. C., et al. (2004) Telomerase inhibition with an oligonucleotide telomerase template antagonist: in vitro and in vivo studies in multiple myeloma and lymphoma. *Blood* **103,** 258–266.

12. Akiyama, M., Hideshima, T., Shammas, M. A., et al. (2003) Effects of oligonucleotide N3′→P5′ thio-phosphoramidate (GRN163) targeting telomerase RNA in human multiple myeloma cells. *Cancer Res.* **63,** 6187–6194.

13. Kim, N. W., Piatyszek, M. A., Prowse, K. R., et al. (1994) Specific association of human telomerase activity with immortal cells and cancer. *Science* **266,** 2011–2015.

14. Wright, W. E., Shay, J. W., and Piatyszek, M. A. (1995) Modifications of a telomeric repeat amplification protocol (TRAP) result in increased reliability, linearity and sensitivity. *Nucleic Acids Res.* **23,** 3794–3795.

15. Allsopp, R. C., Vaziri, H., Patterson, C., et al. (1992) Telomere length predicts replicative capacity of human fibroblasts. *Proc. Natl. Acad. Sci. USA* **89,** 10,114–10,118.

16. Allshire, R. C., Dempster, M., and Hastie, N. D. (1989) Human telomeres contain at least three types of G-rich repeats distributed non-randomly. *Nucleic Acids Res.* **17,** 4611–4627.

17. Harley, C., Futcher. A., and Greider., C. (1990) Telomeres shorten during ageing of human fibroblasts. *Nature* **345,** 458–460.

18. de Lange, T., Shiue, L., Myers, R. M., et al. (1990) Structure and variability of human chromosome ends. *Mol. Cell Biol.* **10,** 518–527.

19. Feng, Y. R., Biggar, R. J., Gee, D., Norwood, D., Zeichner, S. L., and Dimitrov, D. S. (1999) Long-term telomere dynamics: modest increase of cell turnover in HIV-infected individuals followed for up to 14 years. *Pathobiology* **67,** 34–38.

20. Norwood, D. and Dimitrov, D. S. (1998) Sensitive method for measuring telomere lengths by quantifying telomeric DNA content of whole cells. *Biotechniques* **25,** 1040–1045.

21. Rufer, N., Dragowska, W., Thornbury, G., Roosnek, E., and Lansdorp, P. M. (1998) Telomere length dynamics in human lymphocyte subpopulations measured by flow cytometry. *Nat. Biotechnol.* **16,** 743–747.

22. Baerlocher, G. M., Mak, J., Tien, T., and Lansdorp, P. M. (2002) Telomere length measurement by fluorescence in situ hybridization and flow cytometry: tips and pitfalls. *Cytometry* **47,** 89–99.

23. Lauzon, W., Dardon, S. J., Cameron, D. W., and Badley, A. D. (2000) Flow cytometric measurement of telomere length. *Cytometry* **42,** 159–164.

17

Dendritic Cell/Myeloma Hybrid Vaccine

Dajing Xia, Tim Chan, and Jim Xiang

Summary

Dendritic cell (DC)–tumor fusion hybrid vaccine that facilitates antigen presentation represents a new, powerful strategy in cancer therapy. We investigated the antitumor immunity derived from vaccination of fusion hybrids between wild-type J558 or engineered J558-IL-4 myeloma cells secreting cytokine interleukin-4 (IL-4) and DCs. The design and methods for generation of mature bone marrow-derived DCs, preparation of DC/J558-IL-4 hybrid, and in vivo animal studies of DC/myeloma hybrid vaccine are described. Our data show that the fusion efficiency was approx 20% by using polyethylene glycol. Our data also show that immunization of C57BL/6 mice with engineered DC/J558-IL-4 hybrids elicited stronger J558 tumor-specific cytotoxic T-lymphocyte responses in vitro and induced more efficient protective immunity against J558 tumor challenge in vivo than DC/J558 hybrid vaccines.

Key Words

Dendritic cells; engineered myeloma cells; interleukin-4; cell fusion; hybrid vaccine; antitumor immunity; polyethylene glycol; bone marrow cells; cell culture.

1. Introduction

Dendritic cells (DCs), one of the most potent antigen-presenting cells, are capable of stimulating both naive CD4[+] helper T (Th)-cells and CD8[+] cytotoxic T-lymphocytes (CTLs) *(1)*. The antigen-presenting capability of DCs makes them attractive vehicles for the delivery of therapeutic cancer vaccines *(2,3)*. DCs pulsed with synthetic tumor-derived major histocompatibility complex (MHC) class I-restricted peptides or tumor lysates have been shown to induce significant CTL-dependent antitumor immune responses in vitro as well as in mice in vivo *(4–6)*. Recently, Labeur et al. *(7)* have demonstrated that the induction of antitumor immunity by DC vaccines is correlated with the maturation stages of DCs. However, these DC vaccine strategies are currently

From: *Methods in Molecular Medicine, Vol. 113: Multiple Myeloma: Methods and Protocols*
Edited by: R. D. Brown and P. J. Ho © Humana Press Inc., Totowa, NJ

limited by their dependence on in vitro antigen loading and the availability of appropriate, defined tumor antigens.

Fusion of two different kinds of cells can generate hybrid cells that presumably have phenotypic characteristics of both of the progenitor cells. In a novel approach to tumor cell-based immunization, Guo et al. *(8)* originally showed that the fusion of activated B-cells to tumor cells produced a potent immunogen capable of inducing tumor-specific immunity. The advantages of this novel approach include its ability to correct defects in costimulatory signaling, provide both MHC class I and II epitopes, and not require the identification of tumor antigens. Recently, Gong et al. *(9,10)* have further demonstrated the induction of antitumor activity by immunization with fusions of granulocyte macrophage colony-stimulating factor (GM-CSF)/interleukin-4 (IL-4)-stimulated peripheral blood mononuclear cell (PBMC)-derived DCs and carcinoma cells. More recently, Kugler et al. *(11)* have shown that 41% of patients responded to hybrid cell vaccine with four complete remissions of metastatic renal cell carcinoma. However, the maturation of GM-CSF/IL-4-stimulated PBMC-derived DCs is not stable and needs to be stabilized in macrophage-conditioned medium *(12)*. Sometimes, these PBMC-derived DCs also display immature phenotypes in a medium containing GM-CSF/IL-4 *(13)*. Therefore, the potential effect of DC maturation stages on the antitumor efficiency of hybrid vaccines should be seriously considered.

The induction of stronger CTL responses has become a major goal of current cancer vaccine strategies. IL-4 is a cytokine that stimulates the differentiation and maturation of DCs *(14,15)*. Vaccines using tumor cells engineered to secrete IL-4 enhanced infiltration of DCs and their indirect antigen presentation; this has been shown to enhance the antitumor immunity mediated by CD8[+] T-cells *(16,17)*. To enhance the potential vaccine efficiency of fusion hybrids, we proposed a novel approach of engineered fusion hybrid DC/J558-IL-4 *(18)* derived from the fusion of DCs with an engineered J558-IL-4 myeloma cell line secreting cytokine IL-4 *(19)*. We assume that the secreted IL-4 will stimulate maturation of fusion hybrids in an autocrine fashion, leading to enhanced tumor antigen presentation and antitumor immunity. In addition, we also investigated the antitumor immunity derived from vaccination of the fusion hybrid in animal studies.

In this chapter, we describe the design and methods for generation of mature bone marrow-derived DCs, preparation of DC/J558-IL-4 hybrid, and in vivo animal studies of DC/myeloma hybrid vaccine. The principle and methods are also applicable to DC hybrids between DCs and other kinds of tumor cells.

2. Materials

1. DC culture medium: Dulbecco's modified essential medium (DMEM) plus 10% fetal calf serum (FCS), GM-CSF (10 ng/mL), and IL-4 (10 ng/mL).

2. Rat anti-mouse CD11c antibody (5 µg/mL) (e.g., BD PharMingen, Mississauga, Ontario, Canada).
3. Fluorescein isothiocyanate (FITC)-conjugated goat anti-rat IgG antibody (1:60) (e.g., Cedarlane Lab, Hornby, Ontario, Canada).
4. DMEM (Gibco, Gaithersburg, MD).
5. GM-CSF (10 ng/mL) (R&D Systems, Minneapolis, MN).
6. J558: This is a poorly immunogenic myeloma cell line of Balb/c (H-2K^d) mouse origin (American Type Culture Collection, Rockville, MD) that is maintained in DMEM plus 10% FCS.
7. J558-IL-4 *(15)*: This cell line was engineered by retroviral infection to secrete IL-4 and is maintained in DMEM plus 10% FCS and G418 (0.5 mg/mL) (Gibco).

3. Methods

3.1. Preparation of Murine Bone Marrow Cells

Although bone marrow cells can be obtained from any of the long bones, the femur and tibia are usually used because they give the best yields.

1. Kill mice by CO_2 inhalation and dip them in 70% ethanol.
2. Place the mice on their backs and make a long transverse incision through the skin in the middle of the abdominal area of each mouse. Retract the skin completely from the hindquarters, including the hind legs.
3. Flood the hind legs with 70% ethanol.
4. While grasping the hind legs with mouse tooth forceps, cut away as much muscle as possible with scissors.
5. Separate the legs from the body at the hip joint and remove the feet. Place the legs in a culture dish containing phosphate-buffered saline (PBS) (*see* **Note 1**).
6. Begin removing the adherent muscle tissue from the femur and tibia by grasping the bones with mouse tooth forceps and scraping them with flat forceps. Transfer the partially cleaned bones to another culture dish containing PBS.
7. Separate the tibia and femur with scissors.
8. Remove the epiphyses with scissors and puncture the bone ends with a 20-gage needle (*see* **Note 2**).
9. Using a syringe with a 25-gage needle attached, expel the marrow by pushing PBS through the center of the bones. Draw the marrow in and out of the needle and syringe to obtain a single-cell suspension.

3.2. Generation of DCs

1. Deplete red blood cells by resuspending bone marrow cell pellets in 10 mL of 0.84% ammonium chloride in a 50-mL tube for bone marrow cells obtained from one mouse.
2. Incubate for 5 min at room temperature.
3. Add 10 mL of PBS to the tube and spin for 10 min at 800*g*.

4. After centrifugation, plate the cells from one bone marrow in a six-well plate with 3 mL of DMEM (Gibco) plus 10% FCS and GM-CSF (10 ng/mL) (R&D Systems) in each well.
5. On d 3, gently remove the nonadherent granulocytes and T- and B-cells, and add DC culture medium (DMEM plus 10% FCS, GM-CSF [10 ng/mL], and IL-4 [10 ng/mL]) (*see* **Note 3**).
6. On d 5, dislodge the loosely adherent proliferating DC aggregates and replate by using DC culture medium.
7. On d 7, harvest the nonadherent DCs and use for in vitro fusion with J558 or J558-IL-4 (*see* **Note 4**).

The mature DCs generated in this manner should display: typical morphological features of DCs (i.e., numerous dendritic processes) and significant expression of MHC class I and II antigens, costimulatory molecules (CD80 and CD86), and adhesion molecules (intercellular adhesion molecular-1, CD11b, CD11c, and CD40).

3.3. Tumor Cell Culture

1. Thaw one vial of frozen low-passage J558 or J558-IL-4 cells in a 37°C water bath.
2. Transfer the cells in a dropwise fashion into a T75 tissue culture flask containing 15 mL of DMEM plus 10% FCS.
3. Maintain the cells at 37°C in an atmosphere of 5% CO_2. For 5 h after incubation, centrifuge the cells at 800g for 10 min and change the medium once to remove any traces of the freezing medium from the cells.
4. Incubate at 37°C for 2 to 3 d (depending on cell density), dilute the mixture in growth medium, and distribute to three flasks for further incubation.
5. When preparing J558 or J558-IL-4 cells in T75 flasks for fusion, use one flask for each fusion. Cells are ready for fusion when they are in the logarithmic phase of growth. Replace the medium with fresh DMEM consisting of 10% FCS 24 h prior to fusion.

3.4. Mice

Female Balb/c (H-2K^d) mice, 6–8 wk old, are obtained from the animal resources center of the University of Saskatchewan and housed in specific pathogen-free conditions of the animal facility at the Saskatoon Cancer Center.

3.5. Preparation of DC/Myeloma Hybrid

3.5.1. Generation of DC/J558-IL-4 Hybrid

DCs derived from bone marrow cell culture are fused with tumor cells at a 6:1 (DC:tumor cell) ratio using polyethylene glycol (PEG) (mol wt = 1450)/dimethyl sulfoxide solution (Sigma, St. Louis, MO). The fusion hybrids between DCs with J558-IL-4 cells and J558 cells are termed DC/J558-IL-4 and DC/J558, respectively.

1. Mix 6×10^6 DCs with 1×10^6 tumor cells and wash with serum-free DMEM.
2. Remove the medium and add 1 mL of PEG to the cell pellet while resuspending the cells by stirring for 2 min.
3. Add an additional 10 mL of DMEM to the cell suspension over the next 3 min with constant stirring (*see* **Note 5**).
4. Centrifuge the cells at 400g for 5 min to remove the PEG, further wash the cells with PBS three times, and then resuspend them in PBS for immunization of mice (*see* **Note 6**).

3.5.2. Evaluation of Fusion Efficiency

To evaluate fusion efficiency, myeloma cells are labeled with the fluorescence dye before being fused with DCs.

1. Resuspend J558-IL-4 or J558 cells in DMEM at 1×10^6 cells/mL, and incubate them with tetramethyl rhodamine (TRITC; Sigma) (0.5 μg/mL) at 37°C for 45 min.
2. Wash the labeled cells with PBS three times, and further stain the fusion preparations with rat anti-mouse CD11c antibody (5 μg/mL) (BD PharMingen) on ice for 30 min.
3. After three washes with PBS, incubate the cells with FITC-conjugated goat anti-rat IgG antibody (1:60) (Cedarlane Lab) on ice for another 30 min.
4. Wash the cells with PBS three times, and then observe the cell suspensions by fluorescence microscopy.

Single tumor cells or DCs are stained with the red fluorescence TRITC and the green fluorescence FITC, respectively, whereas the fused hybrid cells simultaneously display the red TRITC and the green FITC fluorescences in their cytoplasms and on their cell-surface membranes (**Fig. 1**). After randomly picking up 12 high-power fields (×400) for counting fused vs unfused cells in three independent experiments, the fusion efficiency of DC hybrids is estimated to be about 20%.

3.6. DC/Myeloma Hybrid Vaccine

For evaluation of the antitumor efficiency induced by DC/myeloma hybrids, animal studies are conducted to examine whether the immunized mice have immunopreventive effects against the rechallenge of parental J558 tumor cells.

1. Irradiate (8000 rad) DC/J558-IL-4, DC/J558, J558-IL-4, or J558 cells.
2. Inject subcutaneously 1.4×10^6 irradiated DC/J558-IL-4 or DC/J558 fusion hybrid cells into the right thighs of Balb/c mice. For controls, vaccinate mice with 1.4×10^6 irradiated mixed cells (1.2×10^6 DCs and 0.2×10^6 J558-IL-4 cells) or 0.2×10^6 irradiated J558-IL-4 cells or PBS.
3. Ten days later, inject subcutaneously 1×10^6 (high dose) J558 wild-type tumor cells into the left thighs of the immunized mice.

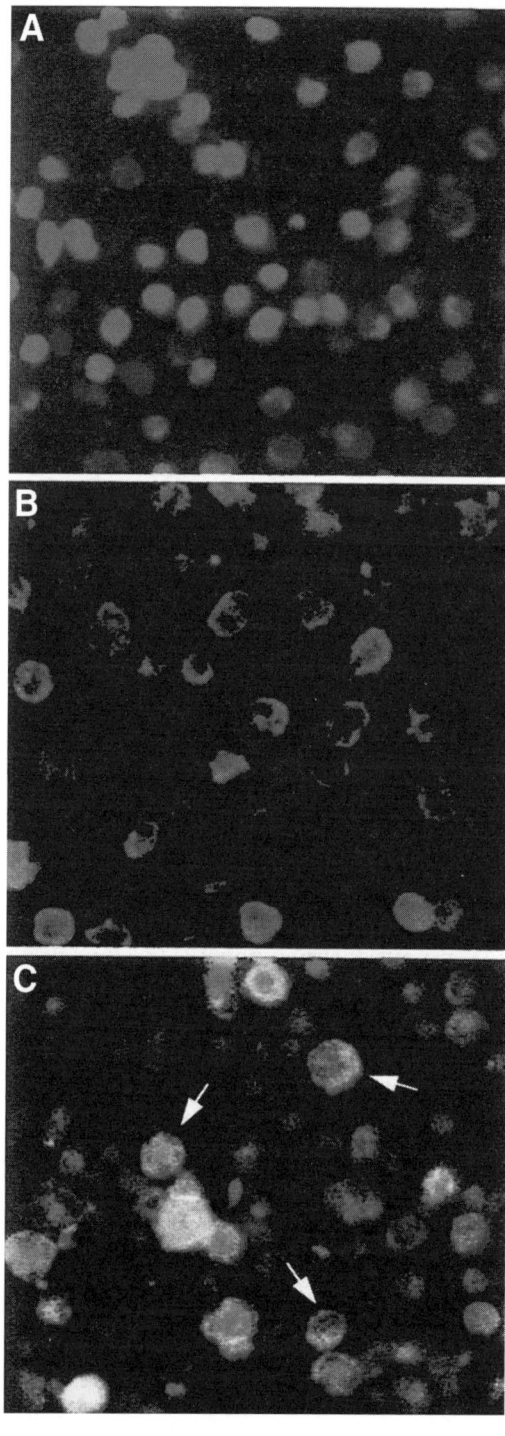

Table 1
Tumor Growth of J558 Myeloma Cells
in Balb/c Vaccinated Mice[a]

Vaccination	Tumor incidence
DC/J558	7/10
DC/J558-IL-4	0/10
DC and J558-IL-4	10/10
J558-IL-4	10/10
PBS	10/10

[a]Mice were subcutaneously vaccinated with 1.4×10^6 irradiated DC/J558-IL-4 or DC/J558 fusion hybrid cells. As controls, mice were vaccinated with 1.4×10^6 irradiated mixed cells (1.2×10^6 DCs and 0.2×10^6 J558-IL-4 cells) or 0.2×10^6 irradiated J558-IL-4 cells or PBS. Ten days after vaccination, mice were subcutaneously injected with 1×10^6 J558 tumor cells and monitored for tumor growth.

4. After tumor inoculation, monitor tumor growth by measuring the length and width of each tumor mass with a caliper every other day for up to 10 wk; for ethical reasons, sacrifice all mice with tumors that achieve a size of 1.5 cm in diameter.

Our data show that vaccination of mice with DC/J558-IL-4 hybrid resulted in more efficient protection (100%) against second challenge of J558 tumor cells than DC/J558 hybrid (30%), a mixture of DC and J558-IL-4 (0%), and J558-IL-4 alone (0%) **(Table 1)**. Our results indicate that an engineered fusion hybrid vaccine of IL-4 gene-modified myeloma and DCs significantly enhanced antitumor immunity.

4. Notes
1. Autoclaved solutions should be used during the whole experimental process to ensure that cells are free of microbial contamination.
2. To obtain enough bone marrow cells, retain the two ends of joints of tibia and femur as much as possible when separating the legs from the body.

Fig. 1. *(see opposite page)* Fluorescence photomicrographs of J558-IL-4 and DC fusion preparations. **(A)** J558-IL-4 cells were stained with TRITC. The TRITC-labeled J558-IL-4 cells were fused with DCs using PEG. **(B)** DCs and **(C)** DC/J558-IL-4 fusion preparation were then stained with rat anti-CD11c antibody followed by goat anti-rat IgG-FITC antibody. Arrows represent the fusion hybrids (DC/J558-IL-4) (magnification: ×400).

3. To generate DCs with high purity, gently wash each well of the plate with cells three times with prewarmed PBS on d 3, so that the majority of the nonadherent granulocytes T- and B-cells are removed.

4. In general, we can obtain 8×10^6 and 12×10^6 DCs from one Balb/c and one C57BL/6 mouse 2–4 mo of age, respectively. DCs will be fewer in mice younger or older than these ages.

5. The fusion between DC and tumor cells is the key step for producing DC/myeloma hybrid. To obtain efficient DC hybrids, add the 1 mL of PEG to the mixed cells drop by drop over 2 min (about one drop every 5 s) while gently resuspending the cells synchronously.

6. To remove completely the PEG after the fusion, centrifuge the fusion samples at 400g for 5 min and then further wash with PBS an additional three times. The speed of the centrifugation must not exceed 400g; otherwise, the DC/myeloma hybrids will be agglomerated.

References

1. Banchereau, J., Briere, F., Caux, C., et al. (2000) Immunobiology of dendritic cells. *Annu. Rev. Immunol.* **18,** 767–811.

2. Bubenik, J. (2001) Genetically engineered dendritic cell-based cancer vaccines. *Int. J. Oncol.* **18,** 475–478.

3. Schreurs, M. W., Eggert, A. A., de Boer, A. J., et al. (2000) Dendritic cells break tolerance and induce protective immunity against a melanocyte differentiation antigen in an autologous melanoma model. *Cancer Res.* **60,** 6995–7001.

4. Mayordomo, J., Zorina, T., Storkus, W., et al. (1995) Bone marrow-derived dendritic cells pulsed with synthetic tumor peptide elicit protective and therapeutic antitumor immunity. *Nat. Med.* **1,** 1297–1302.

5. Asheley, D., Faiola, B., Nair, S., Hale, L., Bigner, D., and Gilbao, E. (1997) Bone marrow–generated dendritic cells pulsed with tumor extracts or tumor RNA induced antitumor immunity against central nervous system tumors. *J. Exp. Med.* **186,** 1177–1182.

6. Nestle, F., Alijagic, S., Gilliet, M., et al. (1998) Vaccination of melanoma patients with peptide- or tumor lysate–pulsed dendritic cells. *Nat. Med.* **4,** 328–332.

7. Labeur, M., Roters, B., Pers, B., et al. (1999) Generation of tumor immunity by bone marrow-derived dendritic cells correlates with dendritic cell maturation stage. *J. Immunol.* **162,** 168–175.

8. Guo, Y., Wu, M., Chen, H., Wang, X., et al. (1994) Effective tumor vaccine generated by fusion of hepatoma cells with activated B cells. *Science* **263,** 518–520.

9. Gong, J., Chen, D., Kashiwaba, M., and Kufe, D. (1997) Induction of antitumor activity by immunization with fusion of dendritic and carcinoma cells. *Nat. Med.* **3,** 558–560.

10. Gong, J., Chen, D., Kashiwaba, M., et al. (1998) Reversal of tolerance to human MUC1 antigen in MUC1 transgenic mice immunized with fusions of dendritic and carcinoma cells. *PNAS* **95,** 6279–6283.

11. Kugler, A., Stuhler, G., Walden, P., et al. (2000) Regression of human metastatic renal cell carcinoma after vaccination with tumor cell-dendritic cell hybrids. *Nat. Med.* **6**, 332–336.
12. Bender, A., Sapp, M., Schuler, G., Steinman, R., and Bhardwaj, N. (1996) Improved methods for the generation of dendritic cells from nonproliferating progenitors in human blood. *J. Immunol. Methods* **196**, 121–135.
13. Caron, G., Delneste, Y., Roelandts, E., et al. (2001) Histamine induces CD86 expression and chemokine production by human immature dendritic cells. *J. Immunol.* **166**, 6000–6006.
14. Lutz, M., Suri, R., Niimi, M., Ogilvie, A., Kukutsch, N., and Robner, S. (2000) Immature dendritic cells generated with low doses of GM-CSF in the absence of IL-4 are maturation resistant and prolong allograft survival in vivo. *Eur. J. Immunol.* **30**, 1813–1820.
15. Jonuleit, H., Knop, J., and Enk, A. (1996) Cytokines and their effects on maturation, differentiation and migration of dendritic cells. *Arch. Demertol. Res.* **289**, 1–8.
16. Stoppacciato, A., Pagilia, P., Lombardi, L., Parmiani, G., Baroni, D., and Colombo, M. (1997) Genetic modification of a carcinoma with IL-4 gene increase the influx of dendritic cells relative to other cytokines. *Eur. J. Immunol.* **27**, 2375–2382.
17. Cayeux, S., Richter, G., Noffz, G., Dorken, B., and Blackenstein, T. (1997) Influence of gene-modified (IL-7, IL-4 and B7) tumor cell vaccines on tumor antigen presentation. *J. Immunol.* **158**, 2834–2841.
18. Liu, Y., Zhang, W., Chan, T., Saxena, A., and Xiang, J. (2002) Engineered fusion hybrid vaccine of IL-4-gene-modified myeloma and relative mature dendritic cells enhances antitumor immunity. *Leukemia Res.* **26**, 757–763.
19. Hock, H., Dorsch, M., Kunzendorf, U., Qin, Z., Diamantstein, T., and Blankenstein, T. (1993) Mechanisms of rejection induced by tumor cell–targeted gene transfer of interleukin 2, interleukin 4, interleukin 7, tumor necrosis factor and interferon gamma. *PNAS* **90**, 2774–2778.

18

Genetically Engineered Myeloma Cell Vaccine

Siguo Hao, Tim Chan, and Jim Xiang

Summary

Tumor cells engineered to express immunogenes have been used for cancer vaccines to induce antitumor immunity and to study the antitumor immune mechanisms derived from immunogene expression. In this chapter, we describe the design and methods for cloning a cDNA gene coding for the mouse CD40L molecule and for construction of the expression vector pcDNA-CD40L, as well as the methods for generation of engineered myeloma cells J558/CD40L expressing CD40 ligand. We also demonstrate that the engineered J558/CD40L tumor cells lose their tumorigenicity in syngeneic mice, and that the inoculation of J558/CD40L tumor cells further leads to protective immunity against wild-type J558 tumors.

Key Words

Genetic engineering; CD40 ligand; gene cloning; reverse transcription polymerase chain reaction; expression vector; myeloma cell line; myeloma vaccine; antitumor immune response.

1. Introduction

A number of different approaches have been developed to generate vaccines against tumors. One of these approaches is based on genetically engineered tumor cells that become immunogenic and thereby efficiently stimulate the generation of tumor-specific immune effector cells. The inoculation of cytokine-secreting engineered tumor cells into syngeneic mice can induce tumor regression, which further leads to long-term protective immunity against a second challenge of the parental tumor cells (1–4). The latter immunity is mostly mediated by the tumor-specific and major histocompatibility complex-restricted CD8[+] cytotoxic T-lymphocytes (1,2). However, cancer immunotherapy employing these engineered tumor cells as vaccines is usually unsuccessful in inducing regression of preestablished tumors when the vaccine is administered in sites anatomically distant to the tumor locations (5).

From: *Methods in Molecular Medicine, Vol. 113: Multiple Myeloma: Methods and Protocols*
Edited by: R. D. Brown and P. J. Ho © Humana Press Inc., Totowa, NJ

It is clear the antigen recognition by itself is not sufficient for activation of T-cell effector functions. Second signals such as the costimulatory molecule B7-1 are also critical for generation of T-cell-mediated immunity. Antigen recognition in the absence of these second signals can lead to tolerance or anergy *(6)*. As such, costimulation plays an important role in antitumor immunity *(7,8)*. The cotransfection of engineered tumor cells with genes coding for cytokines and the costimulatory molecule B7-1 significantly increased their efficiency in stimulation of antitumor immune responses *(9,10)*. However, in some animal models, the failure of B7-1 to induce an antitumor response has been reported *(11,12)*, indicating that other costimulatory signals may also be involved in induction of antitumor immune responses.

Costimulatory function can be attributed to various interactions such as CD40/CD40 ligand (CD40L) *(13–15)* besides the dominant CD28/B7-1 pathway. CD40L is a 33-kDa type II membrane protein, a member of the tumor necrosis factor (TNF) gene family, that is preferentially expressed on activated CD4$^+$ T-cells *(16,17)*. The receptor for CD40L is CD40, a member of the TNF receptor family *(18)*. CD40 is expressed on antigen-presenting cells including dendritic cells (DCs). The CD40-CD40L interaction was initially identified in relation to T- and B-cell interactions relevant to humoral immune responses *(19)*. It has recently been reported that stimuli from CD4$^+$ helper T (Th)-cells via the CD40-CD40L interaction is also essential in the activation of DCs with upregulation of costimulatory B7-1 molecule and intercellular adhesion molecule-1, which can then autonomously trigger the CD8$^+$ cytotoxic T-cell responses *(20–22)*. In addition, the CD40-CD40L interaction also induces the production of cytokines that favor the development of Th1-type immune response *(21–23)*. Therefore, we assume (1) that engineered myeloma cells J558/CD40L expressing CD40 ligand will become more immunogenic by activation of DCs and enhancement of tumor antigen presentation to T-cells, and (2) that vaccination of these engineered myeloma cells will induce enhanced antitumor immunity.

In this chapter, we describe the design and methods for cloning a cDNA gene coding for the mouse CD40L molecule and for construction of the expression vector pcDNA-CD40L. We also describe the methods for generation of engineered myeloma cells J558/CD40L expressing CD40 ligand. The principle and methods are also applicable to construction of other kinds of engineered tumor cells.

2. Materials

1. Tris-ammonium chloride solution: 17 m*M* Tris; 0.84% ammonium chloride, pH 7.2.
2. 10X First-strand buffer: 500 m*M* Tris-HCl, pH 8.3; 750 m*M* KCl; 30 m*M* MgCl.

3. 10X Reaction buffer: 200 m*M* Tris-HCl, pH 8.8; 100 m*M* KCl; 100 m*M* (NH$_4$)$_2$SO$_4$; 20 m*M* MgSO$_4$; 1% Triton X-100; 1 mg/mL of nuclease-free bovine serum albumin (BSA).

4. RNase Block Ribonuclease Inhibitor, dNTPs, Stratascript Reverse Transcriptase, Oligo dt primer, and *pfu* DNA polymerase (Stratagene, La Jolla, CA).

5. *Hind*III and *Xba*I restriction enzymes (Gibco/BRL, Burlington, Ontario, Canada).

6. pcDNA3.1/neo vector and pCR-Blunt vector (Invitrogen, Carlsbad, CA).

7. J558 cell line (American Type Culture Collection [ATCC], Rockville, MD): This is maintained in Dulbecco's modified essential medium (DMEM) plus 10% fetal calf serum (FCS) (Gibco, Gaithersburg, MD).

8. Qiagen RNeasy Mini Kit and QIAshredder spin column (Qiagen, Mississauga, Ontario, Canada).

9. TwinBlock thermocycler (Ericomp, San Diego, CA).

10. Bio-Rad Gene Pulser II apparatus (Bio-Rad, Hercules, CA).

11. G418 (Gibco).

3. Methods

3.1. Construction of Expression Vector pcDNA-CD40L

3.1.1. Generation of a cDNA Library of Concanavalin A-Stimulated Mouse Spleen T-Cells

Balb/c mouse spleen T-cells are cultured in the presence of the T-cell mitogen, concanavalin A (ConA), to stimulate the T-cells to become T-cell blasts.

3.1.1.1. PREPARATION OF CONA-STIMULATED SPLEEN T-CELLS

1. Euthanize a Balb/c mouse and spray with 70% ethanol.

2. Using aseptic techniques, remove the spleen with scissors and forceps, and then place in a Petri dish containing phosphate-buffered saline (PBS).

3. Place the spleen on a mesh screen and cut into smaller portions using scissors. Take the plunger from a 5-mL syringe, and press the spleen fragments through the mesh screen to prepare a single-cell suspension.

4. Rinse the mesh screen using PBS and then transfer the cells to a 50-mL tube.

5. Centrifuge at 800*g* for 10 min.

6. Add 5–10 mL of Tris-ammonium chloride solution, and incubate at room temperature for 5 min to lyse the red blood cells.

7. Dilute with PBS and centrifuge at 800*g* for 10 min.

8. Resuspend the cell pellet in 10–20 mL of DMEM + 10% FCS, and count the cells using a hemacytometer to obtain a final concentration of 2×10^6 cells/mL.

9. Add 0.6 µg of ConA/mL (5 mg/mL stock solution) (Sigma, St. Louis, MO) to the cell suspension.

10. Place the cell suspension into tissue culture flasks in a vertical position, and maintain the culture in a 37°C incubator with a 5% CO$_2$ atmosphere. After 2 to 3 d, the T-cells will become blast cells.

3.1.1.2. PREPARATION OF A cDNA LIBRARY

1. Harvest T-cells from the flask and centrifuge at 800*g* for 10 min.
2. Isolate the total RNA from the ConA-stimulated T-cells using a Qiagen RNeasy Mini Kit and QIAshredder spin column (Qiagen) according to the manufacturer's instructions (*see* **Note 1**).
3. Read the absorbance at 260 and 280 nm to determine the concentration and purity of the RNA sample (*see* **Note 2**). For long-term storage, place the RNA sample in liquid nitrogen (*see* **Note 3**).
4. Add 5 µg of total RNA resuspended in a total volume of 38 µL using diethyl-pyrocarbonate-treated distilled water.
5. Mix 300 ng of Oligo dT primer (Stratagene), incubate at 65°C for 5 min, then slowly cool to room temperature.
6. In the following order, add 5 µL of 10X first-strand buffer (500 m*M* Tris-HCl, pH 8.3; 750 m*M* KCl; 30 m*M* MgCl), 40 U of RNase Block Ribonuclease Inhibitor (Stratagene), 200 m*M* dNTPs (Stratagene), and 50 U of Stratascript Reverse Transcriptase (Stratagene) to the sample. Incubate the sample at 37°C for 1 h.
7. Heat the sample to 95°C for 5 min to heat-inactivate the enzyme, and then store at 4°C until further use.

3.1.2. Cloning of CD40L Gene

A 1-kb cDNA fragment coding for the full open reading frame of mouse CD40L gene is cloned by reverse transcriptase polymerase chain reaction (RT-PCR) from a cDNA library of ConA-stimulated mouse spleen T-cells using *pfu* polymerase (*see* **Note 4**). Two PCR primers (1 and 2) are used: the sense primer (5′ ctcca ttggc tctag attcc 3′) and the antisense primer (5′ cctca tgagc cacat aatac 3′). The method for PCR cloning of CD40L gene is as follows:

1. Add 0.1 µg of cDNA library DNA to a sterile 500-µL microcentrifuge tube.
2. Add 1 µL of the primers (1 mg/mL; primers 1 and 2) to the tube.
3. Add 10 µL of 10X reaction buffer (200 m*M* Tris-HCl, pH 8.8; 100 m*M* KCl; 100 m*M* [NH$_4$]$_2$SO$_4$; 20 m*M* MgSO$_4$; 1% Triton X-100; 1 mg/mL of nuclease-free BSA) to the tube.
4. Add 0.8 µL of 100 m*M* dNTP (Stratagene) to the tube.
5. Add sterile water to a final volume of 99 µL.
6. Place the tube in a TwinBlock thermocycler (Ericomp). Heat the reaction to 94°C for 5 min, and then immediately cool the reaction to 54°C for 5 min.
7. Briefly microcentrifuge the sample, and then add 1 µL of *pfu* DNA polymerase (2.5 U/µL). Microcentrifuge the sample again.
8. Carefully overlay the reaction mixture with a drop of mineral oil to prevent evaporation from the reaction during the amplification procedure.
9. Place the tube back in the thermocycler and program the heating block for 30 cycles (94°C for 1 min, 54°C for 1 min, and 68°C for 1 min) followed by one cycle at 68°C for 10 min.

10. After amplification, visualize the CD40L gene fragment on an ethidium bromide-stained 1% (w/v) agarose gel.

3.1.3. Construction of Expression Vector pcDNA-CD40L

The cloned cDNA fragment is first ligated into the pCR-Blunt vector (Invitrogen) to form pCR-Blunt-CD40L. The CD40L gene fragment (*see* **Note 5**) is digested with *Hin*dIII and *Xba*I restriction enzymes (Gibco/BRL) respectively. Briefly, microgram quantities of pCR-Blunt-CD40L DNA are digested with 5–25 U of restriction enzymes in a volume of 10–50 μL of 1X digestion buffer solution (Gibco/BRL) appropriate for the DNA and endonuclease being used. The reaction mixtures are incubated at 37°C for 1 to 2 h. The DNA fragment of CD40L (*Hin*dIII/*Xba*I) from the pCR-Blunt-CD40L is further ligated into the *Hin*dIII/*Xba*I sites of pcDNA3.1/neo vector (Invitrogen) to form pcDNA3.1/neo-CD40L (pcDNA-CD40L). Briefly, the purified CD40L (*Hin*dIII/*Xba*I) fragment is mixed with the vector-digested pcDNA (*Hin*dIII/*Xba*I) DNA at a molar ratio of approx 1:1 in 10 μL of solution containing 50 mM Tris-HCl, pH 7.6; 10 mM MgCl$_2$; 10 mM dithiothreitol; 1 mM adenosine triphosphate; and 5 U of T4 DNA ligase. The mixture is incubated at 16°C for at least 2 h. Optimal results are obtained by incubating the reaction overnight.

3.2. Engineering of J558 Myeloma Cells With pcDNA-CD40L

3.2.1. Tumor Cell Culture

J558 is a poorly immunogenic myeloma line of Balb/c (H-2K^d) mouse origin. This cell line is obtained from ATCC and maintained in DMEM plus 10% FCS (Gibco).

1. Thaw one vial of the frozen low-passage J558 cells in a 37°C water bath.
2. Transfer cells dropwise into a T75 tissue culture flask containing 15 mL of DMEM plus 10% FCS.
3. Maintain the cells at 37°C in an atmosphere of 5% CO$_2$. Five hours after incubation, collect and centrifuge the cells at 800g for 10 min, and change the medium once to remove any traces of the freezing medium from the cells.
4. Incubate at 37°C for 2 to 3 d (depending on cell density), dilute the mixture in growth medium, and distribute to three flasks for further incubation.
5. When preparing J558 cells for electroporation, use the myeloma cells when they are in the logarithmic phase of growth. Replace the medium with fresh DMEM consisting of 10% FCS 24 h prior to electroporation.

3.2.2. Electroporation

1. Resuspend 20 million J558 cells in 0.7 mL of PBS and mix with 0.3 mL of PBS containing 10 μg of pcDNA-CD40L DNA.

2. Transfect the tumor cells with pcDNA-CD40L using a Bio-Rad Gene Pulser II apparatus with parameters of 250 V and 125 μF capacitance (*see* **Note 6**).

3. Select the transfected cells for growth in DMEM plus 10% FCS plus 3 mg/mL of G418 (Gibco) (*see* **Notes 7** and **8**).

4. Maintain the selected J558/CD40L clone in DMEM plus 10% FCS with 0.5 mg/mL of G418 (*see* **Note 9**). The clone is used for in vitro analysis of CD40L expression by RT-PCR and for in vivo animal studies.

3.3. Expression of Transgene CD40L

To examine CD40L expression, total RNA is extracted from J558/CD40L tumor cells using the guanidinium thiocyanate–phenol–chloroform extraction method or a similar method. Synthesis and amplification of mCD40L cDNA or the control glyceraldehyde-3-phosphate dehydrogenase (GAPDH) cDNA are done using the one-step RT-PCR system (Boehringer Mannheim, Indianapolis, IN). The cDNA is amplified with primers specific for either CD40L or GAPDH transcripts. Primers 3 (5′ atgat agaaa catac agcca acct 3′) and 4 (5′ tcaga gtttg agtaa gccaa aaga 3′) are for CD40L, and primers 5 (5′ atggt gaagg tcggt gtgaa cgga 3') and 6 (5' ttact ccttg gaggc catgt aggc 3′) are for GAPDH. Synthesis and amplification conditions using *Taq* polymerase and 1 cycle of 50°C for 30 min and 94°C for 2 min; 30 cycles of 94°C for 1 min, 55°C for 1 min, and 72°C for 1 min; followed by 1 cycle of 72°C for 7 min. Each RT-PCR reaction is done using 1 μg of total RNA in a final volume of 100 μL, and resolving 8 μL of the PCR products on a 1% agarose gel. As shown in **Fig. 1**, the engineered J558-CD40L cells display significant amounts of CD40L mRNA expression, whereas the parental J558 myeloma cells show no expression of CD40L molecule.

3.4. Engineered Myeloma Cell Vaccine

3.4.1. Mice

Female Balb/c (H-2K^d) mice, 6–8 wk old, are obtained from the animal resources center of the University of Saskatchewan and housed in specific pathogen-free conditions of the animal facility at the Saskatoon Cancer Center.

3.4.2. Tumorigenicity of J558/CD40L Cells

To evaluate the tumorigenicity of J558/CD40L cells, naive Balb/c mice (eight per group) are subcutaneously inoculated into their right thighs with 0.3×10^6 J558-CD40L and parental J558 myeloma cells, respectively. Mice are then monitored for tumor progression or regression daily. Animals are sacrificed 2 wk after tumor inoculation. As shown in **Table 1**, the parental J558 myeloma cells grow aggressively in all mice, whereas none of the mice inoculated with J558-CD40L tumor cells has tumor growth. This indicates that the

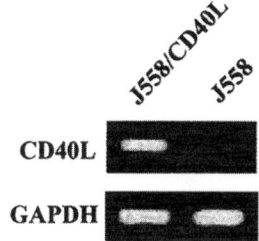

Fig. 1. Expression of CD40L molecule by RT-PCR analysis. RNA was extracted from J558/CD40L and J558 cells. RT was used to synthesize the first-strand cDNA. PCRs were conducted using primer sets for CD40L and the control housekeeping gene, GAPDH.

engineered J558-CD40L myeloma cells become immunogenic and lose their tumorigenicity in syngeneic Balb/c mice.

3.4.3. J558-CD40L Tumor Cell Vaccine

To evaluate the antitumor efficiency induced by J558-CD40L, animal studies are conducted to examine whether the immunized mice have immunopreventive effects against the rechallenge of the parental J558 myeloma cells.

1. Irradiate J558-CD40L and J558 cells (8000 rad).
2. Inject subcutaneously 0.3×10^6 irradiated J558-CD40L or J558 cells into the right thighs of Balb/c mice. For controls, inject mice with PBS.
3. Ten days later, inject subcutaneously 0.3×10^6 parental J558 myeloma cells into the left thighs of the immunized mice.
4. After tumor inoculation, monitor the tumor growth by measuring the length and width of each tumor mass with calipers every other day for up to 10 wk. For ethical reasons, sacrifice all mice with tumors reaching a diameter of 1.5 cm.

Our data show that all the mice (8/8) that we vaccinated with engineered J558-CD40L tumor cells developed immune protection against the challenge of parental J558 myeloma cells. Meanwhile, none of the mice (0/8) immunized with irradiated J558 myeloma cells induced a strong antitumor immune response to protect the mice from J558 myeloma challenge (**Table 1**). Our results indicate that vaccination using engineered J558-CD40L myeloma cells can induce enhanced antimyeloma immunity against the challenge of the parental myeloma J558 cells.

4. Notes

1. Maintain an RNase-free environment to avoid RNase contamination from cells throughout the course of the total RNA extraction procedure.

Table 1
Tumor Growth and Protective Immunity After Inoculation of J558/CD40L Cells in Balb/c Mice

| Tumor cells | Fraction of tumor-bearing mice (%) | |
	Primary injection[a]	Challenged with J558 wt tumor[b]
J558	8/8 (100)	—
J558/CD40L	0/8 (0)	—
Irradiated J558	—	8/8 (100)
Irradiate J558/CD40L	—	0/8 (0)
Control	—	8/8 (100)

[a]Primary injection represents the relative number of tumor-bearing mice (%) observed 2 wk following the injection of 0.3×10^6 J558 and J558/CD40L, respectively. Tumors were removed and confirmed by histological analysis 2 wk after tumor inoculation. Mice without tumor growth were continually monitored for an additional 2 mo.

[b]Mice were immunized with 0.3×10^6 irradiated J558 or J558/CD40L tumor cells followed by tumor challenge with 0.3×10^6 J558 cells. Mice were continually monitored up to 10 wk from initial tumor challenge. Tumors were removed and examined for histological analysis.

2. The purity of RNA is determined using the ratio of the absorbance readings at 260 and 280 nm (260/280), which is between 1.8 and 2.0. If the ratio is lower than 1.8, it indicates DNA contamination.

3. To avoid RNA degradation, the RNA sample can be stored at –80°C or in liquid nitrogen for long-term storage.

4. To avoid mutations when amplifying the CD40L gene fragment, *pfu* DNA polymerase is used instead of *Taq* DNA polymerase. *pfu* DNA polymerase is a thermostable polymerase isolated from *Pyrococcus furiosus* that contains $3'–5'$ exonuclease (proofreading) activity. This provides a lower error rate when compared with other thermostable DNA polymerases and makes it an ideal choice for high-fidelity DNA amplification by PCR.

5. The entire gene must be sequenced to confirm the presence of the gene and to detect any mutations within the cloned gene compared to the sequence obtained from the NCBI database.

6. The parameter setting using the Bio-Rad Gene Pulser II system has been optimized for J558 cells. When using other cells, the parameters need to be optimized by changing the voltage and capacitance so that there is approx 80% cell viability 24 h after electroporation.

7. The dose of G418 added to transfected cells 24 h after electroporation varies with different cells. The dose is determined by plating the cells in duplicates in a six-well plate and then adding media containing various concentrations of G418. The cells are cultured for several days and examined to determine the minimal dose that causes all of the cells to die.

8. To increase the growth of positive clones in selection medium, we usually reduce the G418 concentration in the selection medium in each well 3 d after adding the selection medium. This can be easily done by carefully aspirating of 150 µL of the selection medium in each well and replacing with 150 µL of DMEM plus 10% FCS.
9. The J558/CD40L cells must be continually cultured in growth medium containing 0.5 mg/mL of G418 to maintain selective pressure for transgene CD40L expression.

References

1. Blankenstein, T., Qin, Z., Uberla, K., et al. (1991) Tumor suppression after tumor cell-targeted tumor necrosis factor gene transfer. *J. Exp. Med.* **173,** 1047–1052.
2. Qi, Y., Chen, Y., and Xiang, J. (1996) Mouse myeloma cell line secreting bifunctional fusion protein RM4/IFN elicits antitumor CD8 MHC class I-restricted T cells that are cytolytic in vitro and tumoricidal in vivo. *J. Interferon Cytokine Res.* **16,** 771–776.
3. Koshita, Y., Lu, Y., Fujii, S., et al. (1995) Efficiency of TNF-α gene-transduced tumor cells in treatment of established in vivo tumor. *Int. J. Cancer* **63,** 130–135.
4. Colombo, M., Ferrari, G., Stoppacciaro, A., et al. (1991) Granulocyte colony-stimulating factor gene transfer suppresses tumorigenicity of a murine adenocarcinoma in vivo. *J. Exp. Med.* **173,** 889–897.
5. Allione, A., Consalvo, M., Manni, P., Cavallo, F., Giovarelli, M., and Forni, G. (1994) Immunizing and curative potential of replicating and nonreplicating murine mammary adenocarcinoma cells engineered with IL-2, IL-4, IL-6, IL-7, IL-10, TNF, GMCSF and IFN gene or admixed with conventional adjuvants. *Cancer Res.* **54,** 6022–6026.
6. Linsley, P. and Ledbetter, J. (1993) The role of CD28 receptor during T cell responses to antigen. *Annu. Rev. Immunol.* **11,** 191–212.
7. Schwartz, R. (1992) Costimulation of T lymphocytes: the role of CD28, CTLA-4 and 41BBL in IL-2 production and immunotherapy. *Cell* **71,** 1065–1072.
8. Hathcock, K., Laszlo, C., Pucillo, C., Linsley, P., and Hodes, R. (1994) Comparative analysis of B7-1 and B7-2 costimulatory ligands: expression and function. *J. Exp. Med.* **180,** 631–640.
9. Cayeux, S., Beck, C., Dorken, B., and Blankenstein, T. (1996) Coexpression of IL-4 and B7-1 in murine tumor cells leads to improved tumor rejection and vaccine effect compared to single gene transfectants and a classical adjuvant. *Hum. Gene Ther.* **7,** 525–529.
10. Cayeux, S., Richter, G., Noffz, G., Dorken, B., and Blankenstein, T. (1997) Influence of gene-modified (IL-7, IL-7 and B7-1) tumor cell vaccines on tumor antigen presentation. *J. Immunol.* **158,** 2834–2841.
11. Wu, T. C., Huang, A., Jaffee, E., Levitsky, H., and Pardoll, D. (1995) A reassessment of the role of B7-1 expression in tumor rejection. *J. Exp. Med.* **182,** 1415–1421.

12. Restifo, N. P., Esquivel, F., Asher, A. L., et al. (1991) Defective presentation of endogenous antigens by a murine sarcoma: implications for the failure of an anti-tumor response. *J. Immunol.* **147,** 1453–1459.

13. Van Essen, D., Kikutani, H., and Gray, D. (1995) CD40 preferentially costimu-lates activation of T cell in the development of helper function. *Nature* **378,** 620–622.

14. Blotta, M. H., Marshall, J. D., DeKruyff, R., and Umetsu, D. T. (1996) Crosslinking of the CD40 ligand on human CD4+ T lymphocytes generates a co-stimulatory signal that up-regulates IL-4 synthesis. *J. Immunol.* **156,** 3133–3142.

15. Grewal, I. S., Xu, J., and Flavell, R. A. (1995) Impairment of antigen specific T cell priming in mice lacking CD40 ligand. *Nature* **378,** 617–623.

16. Roy, M., Waldschmidt, T., Aruffo, A., Ledbetter, J.A., and Noelle, R. J. (1993) The regulation of the expression of gp39, the CD40 ligand on normal and cloned CD4 T cells. *J. Immunol.* **151,** 497–2510.

17. Grewal, I. and Flavell, R. (1998) CD40 and CD154 in cell-mediated immunity. *Annu. Rev. Immunol.* **16,** 111–135.

18. Smith, C., Farrah, T., and Goodwin, R. (1994) The TNF receptor superfamily of cellular and viral proteins: activation, costimulation and death. *Cell* **76,** 959–962.

19. Foy, T. M., Shepherd, D. M., Durie, F. H., Aruffo, A., Ledbetter, J. A., and Noelle, R. J. (1993) In vivo CD40-gp39 interactions are essential for thymus-dependent humoral immunity. II. Prolonged suppression of the humoral immune response by an antibody to the ligand for CD40, gp39. *J. Exp. Med.* **178,** 1567–1575.

20. Schoenberger, S. P., Toes, R. E., van der Voort, E. I., Offringa, R., and Melief, C. J. (1998) T-cell help for cytotoxic T lymphocytes is mediated by CD40-CD40L interactions. *Nature* **393,** 480–483.

21. Caux, C., Massacrier, C., and Vanbervliet, B. (1994) Activation of human den-dritic cells through CD40 cross-linking. *J. Exp. Med.* **180,** 1263–1272.

22. Cella, M., Scheidegger, D., Palmer-Lehmann, K., Lane, P., Lanzavecchia, A., and Alber, G. (1996) Ligation of CD40 on dendritic cells triggers production of high levels of IL-12 and enhances T cell stimulatory capacity: T-T help via APC acti-vation. *J. Exp. Med.* **184,** 747–752.

23. Koch, F., Stanzl, U., Jennewein, P., et al. (1996) High level IL-12 production by murine dendritic cells: upregulation via MHC class II and CD40 molecules and downregulation by IL-4 and IL-10. *J. Exp. Med.* **184,** 741–746.

19

An In Vitro Osteoclast-Forming Assay to Measure Myeloma Cell-Derived Osteoclast-Activating Factors

Andrew C. W. Zannettino, Amanda N. Farrugia, L. Bik To, and Gerald J. Atkins

Summary

Much of the morbidity and mortality associated with the plasma cell (PC) malignancy, multiple myeloma (MM), is owing to the severe osteolytic bone disease seen in patients with this disease. Although the molecular mechanisms responsible for osteolysis remain to be fully elucidated, it is clear from numerous studies that it is owing, in part, to an increase in osteoclastic bone resorption. Several known osteoclast (OC)-activating factors (OAFs) are produced by myeloma PCs (MPCs), or by stromal cells in response to MPCs and include interleukin-1β (IL-1β); tumor necrosis factor-α (TNF-α); IL-6; parathyroid hormone-related protein; macrophage inflammatory protein-1α; and, most recently, the TNF-ligand family member receptor activator of nuclear factor-κB ligand (RANKL). The identification and significance of any one of these myeloma-derived OAFs is dependent on robust and reliable assays that measure the *de novo* formation and activation of OCs. A number of in vitro assay systems have been described that examine the requirements for normal OC formation and are easily adaptable for examining which MM-derived OAF and to what extent it is responsible for the bone loss observed in individuals with myeloma. This chapter describes one such in vitro model system.

Key Words

Osteoclast; myeloma plasma cell; bone resorption; osteoclast activating factor; in vitro assay.

1. Introduction

A predominant clinical feature in patients with multiple myeloma (MM) is bone destruction, which accounts for much of the morbidity and mortality associated with this disease *(1,2)*. The precise molecular mechanisms responsible for osteolysis are unknown; however, it is clear from histomorphometric studies that it is owing to an uncoupling of the normal process of bone remodeling leading to an increase in osteoclast (OC) activity and bone resorption *(1,3)*.

From: *Methods in Molecular Medicine, Vol. 113: Multiple Myeloma: Methods and Protocols*
Edited by: R. D. Brown and P. J. Ho © Humana Press Inc., Totowa, NJ

Several known OC-activating factors (OAFs) are produced by myeloma plasma cells (MPCs), or by stromal cells in response to MPC *(1,4,5)* including lymphotoxin *(6,7)*; interleukin-1 (IL-1) *(8–10)*; tumor necrosis factor-α (TNF-α) *(10)*; IL-6 *(11,12)*, parathyroid hormone-related protein *(13,14)*; macrophage inflammatory protein-1α *(15)*; and, most recently, the TNF-ligand family member receptor activator of nuclear factor-κB ligand (RANKL) *(16–18)*. The identification and significance of any myeloma-derived OAF is therefore dependent, in part, on robust and reliable in vitro assays that measure the *de novo* formation and activation of OCs. A number of assay systems have been described *(19–26)* that examine the requirements for normal OC formation and are easily adaptable for examining which OAF is responsible for the bone loss observed in individuals with myeloma and to what extent. Because of their low cost and relative ease of establishment, these assays represent a useful tool to examine not only basic OC biology, but also potential therapies directed at reducing OC-mediated bone loss.

2. Materials

1. Sodium heparin (1000 U/mL).
2. Ficoll-Hypaque (Lymphoprep, 1.077 g/dL; Nycomed Pharma AS, Oslo, Norway).
3. Hank's balanced salt solution (HBSS).
4. Fetal bovine serum (FBS).
5. Biotinylated goat anti-mouse IgG, γ-chain specific (Southern Biotechnology, Birmingham, UK).
6. Streptavidin microbeads and magnetic activated cell sorting (MACS) Columns (Miltenyi Biotec; Bergisch Gladbach, Germany).
7. Anti-CD38 directly conjugated to phycoerythrin (PE); anti-CD45 directly conjugated to fluorescein isothiocyanate (FITC) (BD Pharmingen, San Diego, CA).
8. Low-speed saw (e.g., Isomet; Buehler, IL).
9. α-Modified minimal essential medium (α-MEM) (JRH Biosciences, Lenexa, KS).
10. Iscove's modified Eagle's medium (IMDM) (JRH Biosciences, Lenexa, KS).
11. Recombinant human macrophage colony-stimulating factor (rhM-CSF) (Pepro-tech, Rocky Hill, NJ).
12. Recombinant human RANKL (rhRANKL) (R&D Systems, Minneapolis, MN).
13. Leukocyte Acid Phosphatase kit (Sigma, St. Louis, MO).
14. HHF wash buffer: HBSS (Gibco/BRL, Glen Waverley, Victoria, Australia) supplemented with 20 mM HEPES, pH 7.35, and 5% (v/v) FBS (CSL Limited, Victoria, Australia).
15. Blocking buffer: HHF supplemented with 5% (v/v) normal human serum and 1% (v/v) bovine serum albumin (BSA).
16. FMC-17: a kind gift from Prof. Peter McCardle, Flinders Medical Centre, Bedford Park, South Australia, Australia.
17. MACS buffer: Ca^{2+}- and Mn^{2+}-free phosphate-buffered saline (PBS) supplemented with 1% BSA in PBS, 5 mM EDTA, and 0.01% sodium azide.

18. Fluorescence-activated cell sorting (FACS) fix: 1% (v/v) formalin, 0.1 M D-glucose, 0.02% sodium azide in PBS.
19. Thaw medium: IMDM (JRH Biosciences) supplemented with 20% (v/v) FCS and 50 Kunitz U/mL of Dnase-1.
20. Complete growth medium: α-MEM (JRH Biosciences) supplemented in 10% (v/v) FBS, 2 mM L-glutamine, 2 mM each of gentamycin and penicillin, 1×10^{-8} M dexamethasone (Sigma), 1×10^{-7} M 1,25 (OH)$_2$ vitamin D$_3$ (Hoffman La Roche, Nutley, NJ), and 25 ng/mL of rhM-CSF (Peprotech).

3. Methods

The methods described outline the preparation of the peripheral blood-derived OC precursor population, the preparation of the phenotypically defined subpopulations of patient-derived MPCs, the establishment of the MPC:OC co-culture, the assessment of *de novo* OC formation, and the measurement of in vitro OC activity.

3.1. Preparation of Human Peripheral Blood-Derived OC Precursors

A number of studies have clearly demonstrated that circulating human OC precursors are found exclusively within the fraction of peripheral blood mononuclear cells (PBMCs) that express the glycosyl phosphatidylinositol (GPI)-linked monocyte/macrophage marker, CD14 *(27)*. These peripheral blood-derived CD14$^+$ cells originate from CD34$^+$ hemopoietic stem cells found in the bone marrow. The following section describes the methods used to isolate CD14$^+$ cells from peripheral blood.

3.1.1. Preparation of Human Peripheral Blood-Derived Mononuclear Cells

1. Collect 50 mL of normal peripheral blood by aspiration into preservative-free, sodium heparin-containing tubes following informed consent.
2. Prepare low-density PBMCs by centrifuging peripheral blood at 400g over Ficoll-Hypaque for 30 min at room temperature. Then collect the "buffy layer" of cells at the interface with a Pasteur pipet and transfer to a fresh tube.
3. Wash the PBMCs three times by centrifugating at 4°C in wash buffer (HHF), in preparation for CD14$^+$ monocyte isolation by MACS.

3.1.2. Isolation of CD14$^+$ Monocytes Using MACS

1. Prior to immunolabeling, resuspend the PBMCs (approx 0.5×10^8 cells) in 0.5 mL of blocking buffer, and incubate for 30 min on ice to block possible Fc receptor-mediated binding of antibodies.
2. Add 500 μL of the anti-CD14 monoclonal antibody (MAb), FMC-17 previously diluted to a concentration of 20 μg/mL in blocking buffer, to the PBMCs and incubate for 60 min at 4°C with occasional, gentle mixing (*see* **Note 1**).
3. Wash the PBMCs twice in HBSS/5% FBS, resuspend in 0.5 mL of HHF containing biotinylated goat anti-mouse IgG (γ-chain specific) at a 1/50 dilution, and incubate at 4°C for 45 min.

4. Wash the PBMCs three times in MACS buffer, and resuspend in 450 µL of MACS buffer to which 50 µL of streptavidin microbeads are added (10 µL of microbeads/10^7 cells in 90 µL of MACS buffer). Incubate the mixture at 4°C for 15 min.

5. To monitor the purification process (optional), add streptavidin-PE conjugate (1/50) (Caltag, San Francisco, CA) directly to the cell suspension for an additional 5 min.

6. After one wash in ice-cold degassed MACS buffer, remove a small aliquot of cells for flow cytometric analysis (presample). Then place the remaining cells onto a mini MACS column (column capacity of 10^8 cells). The CD14$^-$ cells (negative fraction) are not retained within the column and pass through, under gravity, into the effluent, while the CD14$^+$ cells remain attached to the magnetized matrix.

7. Wash the column three times with 0.5 mL of degassed MACs buffer to remove any nonspecifically bound CD14$^-$ cells.

8. Recover the CD14$^+$ cells (positive fraction) by flushing the column with MACS buffer after withdrawing the column from the magnetic field. Remove small samples from each of the pre, negative, and positive fractions, fix in FACS fix, and subsequently analyze by flow cytometry in order to assess purity and recovery. An example is shown in **Fig. 1** (*see* **Note 2**).

3.2. Preparation of Human MPCs

Although many groups identify and isolate MPCs using antibodies to the widely accepted marker CD138 or syndecan-1, our experience, as well as that of several other groups, shows that CD138 is variably expressed and sometimes lacking in patients with significant MPC burden *(28)*. With this in mind, we routinely use high expression of CD38 to isolate bone marrow-derived MPCs. An additional issue requiring consideration is the fact that primary MPCs do not have the capacity to divide or survive for extended periods in vitro. Because the co-culture assay described in **Subheading 3.3.** represents a 21-d assay, and given the poor survival characteristics of MPCs, we have found it necessary to isolate more immature MPCs with the phenotype CD38^{+++} CD45$^+$ to ensure adequate *de novo* OC formation.

3.2.1. Preparation of Human MPCs Prior to Flow Cytometric Cell Sorting

1. All bone marrow samples from patients with MM are collected by the Therapeutic Product Facility (Institute of Medical and Veterinary Science, South Australia). Bone marrow mononuclear cells (BMMNC) are prepared essentially as described in **Subheading 3.1.** and cryopreserved in FBS supplemented with 10% (v/v) dimethyl sulfoxide (AnalaR; Merck). To ensure adequate recovery of MPCs from cryopreserved samples, rapidly thaw BMMNC preparations from patients with MM by resuspending 2×10^7 MM BMMNC in 10 mL of thaw medium and then wash twice by centrifugating at 4°C in HHF wash buffer.

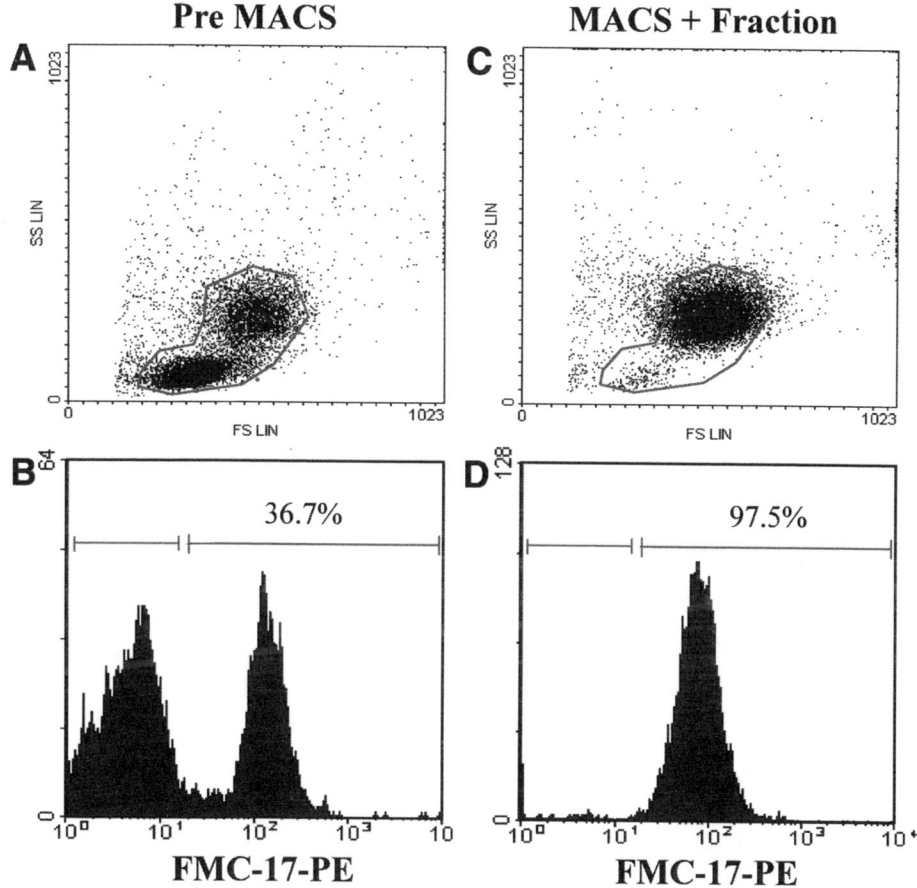

Fig. 1. CD14+ pre-OCs were purified by CD14 MACS. An unfractionated or "pre-" sample (**A,B**) and an MACS positive fraction (**C,D**) were assessed by flow cytometry. The homogeneous light scatter characteristics and uniform expression of CD14 indicate successful enrichment of the CD14+ pre-OC population (**C,D**).

3.2.2. Isolation of CD38+++CD45+ MPCs Using FACS

1. Prior to immunolabeling, resuspend MM bone marrow mononuclear cells (routinely $0.2 - 1 \times 10^8$ cells) in 0.5 mL of blocking buffer, and incubate for 30 min on ice to block possible Fc receptor-mediated binding of antibodies.
2. For two-color immunofluorescence (*see* **Fig. 2**), add anti-CD38 directly conjugated to phycoerythrin (PE) and anti-CD45 directly conjugated to FITC or appropriate isotype-matched controls (BD Pharmingen) to the cell pellet at a ratio of 5 μL of antibody to 1×10^6 cells, and incubate at 4°C for 1 h.
3. Wash the bone marrow mononuclear cells as described previously, and resuspend at a concentration of 1×10^7 cells/mL prior to sorting on any sorter fitted with a

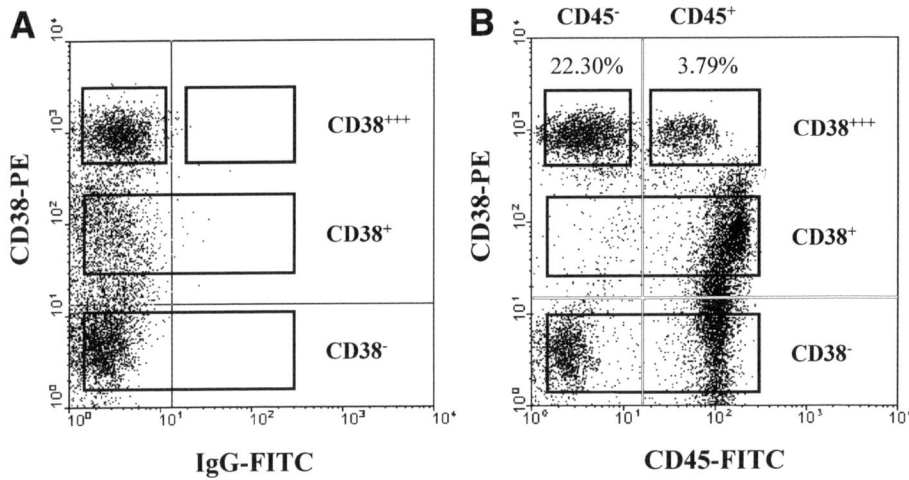

Fig. 2. Patient-derived bone marrow was stained with CD38 and CD45 (or IgG control, [**A**]), MAbs, and sort gates were drawn, as indicated, to generate CD38⁻, CD38⁺ (both independent of CD45 expression), CD38^{+++}45⁻, and CD38^{+++}45⁺ populations. The CD38^{+++}45⁺ subpopulation exhibits the longest life-span in culture and was therefore co-cultured with normal human PBMCs, as described in the text. The percentage of cells in each subpopulation is indicated and differs between patients.

250-mW argon laser emitting light at a wavelength of 488 nm able to simultaneously detect FITC and PE. Sorted bone marrow mononuclear cells may then be used immediately for culture (discussed later) or cryopreserved for later use.

3.3. Establishment of a MPCs and OC Coculture Assay

As discussed in **Subheading 3.2.**, primary MPCs display a limited capacity for survival in vitro, necessitating the development of an assay system that in its later stages is dependent on the addition of low concentrations of the potent pro-osteoclastogenic molecule, RANKL. This ensures survival and activation of any preformed OCs present within the culture.

3.3.1. Preparation of OC Substrate: Dentine Slices

1. Cut 150-μ*M* transverse slices of dentine using a low-speed saw (e.g., Isomet; Buehler), and then cut the resultant "sheets" into 4-mm squares.
2. Mark one side of each dentine slice with an "F" in lead pencil to ensure the correct orientation.
3. Sterilize the dentine slices by submerging in 70% ethanol for 30 min. Place the slices in a sterile Petri dish and ultraviolet irradiate in a biohazard cabinet (e.g., Class II Biohazard hood; Gelman Sciences, Australia) for 1 h on each side. The slices can be stored indefinitely in a sterile vessel at –20°C.

4. Immediately prior to use, wash the slices four times in sterile PBS and incubate in complete culture medium containing 10% FBS for 1 h at 37°C (*see* **Note 3**).

3.3.2. Culture of CD14⁺ Cells on Dentine Slices

Several appropriate controls should always be used in each experiment including a negative control in which CD14⁺ cells are cultured in the absence of sorted cells, which will provide a baseline level of spontaneous OC formation attributed to these cells alone; a positive control, in which CD14⁺ cells are cultured in the presence of 50 ng/mL of soluble rhRANKL in complete growth medium from d 7 of culture; and co-cultures in which rhRANKL has not been added in order to assess baseline MPC-mediated OC formation. In addition, irrespective of condition, the medium must be changed every 3 d for the duration of 21 d.

1. Place the dentine slices "F" side down in each well of a tissue culture 96-well microtiter plate containing 100 μL of complete growth medium (*see* **Subheading 2., item 20**).
2. Resuspend CD14⁺ monocytes (prepared in **Subheading 3.1.2.**) at a density of 0.4×10^5 cells/mL in complete growth medium and seed 100 μL onto each dentine slice. Culture the monocytes at 37°C in 5% CO_2 in a humidified incubator for 7 d. Aspirate the medium and replace every 3 d with fresh complete growth medium. In accordance with the observations of Nicholson et al. *(29)*, a source of human RANKL is not required and therefore not included for the first 7 d of culture.
3. On d 7, add purified populations of sorted MM-derived MPCs (CD38⁺⁺⁺45⁺⁻ prepared as described in **Subheading 3.2.2.** and **Fig. 2**) to at least four replicate wells at a concentration of 2×10^4 cells/well (*see* **Note 4**).
4. Owing to the poor viability of the sorted MPC subpopulations, add additional freshly sorted MPCs at d 16 of culture. Alternatively, add rhRANKL (R&D Systems) at a concentration of 2 ng/mL. Although unable to support *de novo* OC formation, the addition of low concentrations of rhRANKL will ensure activation of any preformed multinucleated OCs in the culture.

3.4. Assessment of De Novo OC Formation

A number of key markers and phenotypic characteristics identify cells as bona fide OCs. These include expression of the calcitonin receptor (CTR) *(30)*, cathepsin *(31)*, carbonic anhydrase II *(32)*, αvβ3 integrin *(33)*, and tartrate-resistant acid phosphatase (TRAP) *(34)*, specifically, the 5b isoform *(35)*. Recently, expression of the RANKL receptor, RANK, on mature OCs has also been confirmed *(36)*. Expression of most of these can be confirmed by reverse transcriptase polymerase chain reaction *(37)*, or in the case of CTR, radiolabeled calcitonin can also be used to identify OCs *in situ* *(30)*. Histochemical staining for TRAP and the multinuclearity of the OCs are commonly used as sole identifiers of OC formation. Although convenient when small numbers of

OCs are formed, it is not considered reliable in in vitro culture systems *(38)*. Perhaps the single most definitive criterion for OC formation is the ability of the resulting OC to form classic resorption lacunae on mineralized substrates, such as cortical bone or dentine. Preferably, a number of criteria are used in concert to identify OCs. The appearance of large, multinucleated cells staining positive for TRAP and capable of resorption lacunae formation is reliably indicative of the formation of OCs in coculture. The following sections describe the method used to identify and enumerate OCs.

3.4.1. TRAP Staining

1. Wash the cells once in PBS, and fix for 10 min in 4% (v/v) glutaraldehyde in PBS.
2. Following fixation, wash the cells four times in distilled water and stain using a commercially available Leukocyte Acid Phosphatase kit (Sigma) according to the manufacturer's instructions.
3. Remove excess TRAP stain by washing the cells four times in distilled water.
4. Counterstain the cells with 0.05% (w/v) Methylene green (optional step). An example is shown in **Fig. 3**.

3.5. Assessment of OC Activity

Several alternatives exist for assessing resorption lacunae or pit formation, including light microscope imaging of dentine slices stained with India ink or negatively stained with protein dyes such as Toluidine Blue, or by our preferred method because of its superior accuracy—scanning electron microscopy (SEM).

3.5.1. Identification of Resorption Pit Formation

1. Wash slices twice in PBS, place in 6 M NH_4OH for at least 2 h, and then sonicate in a sonicating water bath (e.g., Branson B15100; Branson Ultrasonics, Danbury, CT) for 30 min.
2. Remove cell debris with an artist's brush and redraw the "F"s to ensure maintenance of correct orientation of the dentine slice for analysis.
3. Thoroughly remove excess salt by washing the slices five times in deionized water.
4. Sequentially dehydrate the slices by submerging in 70% and then absolute ethanol for 5 min. Leave the slices to air-dry for several hours, and then mount in the correct orientation ("F" side down) onto metal stubs for SEM analysis. Then "dag" each slice using carbon paint to ensure conductivity of the dentine surface.
5. Coat the stubs with carbon/gold for analysis under a scanning electron microscope (e.g., a Philips XL-20) *(22,37)*.

3.5.2. Calculation of Resorption Pit Area

Although several computer packages may be used to assess the area of resorption on the digital SEM images, we use the Scion Image software (Scion,

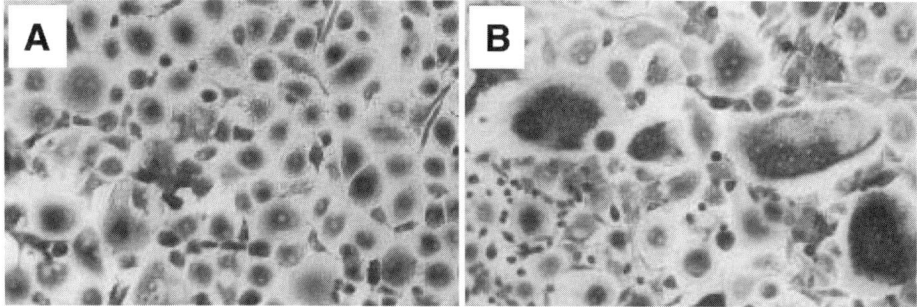

Fig. 3. The numbers of TRAP$^+$ cells were scored by light microscopic analysis of stained cells after 21 d of culture. TRAP$^+$ cells with three or more nuclei are scored as positive. A sample in which CD38^{+++}45$^+$ were omitted (**A**) and added (**B**) to the pre-OCs is shown.

Frederick, MD). This software is available free from Scion's Web site (http://www.scioncorp.com) and allows the user to measure accurately the dimensions/area of resorption, as shown in **Fig. 4B**.

4. Notes

1. Alternative, commercially available anti-CD14 MAbs may be used, but we have not tested them.
2. If CD14 selection is not possible or desired, PBMCs may be plated onto the dentine slice at a concentration of 0.5×10^6 cells/slice, allowed to adhere for 1 h at 37°C, and the nonadherent cells removed by washing three times in basal α-MEM without serum.
3. Although we use elephant tusk dentine, whale dentine or femoral cortical may serve as alternative resorptive media to measure OC activity. This material can usually be obtained via customs departments at large international airports. Government approval is usually required and will vary from country to country. Alternative, commercially available mineralized collagen assay plates are now available for assessment of OC activity, but we have not tested them.
4. The assay system described is amenable to the addition of function blocking antibodies, antagonists, purified proteins, growth factors, and so on. This will enable workers to establish the biological significance of molecules of choice.

Acknowledgments

We wish to thank Prof. P. McCardle for providing the anti-CD14 MAb. We also thank P. Kostakis, Christopher Holding, and Beiqing Pan for their technical assistance and Prof. D Findlay for his constant support and advice. This work was supported by National Health and Medical Council of Australia grants 150401, 157984, and 298935.

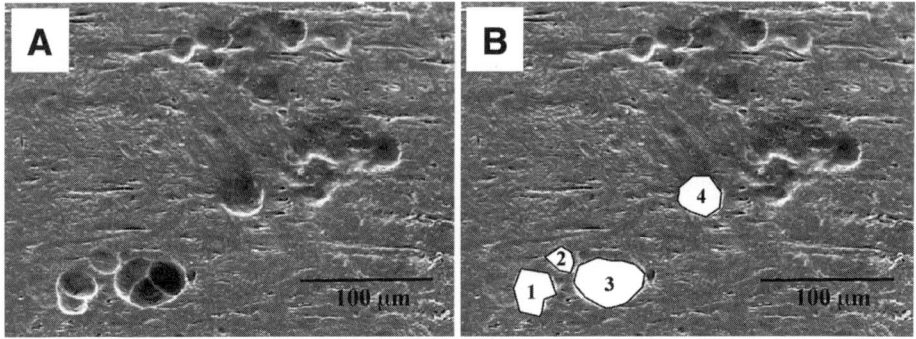

Fig. 4. (**A**) Scanning electron micrograph showing bone resorption mediated by multinucleated TRAP$^+$ OCs generated by culturing CD38^{+++}45$^+$ MPC cells with CD14$^+$ peripheral blood–derived OC precursors. (**B**) A single resorption lacuna is defined as a region of contiguous resorption. The area of resorption (defined as region 1, 2, 3, 4) can be calculated using area analysis software as described in the text.

References

1. Roodman, G. D. (1997) Mechanisms of bone lesions in multiple myeloma and lymphoma. *Cancer* **80,** 1557–1563.
2. Mundy, G. R. (1997) Mechanisms of bone metastasis. *Cancer* **80,** 1546–1556.
3. Bataille, R., Chappard, D., Marcelli, C., et al. (1991) Recruitment of new osteoblasts and osteoclasts is the earliest critical event in the pathogenesis of human multiple myeloma. *J. Clin. Invest.* **88,** 62–66.
4. Lichtenstein, A., Berenson, J., Norman, D., Chang, M. P., and Carlile, A. (1989) Production of cytokines by bone marrow cells obtained from patients with multiple myeloma. *Blood* **74,** 1266–1273.
5. Croucher, P. I. and Apperley, J. F. (1998) Bone disease in multiple myeloma. *Br. J. Haematol.* **103,** 902–910.
6. Garrett, I. R., Durie, B. G., Nedwin, G. E., et al. (1987) Production of lymphotoxin, a bone-resorbing cytokine, by cultured human myeloma cells. *N. Engl. J. Med.* **317,** 526–532.
7. Bataille, R., Klein, B., Jourdan, M., Rossi, J. F., and Durie, B. G. (1989) Spontaneous secretion of tumor necrosis factor-beta by human myeloma cell lines. *Cancer* **63,** 877–880.
8. Cozzolino, F., Torcia, M., Aldinucci, D., et al. (1989) Production of interleukin-1 by bone marrow myeloma cells. *Blood* **74,** 380–387.
9. Yamamoto, I., Kawano, M., Sone, T., et al. (1989) Production of interleukin 1 beta, a potent bone resorbing cytokine, by cultured human myeloma cells. *Cancer Res.* **49,** 4242–4246.
10. Sati, H. I., Greaves, M., Apperley, J. F., Russell, R. G., and Croucher, P. I. (1999) Expression of interleukin-1beta and tumour necrosis factor-alpha in plasma cells from patients with multiple myeloma. *Br. J. Haematol.* **104,** 350–357.

11. Barille, S., Bataille, R., and Amoit, M. (2000) The role of interleukin-6 and interleukin-6/interleukin-6 receptor-alpha complex in the pathogenesis of multiple myeloma. *Eur. Cytokine Netw.* **11,** 546–551.
12. Sati, H. I., Apperley, J. F., Greaves, M., et al. (1998) Interleukin-6 is expressed by plasma cells from patients with multiple myeloma and monoclonal gammopathy of undetermined significance. *Br. J. Haematol.* **101,** 287–295.
13. Suzuki, A., Takahashi, T., Okuno, Y., et al. (1994) Production of parathyroid hormone-related protein by cultured human myeloma cells. *Am. J. Hematol.* **45,** 88–90.
14. Otsuki, T., Yamada, O., Kurebayashi, J., et al. (2001) Expression and in vitro modification of parathyroid hormone-related protein (PTHrP) and PTH/PTHrP-receptor in human myeloma cells. *Leuk. Lymphoma* **41,** 397–409.
15. Han, J.-H., Choi, S. J., Kurihara, N., Koide, M., Oba, Y., and Roodman, G. D. (2001) Macrophage inflammatory protein-1a is an osteoclastogenic factor in myeloma that is independent of receptor activator of nuclear factor kB ligand. *Blood* **97,** 3349–3353.
16. Farrugia, A. N., Atkins, G. J., To, L. B., et al. (2003) Receptor activator of nuclear factor-kappaB ligand expression by human myeloma cells mediates osteoclast formation in vitro and correlates with bone destruction in vivo. *Cancer Res.* **63,** 5438–5445.
17. Sezer, O., Heider, U., Jakob, C., et al. (2002) Immunocytochemistry reveals RANKL expression of myeloma cells. *Blood* **99,** 4646, 4647; discussion 4647.
18. Heider, U., Langelotz, C., Jakob, C., et al. (2003) Expression of receptor activator of nuclear factor kappaB ligand on bone marrow plasma cells correlates with osteolytic bone disease in patients with multiple myeloma. *Clin. Cancer Res.* **9,** 1436–1440.
19. Haynes, D. R., Atkins, G. J., Loric, M., Crotti, T. N., Geary, S. M., and Findlay, D. M. (1999) Bidirectional signaling between stromal and hemopoietic cells regulates interleukin-1 expression during human osteoclast formation. *Bone* **25,** 269–278.
20. Shalhoub, V., Elliott, G., Chiu, L., et al. (2000) Characterization of osteoclast precursors in human blood. *Br. J. Haematol.* **111,** 501–512.
21. Quinn, J. M., Elliott, J., Gillespie, M. T., and Martin, T. J. (1998) A combination of osteoclast differentiation factor and macrophage-colony stimulating factor is sufficient for both human and mouse osteoclast formation in vitro. *Endocrinology* **139,** 4424–4427.
22. Atkins, G. J., Haynes, D. R., Geary, S. M., Loric, M., Crotti, T. N., and Findlay, D. M. (2000) Coordinated cytokine expression by stromal and hematopoietic cells during human osteoclast formation. *Bone* **26,** 653–661.
23. James, I. E., Lark, M. W., Zembryki, D., et al. (1999) Development and characterization of a human in vitro resorption assay: demonstration of utility using novel antiresorptive agents. *J. Bone Miner. Res.* **14,** 1562–1569.
24. Kudo, O., Sabokbar, A., Pocock, A., Itonaga, I., and Athanasou, N. A. (2002) Isolation of human osteoclasts formed in vitro: hormonal effects on the bone-resorbing activity of human osteoclasts. *Calcif. Tissue Int.* **71,** 539–546.

25. Joyner, C. J., Quinn, J. M., Triffitt, J. T., Owen, M. E., and Athanasou, N. A. (1992) Phenotypic characterisation of mononuclear and multinucleated cells of giant cell tumour of bone. *Bone Miner.* **16,** 37–48.

26. Fujikawa, Y., Quinn, J. M., Sabokbar, A., McGee, J. O., and Athanasou, N. A. (1996) The human osteoclast precursor circulates in the monocyte fraction. *Endocrinology* **137,** 4058–4060.

27. Massey, H. M. and Flanagan, A. M. (1999) Human osteoclasts derive from CD14-positive monocytes. *Br. J. Haematol.* **106,** 167–170.

28. Pope, B., Brown, R. D., Gibson, J., Yuen, E., and Joshua, D. (2000) B7-2-positive myeloma: incidence, clinical characteristics, prognostic significance, and implications for tumor immunotherapy. *Blood* **96,** 1274–1279.

29. Nicholson, G. C., Aitken, C. J., Hodge, J. M., et al. (2001) Limited RANKL exposure in vitro induces osteoclastogenesis in human PBMC. *Bone* **28(Suppl.),** P271 (abstract).

30. Nicholson, G. C., Moseley, J. M., Sexton, P. M., Mendelsohn, F. A., and Martin, T. J. (1986) Abundant calcitonin receptors in isolated rat osteoclasts: biochemical and autoradiographic characterization. *J. Clin. Invest.* **78,** 355–360.

31. Drake, F. H., Dodds, R. A., James, I. E., et al. (1996) Cathepsin K, but not cathepsins B, L, or S, is abundantly expressed in human osteoclasts. *J. Biol. Chem.* **271,** 12,511–12,516.

32. Vaananen, H. K. (1984) Immunohistochemical localization of carbonic anhydrase isoenzymes I and II in human bone, cartilage and giant cell tumor. *Histochemistry* **81,** 485–487.

33. Davies, J., Warwick, J., Totty, N., Philp, R., Helfrich, M., and Horton, M. (1989) The osteoclast functional antigen, implicated in the regulation of bone resorption, is biochemically related to the vitronectin receptor. *J. Cell Biol.* **109,** 1817–1826.

34. Minkin, C. (1982) Bone acid phosphatase: tartrate-resistant acid phosphatase as a marker of osteoclast function. *Calcif. Tissue Int.* **34,** 285–290.

35. Halleen, J. M., Alatalo, S. L., Suominen, H., Cheng, S., Janckila, A. J., and Vaananen, H. K. (2000) Tartrate-resistant acid phosphatase 5b: a novel serum marker of bone resorption. *J. Bone Miner. Res.* **15,** 1337–1345.

36. Hsu, H., Lacey, D. L., Dunstan, C. R., et al. (1999) Tumor necrosis factor receptor family member RANK mediates osteoclast differentiation and activation induced by osteoprotegerin ligand. *Proc. Natl. Acad. Sci. USA* **96,** 3540–3545.

37. Atkins, G. J., Haynes, D. R., Graves, S. E., et al. (2000) Expression of osteoclast differentiation signals by stromal elements of giant cell tumors. *J. Bone Miner. Res.* **15,** 640–649.

38. Hattersley, G. and Chambers, T. J. (1989) Generation of osteoclastic function in mouse bone marrow cultures: multinuclearity and tartrate-resistant acid phosphatase are unreliable markers for osteoclastic differentiation. *Endocrinology* **124,** 1689–1696.

20

Clonality Detection of Expanded T-Cell Populations in Patients With Multiple Myeloma

Daniel M-Y. Sze

Summary

Expanded T-cell clones in the peripheral blood of patients with multiple myeloma and smoldering myeloma are usually CD8 positive and persist over long periods, suggesting that they are the result of chronic antigenic stimulation. The presence of enlarged T-cell clones can be demonstrated as bands other than the germ-line bands on Southern blots probed for the T-cell receptor β gene (Vβ), or defined by anti-TCRVβ monoclonal antibody staining. However, the most sensitive way to demonstrate clonality within a population of T-cells is by analysis of the length of complementarity-determining region 3 of the rearranged TCR gene, followed by sequencing. Furthermore, my colleagues and I have previously shown that the CD57[+] T-cells expressing the "expanded" TCRVβ are monoclonal or biclonal, whereas the CD57[-] cells are usually polyclonal.

Key Words

T-cell; multiple myeloma; polymerase chain reaction; CD57; complementarity-determining region.

1. Introduction

Many groups, including ours, have reported the finding of unusually large ("expanded") CD8[+] T-cell clones in the peripheral blood of patients with multiple myeloma (MM) and smoldering myeloma (*1–3*). These clones have been shown to persist over long periods, suggesting that they are the result of chronic antigenic stimulation (*1*).

The presence of enlarged T-cell clones can be demonstrated as bands other than the germline bands on Southern blots probed for the T-cell receptor (TCR) β gene (Vβ). Another method of detecting the expanded T-cell clone is by using panels of commercially available anti-TCR Vβ monoclonal antibodies, such that there is an increase in the number of cells positively stained by a monoclonal

From: *Methods in Molecular Medicine, Vol. 113: Multiple Myeloma: Methods and Protocols*
Edited by: R. D. Brown and P. J. Ho © Humana Press Inc., Totowa, NJ

antibody to the specific TCR Vβ subfamily expressed by that clone. Several different groups have used this method and detected the presence of abnormally high numbers of T-cells expressing a particular TCR Vβ chain in patients with multiple myeloma (**Note 1**).

Although T-cell expansions, as defined by anti-TCR Vβ monoclonal antibody staining, may account for up to 25% of total T-cells, an excess of TCR Vβ-expressing cells may not necessarily be the result of a clonal expansion. To demonstrate clonality within a population of T-cells, we first analyzed the length of the complementarity-determining region 3 (CDR3) of the rearranged TCR gene, and then followed by sequencing *(2,4)*.

This has been shown to be a very sensitive way to demonstrate clonality. CDR3 length analysis involves polymerase chain reaction (PCR) amplification of cDNA derived from sorted T-cells using a ^{32}P-labeled 5′ primer specific for the relevant TCR Vβ subfamily, together with a 3′ primer from the TCRβ constant region. The PCR products (~250 basepairs) are then electrophoresed through a 6% polyacrylamide gel, and the sizes of the radioactive PCR bands determined by autoradiography.

To improve the sensitivity and specificity of CDR3 length analysis in detecting clonal T-cell populations, cells from MM patients were sorted not only for expression of CD8 and the relevant TCR Vβ, but also for the surface expression of CD57. We have shown the monoclonality of CD57$^+$CD8$^+$-expanded T-cells and confirmed the results by direct DNA sequencing of the PCR product generated by CDR3 length analysis (**Fig. 1**) *(2)*. In contrast, cloning and sequencing of the PCR products from the CD57$^-$-sorted T-cells gives an array of sequences, indicative of a polyclonal population.

2. Materials

2.1. Anti-TCRVβ MAbs

A panel of 21 MAbs is required. These are phycoerythrin (PE)-conjugated anti-TCRVβ1, 2, 3, 5.1, 5.2, 5.3, 7, 8, 9, 11, 12, 13.1, 13.6, 14, 16, 17, 18, 20, 21.3, 22, and 23 (all antibodies are mouse immunoglobulin [Ig] except anti-TCRVβ1, which is a rat IgG1) (Immunotech, Marseille, France). The panel has about 65–70% coverage of normal human TCRVβ repertoire.

2.2. T-Cell Repertoire Assays

The new kit of IO/test beta mark for measuring T-cell repertoire is available from Beckman Coulter. The kit aims at simplifying the TCRVβ repertoire analysis by reducing the number of tubes to analyze (8 instead of 21) and, consequently, the time required to obtain the results. Comparison between the traditional 21-tube panel and this 8-tube panel is further discussed in **Note 2**.

CD57 positive CD57 negative

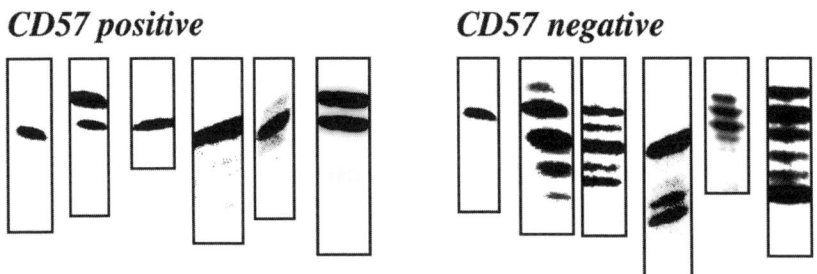

Fig. 1. CDR3 length analysis comparing CD57$^+$ and CD57$^-$ flow-sorted expanded CD8$^+$TCRVβ$^+$ T-cells from six patients with MM. (From **ref. 2**. © American Society of Hematology.)

2.3. Other T-Cell Phenotypic Markers

The following directly conjugated mouse MAbs are useful in further characterization of the T-cell population: anti-CD3, anti-CD4, anti-CD8, and anti-CD57, all fluorescein isothiocyanate (FITC) labeled (Becton Dickinson, San Jose, CA). All these antibodies are also available as PC5 conjugates or PerCP conjugates except anti-CD57.

2.4. Complete Culture Medium (RPMI-10 Medium)

RPMI-1640 containing 10% heat-inactivated fetal calf serum, 1 mM L-glutamine, 100 IU/mL of penicillin, and 160 U/mL (160 mg/mL) of gentamicin.

2.5. Materials for PCR

2.5.1. Preparation of cDNA

1. QuickPrep Micro mRNA Purification Kit (Amersham Pharmacia Biotech, Piscataway, NJ).
2. T-primed First-Strand Kit (Amersham).

2.5.2. Radioactive Labeling of Forward Primers Specific for Various Variable TCRVβ Subfamilies

1. [γ^{32}P]ATP with a specific activity of 3000 Ci/mmol (available from NEN, Boston, MA).
2. T4 Polynucleotide kinase (available from Boehringer Mannheim, Mannheim, Germany).

2.5.3. Polymerase Chain Reaction

1. Thin-walled PCR tubes (0.2 and 0.5 mL).
2. Heat-stable DNA polymerase (10X buffer supplied by manufacturer).
3. 10 mM dNTP (nucleotide) mix.
4. PCR primers (*see* **Table 1**).

Table 1
TCR PCR Primer Sequences

	Primer sequence
TCRVβ subfamilies	
TCRBV1	GCA CAA CAG TTC CCT GAC TTG CAC
TCRBV2	TCA TCA ACC ATG CAA GCC TGA CCT
TCRBV3A	GGG GTA CAG TGT CTC TAG AGA GA
TCRBV3B	GTC TCT AGA GAG AAG AAG GAG CGC
TCRBV5-1	ATA CTT CAG TGA GAC ACA GAG AAA C
TCRBV5-2/3	TTC CCT AAC TAT AGC TCT GAG CTG
TCRBV7	CCT GAA TGC CCC AAC AGC TCT C
TCRBV8	ATT TAC TTT AAC AAC AAC GTT CCG
TCRBV9	CCT AAA TCT CCA GAC AAA GCT CAC
TCRBV13-1	CAA GGA GAA GTC CCC AAT
TCRBV13-2	GGT GAG GGT ACA ACT GCC
TCRVB14	GTC TCT CGA AAA GAG AAG AGG AAT
TCRVB16	AAA GAG TCT AAA CAG GAT GAG TCC
TCRBV17	CAG ATA GTA AAT GAC TTT CAG
TCRBV20	AGC TCT GAG GTG CCC CAG AAT CTC
TCRBVw22	AAG TGA TCT TGC GCT GTG TCC CCA
TCR β-reverse	TTC TGA TGG CTC AAA CAC
TCRVα subfamilies	
TCRVA1	GGC ATT AAC GGT TTT GAG GCT GGA
TCRVA2	CAG TGT TCC AGA GGG AGC CAT TGT
TCRVA3	CCG GGC AGC AGA CAC TGC TTC TTA
TCRVA4	TTG GTA TCG ACA GCT TCA CTC CCA
TCRVA5	CGG CCA CCC TGA CCT GCA ACT ATA
TCRVA6	TCC GCC AAC CTT GTC ATC TCC GCT
TCRVA7	GCA ACA TGC TGG CGG AGC ACC CAC
TCRVA8	CAT TCG TTC AAA TGT GGG CAA AAG
TCRVA9	CCA GTA CTC CAG ACA ACG CCT GCA
TCRVA10	CAC TGC GGC CCA GCC TGG TGA TAC
TCRVA11	CGC TGC TCA TCC TCC AGG TGC GGG
TCRVA12	TCG TCG GAA CTC TTT TGA TGA GCA
TCRVA13	TTC ATC AAA ACC CTT GGG GAC AGC
TCRVA14	CCC AGC AGG CAG ATG ATT CTC GTT
TCRVA15	TTG CAG ACA CCG AGA CTG GGG ACT
TCRVA16	TCA ACG TTG CTG AAG GGA ATC CTC
TCRVA17	TGG GAA AGG CCG TGC ATT ATT GAT
TCRVA18	CAG CAC CAA TTT CAC CTG CAG CTT
TCRVA19	ACA CTG GCT GCA ACA GCA TCC AGG

Table 1 *(continued)*

TCRVA20	TCC	CTG	TTT	ATC	CCT	GCC	GAC	AGA
TCRVA21	AGC	AAA	ATT	CAC	CAT	CCC	TGA	GCG
TCRVA22	CCT	GAA	AGC	CAC	GAA	GGC	TGA	TGA
TCRVAw23	TGC	CTC	GCT	GGA	TAA	ATC	ATC	AGG
TCRVAw24	CTG	GAT	GCA	GAC	ACA	AAG	CAG	AGC
TCRVAw25	TGG	CTA	CGG	TAC	AAG	CCG	GAC	CCT
TCRVAw26	AGC	GCA	GCC	ATG	CAG	GCA	TGT	ACC
TCRVAw27	AAG	CCC	GTC	TCA	GCA	CCC	TCC	ACA
TCRVAw28	TGG	TTG	TGC	ACG	AGC	GAG	ACA	CTG
TCRVAw29	GAA	GGG	TGG	AGA	ACA	GAT	GCG	TCG
TCR α reverse	GTT	GCT	CCA	GGC	CGC	GGC	ACT	GTT

5. Thermo-fast 96-well plate (Advanced Biotechnologies, Epsom, Surrey, UK).
6. Mineral oil.
7. Thermocycler.
8. Ready-to-go PCR beads (Amersham).

2.5.4. Polyacrylamide Gel Electrophoresis

1. Electrophoresis set for polyacrylamide gel including 30-cm outer (front) and thermocore (back) plates, Base Runner™, buffer tanks and MBP 3000ETM power pack, plastic spacer between plates (International Biotechnologies, Connecticut).
2. 6% Acrylamide/bisacrylamide, 7 M Urea and [γ^{32}P]ATP-labeled molecular markers (no. VIII: 23–1115 bp) (Boehringer Mannheim).
3. Ammonium persulfate and TEMED (ICN, OH).
4. Shark's tooth comb, to be placed between the top of two plates (CBS Scientific, Del Mar, CA).
5. 3MM chromatography paper (Whatman, Maidstone, UK).
6. X-ray films (purchased from Eastman Kodak or Super Rx, Fuji, Tokyo, Japan).
7. Intensifying screens (NEN, Boston, MA).
8. Curix 60 film processor (Agfa-GeTCRVAert, Munchen, Germany).
9. 1X TBE buffer.

2.5.5. Agarose Gel Electrophoresis

1. Agarose.
2. Ethidium bromide (10 mg/mL) (Gibco/BRL, Grand Island, NY); handle with caution because it is teratogenic.
3. Molecular weight ladder (preferably 50-bp ladder).
4. 10X Tris-acetate-EDTA (TAE) buffer: 400 mM Tris-acetate; 10 mM EDTA, pH 8.3.
5. 6X Loading buffer: 0.25% (w/v) bromophenol blue and 40% (w/v) sucrose in water.
6. Standard gel electrophoresis chamber and power supply.

2.6. Plasmid Cloning

1. Original TACloning Kit (Invitrogen): The linearized vector supplied in this kit ends with single deoxythymidine (dT) residue that allows PCR inserts to ligate efficiently with the vector, since the nontemplate-dependent activity of Taq polymerase adds a single deoxyadenosine to the 39 ends of PCR products.
2. NucleoSpin kit, for plasmid DNA purification (Macherey-Nagel, Duren, Germany).

3. Methods

3.1. Twenty-One-Tube T-Cell Repertoire Screening

1. For each whole-blood sample, label 22 tubes with the first one for IgG1 isotype control and the rest with individual TCRVβ subfamilies.
2. Pipet the reagents into the corresponding tubes: 100 μL of blood, 20 μL from each of the 21 PE-conjugated anti-TCRVβ antibodies, and 10 μL of FITC conjugate anti-CD3.
3. Incubate the cells for 30 min on ice.
4. After washing once in phosphate-buffered saline (PBS), lyse the cells by adding 2 mL of 0.16 M NH_4Cl at room temperature for 10 min.
5. Wash the cells twice in PBS and resuspend in 200 μL of PBS for analysis.

3.2. Eight-Tube T-Cell Repertoire Screening

1. For each whole-blood sample, label 10 tubes (control tubes 1 and 2) and the rest with vials A–H, respectively.
2. Pipet the reagents into the corresponding tubes containing 100 μL of blood with 20 μL from each of the eight vials (A–H), a cocktail of three MAbs specific for three different TCRVβ subfamilies. These three antibodies have been conjugated with either FITC or PE, or both FITC and PE (*see* **Note 2**).
3. Add 10 μL of IgG1 PC5 conjugate and CD3-PC5 to the first and second control tubes, respectively.
4. Add 10 μL of CD3-PC5 to all remaining eight tubes. Incubate the cells for 30 min on ice.
5. After washing once in PBS, lyse the cells by adding 2 mL of 0.16 M NH_4Cl at room temperature for 10 min.
6. Wash the cells twice in PBS and resuspend in 200 μL of PBS for analysis.

3.3. Staining for Expanded T-Cell Sorting

1. Stain Ficoll-separated cells with biotinylated anti-CD8 and incubate on ice for 20 min.
2. After two washes with PBS, add a cocktail of FITC-conjugated anti-CD57, PE-conjugated anti-TCRVβ, and streptavidin conjugated to Alexa Fluor-594.
3. Incubate the cells for a further 20 min on ice.
4. Wash the stained cells once with PBS, resuspend in 200 μL to 1 mL of PBS containing 0.5 μL of RNase inhibitor, and leave on ice until sorting.

3.4. Flow Sorting

T-cells of specific phenotype can be accurately sorted into tubes containing 1 mL of culture medium with 0.5 μL of RNase inhibitor. For instance, CD57$^+$TCRVβ$^+$ CD8$^+$ and CD57$^-$TCRVβ$^+$CD8$^+$ cells can be sorted into two separate tubes containing RPMI-10 medium. The tubes are kept cool during the sort by means of a FACStar Plus Cytometer (Becton Dickinson).

3.5. Preparation of cDNA Using Commercial Kit

The QuickPrep Micro mRNA Purification Kit with oligo-dT cellulose is used to obtain mRNA from approx 10^3–10^4 sorted cells (Pharmacia). Briefly, the entire procedure can be divided into four main steps: (1) preparation of oligo-dT cellulose, (2) binding of the prepared oligo(dT) cellulose to the cleared cellular homogenate containing the mRNA, (3) multiple washings of the oligo(dT) cellulose in high- and then low-salt buffer solutions to remove unwanted DNA and protein, and (4) elution with prewarmed (65°C) elution buffer to retrieve mRNA.

cDNA is then prepared by means of the T-primed First-Strand Kit, which uses Moloney murine leukemia virus reverse transcriptase and an oligo-dT primer to generate full-length first-strand cDNA from the mRNA template. The cDNA should be stored at –70°C until in vitro amplification of TCR genes.

3.6. Preparation of cDNA Using In-House Methodology for Small Number of Cells

A convenient in-house RNA extraction and cDNA preparation for a small number of cells has been developed.

1. After sorting, transfer the culture medium containing the sorted cells to an Eppendorf tube.
2. Spin the tube at a low setting or 6000g at 4°C for 5 min.
3. Carefully remove the supernatant; no pellet can be seen normally with the small number of sorted cells.
4. Vortex to loosen the pellet.
5. Prepare GUT buffer by pipetting 7.2 μL of mercaptoethanol in 500 μL of guanidinium stock solution.
6. Resuspend the cells in 500 μL of GUT buffer, and use a 26-gage needle for further mixing by drawing up and down 10 times.
7. Add the following sequentially with mixing after each addition: 50 μL of Na acetate (2 M), 500 μL of pheno phase, and 500 μL of chloroform.
8. Vortex the tubes thoroughly for 15 s and incubate on ice for 15 min.
9. Spin the tube at high speed or 10,000g for 10 min at 4°C.
10. Transfer the water (upper) phase to a new tube, and measure the volume (~400 μL).
11. Add 4 μL of glycogen and mix well.

12. Add an equal volume (~400 μL) of isopropanol at –20°C and mix well.
13. Store the tube at –20°C for at least 2 h and preferably overnight.
14. The next day, centrifuge the tube at 15,000g at 4°C for 20 min.
15. Pour off the supernatant and wipe the inside of the tube with a cotton tip but avoid contact with the pellet, which is very often visible as a semitranslucent pellet. Leave the tube on ice.
16. Wash once with 1 mL of 75% alcohol, and spin for 5 min at 15,000g at 4°C. Remove the supernatant again.
17. Allow the pellet to dry on ice for at least 10 min.
18. Resuspend the pellet in RNase-free water with 0.5 μL of RNase inhibitor, and store at –70°C until cDNA synthesis.

3.7. Radioactive PCR Methodology

In vitro amplification of TCR genes is performed with a reverse primer specific for the constant region, which is common to all rearranged β-chain genes, and the forward primer is specific for the variable region of the corresponding Vβ subfamily (**Table 1**). The reverse primer is radioactively end labeled in a solution consisting of 27 MBq (0.73 μCi/mL) of [γ-^{32}P]ATP, and 2.3 μM of T4 polynucleotide kinase (9.6 × 10^2 U/mL). The PCR reaction mix also contains the following components at the final concentrations listed: 2.3 mM forward primer; 0.38 mM deoxy-ATP (dATP), dCTP, dTTP, and dGTP; a 1-in-5 dilution of the 10X PCR reaction buffer with either 1.5 or 3 mM MgCl$_2$; and 0.01 U of Taq polymerase. Five microliters of PCR reaction mix is added to each well of a Thermo-fast 96-well plate containing 5 μL of cDNA. The mixture is then overlaid with 25 μL of mineral oil. PCR amplification is performed in a thermal cycler (Hybaid, Ashford, UK) by means of the following thermocycling protocol: initial denaturation at 95°C for 5 min; followed by 45 cycles of 95°C for 30 s, 55°C for 30 s, and 72°C for 1 min; with a final extension at 72°C for 7 min.

A typical radioactive PCR assay contains the following for ten 10-μL reactions (*see* **Note 3**):

1. Part 1—Preparation of radioactive labeled reverse primer: 2 μL (equivalent to 514 pmol for 10 reactions) of constant-3′(50OD), 3 μL of water, 0.65 μL of 10X polynucleotide kinase buffer, and 0.50 μL of ^{32}P-ATP, for a total of 6.55 μL.
2. Part 2—Preparation of the reaction mix: approx 2 to 3 μL (equivalent to 514 pmol, depending on the specific oligos) of forward primer (50OD); 10.2 μL of 10X PCR buffer with 1.5 mM MgCl$_2$; 0.65 μL of 10X polynucleotide kinase buffer; 15.5 μL of dNTPs; 0.5 μL of Taq polymerase; and approx 15 to 16 μL of water, depending on the volume of forward primer added, for a total of 51.45 μL.

3.8. Preparation of Denaturing Polyacrylamide Gel

1. Make a 50-mL solution containing 6% acrylamide/bisacrylamide (37.5:1 ratio), 7 *M* urea, and 1X TBE in triple distilled water. Filter the solution to remove undissolved urea.
2. For polymerization to occur, add 250 µL of 25% ammonium persulfate and 25 µL of TEMED to the gel solution prior to pouring.
3. Pour the gel solution onto the hydrophobic side of a horizontally level thermocore plate (*see* **Note 4**).
4. Slowly lower the outer plate, spreading the gel solution evenly between the thermocore plate and the outer plate.
5. Clamp the plates together and place a plastic spacer 1 cm into the top of the gel between the plates.
6. Once the gel has polymerized, remove the spacer and clamps, and place the plates on a Base Runner along with the top and bottom buffer tanks, both filled with 1X TBE buffer.
7. Initially prewarm the gel by running it at a current of 20 W for 10 min.
8. Clean the top surface of the gel with a 1-mL pipet using the 1X TBE running buffer.
9. Place a shark's tooth comb between the top of the two plates until it just makes contact with the polyacrylamide gel.

3.9. CDR3 Length Analysis Using Polyacrylamide Gel Electrophoresis (see Note 5)

1. Before loading onto the polyacrylamide gel, dilute the radioactive PCR products twofold with sequencing gel loading buffer and denature for 5 min at 95°C in a thermal cycler, and then snap-chill on ice.
2. To allow estimation of PCR band sizes, electrophorese $[\gamma\text{-}^{32}P]$ATP-labeled molecular weight markers (no. VIII) on the same gel.
3. Electrophorese the PCR products at 900 V for approx 3 h.
4. Following electrophoresis, transfer the gels to 3MM chromatography paper, cover in plastic wrap, and directly expose to X-OMAT AR scientific imaging film overnight at –70°C by means of intensifying screens.
5. Develop the film in a Curix 60 film processor.

3.10. Direct Sequencing of PCR Products of Specific TCRVβ Subfamilies

To obtain PCR products of specific TCRVβ subfamilies for DNA sequencing, PCR is performed with the use of cDNA samples with Ready-to-go PCR beads (Amersham). The PCR amplification conditions are similar to those described previously except that no radioactive label is used.

3.11. Purification of Transformant Plasmid DNA

Where direct sequencing fails, the Original TA Cloning Kit is used to clone the PCR products in plasmid vectors according to the manufacturer's protocol.

1. Pick a few isolated white transformants individually and allow to grow for 12 h at 37°C in 5 mL of Luria-Bertani medium containing 50 mg/mL of ampicillin in a rotary shaking incubator at 225 rpm.
2. Purify the plasmid DNA with a NucleoSpin kit.
3. Perform DNA sequencing employing dye-terminator chemistry with M13 forward and reverse primers on the extracted plasmid DNA.

4. Notes

1. The cutoff point for "expanded" expression of a particular TCRVβ as well as the total coverage of the TCR repertoire by the antibody panels has TCRVA varied among different studies. We have adopted the strict criterion for the expansion based on a cutoff point of the mean plus three standard deviations of the percentage of cells expressing each TCRVβ in our aged-matched control group. The limits for "expanded" TCRVβ expressions are, however, always arbitrary and may include some mildly increased normal T-cell populations in the category of abnormal ones. Clonal T-cells have also been found in healthy individuals *(2)*.
2. The eight-tube anti-TCRVβ panel is a simple and fast repertoire analysis. It aims at reducing the number of tubes required by combining three TCRVβ-specific reagents in a single test but with only two colors. The method is to have one TCRVβ antibody conjugated to FITC, another one to PE, and the third one to both FITC and PE. In this way, the third TCRVβ-stained population shows up in the diagonal of the quadrant 2 in an FL1/FL2 histogram. The stained samples should be acquired within 24 h if stored at 2–8°C in the dark, but optimally within 2 h. For compensation setup, control tube 1 is used for FL1/FL2 compensations in order to obtain optimal compensations of TCRVβ values for the TCRVβ antibody staining, and the FL2/FL4 compensation should be done on control tube 2 for the optimal compensation setting for the antibody used in the third color.
3. It is easiest to make a master mix of all components for the number of tubes except the forward primer because it is different for different expansions. It is also feasible to prepare stock with allowance for an extra 15–20% (i.e., prepare mix for six tubes although you will be pipetting for only five reactions later on).
4. The thermocore plate can be coated with Rain-XTM (Uneldo, Scottsdale, AZ) on one side to produce a hydrophobic surface. The plate should be cleaned with tap water, distilled water, and then with absolute alcohol before coating.
5. We and others have previously shown that cells within the expanded TCRVβ⁺ populations preferentially express CD57, compared with cells within TCRVβ⁺ populations of normal size *(2,4)*. Thus, expression of CD57 will subdivide potential clonal T-cell expansions and the polyclonal population of normal T-cells expressing the "expanded" TCRVβ. In all six MM samples examined, the CD57⁺ T-cells expressing the "expanded" TCRVβ subsets were mono- or biclonal

whereas the CD57⁻ cells were usually polyclonal. The monoclonality of CD57⁺ cells was confirmed by direct DNA sequencing of the PCR product generated by the CDR3 length analysis **(Fig. 1)**. By contrast, cloning and sequencing of the PCR products from the CD57⁻ sorted T-cells gave an array of sequences, indicative of a polyclonal population.

References

1. Raitakari, M., Brown, R. D., Sze, D. M., et al. (2000) T-cell expansions in patients with multiple myeloma have a phenotype of cytotoxic T cells. *Br. J. Haematol.* **110,** 203–209.
2. Sze, D. M.-Y., Giesajtis, G., Brown, R. D., et al. (2001) Clonal cytotoxic T cells are expanded in myeloma and reside in the CD8+CD57+CD28– compartment. *Blood* **98,** 2817–2827.
3. Brown, R. D., Pope, B., Murray, A., et al. (2001) Dendritic cells from patients with myeloma renumerically normal but functionally defective as they fail to upregulate CD80 (B7-1) expression after huCD40LT stimulation due to inhibition by TGF-β1 and IL-10. *Blood* **98,** 2992–2998.
4. Sze, D. M.-Y., Brown, R. D., Yuen, E., et al. (2003) Clonal cytotoxic T cells in myeloma. *Leuk. Lymphoma* **44,** 1667–1674.

21

Detecting Mismatch Repair Defects in Myeloma

Mark Velangi, Elizabeth Matheson, Andrew Hall, and Julie Irving

Summary

Defects in the mismatch repair system are associated with a microsatellite unstable phenotype. In this chapter, we describe the preparation of purified plasma cells using CD138 magnetic microbeads as a source of tumor DNA. We also describe a robust, sensitive method for comparing microsatellite repeat units of tumor to constitutive DNA using polymerase chain reaction and laser scanning of fluorescently labeled amplicons in an automated sequencer in order to assess microsatellite instability in myeloma.

Key Words

Mismatch repair; microsatellite instability; multiple myeloma; capillary electrophoresis; microsatellite analysis.

1. Introduction

During each cell division, the accurate replication of approx 3 billion nucleotides is required to maintain genetic stability. The fidelity of this process is remarkably high: mispairing occurs in normal cells at a frequency of only about 1 in every 2 million bp and is achieved by the proofreading abilities of DNA polymerases and a complex postreplicative mismatch repair pathway (*1*). The components of this pathway detect mismatches and insertion/deletion loops that may arise and initiate degradation and repair of the error-containing strand, improving the fidelity of DNA replication by more than 10-fold. In human cells, the most important proteins appear to be MSH2, MSH3, MSH6, MLH1, and PMS2 (*2*).

There are several approaches to assess the integrity of the mismatch repair pathway. Expression of components of the pathway at either the mRNA or protein level by Western blotting, immunocytochemistry, or immunohistochemistry can be performed. Functional assays include an in vitro assessment of the

From: *Methods in Molecular Medicine, Vol. 113: Multiple Myeloma: Methods and Protocols*
Edited by: R. D. Brown and P. J. Ho © Humana Press Inc., Totowa, NJ

ability of cellular lysates to recognize and repair a heteroduplex and can be performed in both cell lines and clinical material but require large numbers of cells *(3)*. An alternative functional method is to assess the integrity of microsatellites, intergenic sequences with a minimal repetitive unit of 1–5 bp. These polymorphisms are stable during the lifetime of an organism but are more susceptible to slippage of the replication polymerases owing to their repetitive sequences. If slippage occurs in a cell that is mismatch repair deficient, the ensuing insertion/deletion loop is not repaired and the error at the microsatellite is propagated through future cell generations. Thus, microsatellite instability (MSI) is regarded as a hallmark of defective mismatch repair (MMR) *(4–7)*. Fluorescently labeled polymerase chain reaction (PCR) and laser scanning is a sensitive method to assay the integrity of microsatellites in small numbers of tumor cells *(8)*.

2. Materials

1. Ficoll, for density centrifugation.
2. Phosphate-buffered saline (PBS), pH 7.2.
3. May-Grunwald Giemsa (MGG) staining reagents.
4. CD138 Microbeads (Miltenyi Biotec, Bisley). Store at 4°C protected from light.
5. Midimacs magnetic cell separator (Miltenyi Biotec).
6. Magnetic activated cell sorting (MACS) buffer: PBS, pH 7.2, with 0.5% bovine serum albumin and 2 mM EDTA. Use chilled.
7. Midimacs positive selection columns (LS+) (Miltenyi Biotec).
8. Qiamp DNA mini kit (Qiagen).
9. Primer sets: The forward primer of each pair is fluorescently labeled at the 5′ end with a WellRed dye (either D3 or D4) (Research Genetics, Huntsville, AL) (**Table 1**). Store at –20°C protected from light. Aliquot into smaller volumes to reduce multiple freeze-thawing cycles.
10. *Taq* polymerase (Amplitaq Gold) with 10X buffer and $MgCl_2$. Store at –20°C.
11. dNTPs.
12. PCR plates or tubes.
13. Mineral oil.
14. 96-Well plates.
15. Sample loading solution (Beckman Coulter): This contains deionized formamide, which is classified as an R61 compound; that is, it may cause harm to an unborn child.
16. WellRed Dye 1 400-bp standard. Store at –20°C protected from light.

3. Methods

3.1. Preparation of Sample

3.1.1. Source of Constitutive DNA

The absence or low incidence (<5%) of plasma cells (PCs) in the peripheral blood of patients with multiple myeloma (MM) means that this can serve as an appropriate source of "tumor-free" constitutive DNA.

Table 1
Details of Loci, Repeat Type, Range of Amplicon Size,
and Primer Sequences Used for Microsatellite Analyses

Locus	Map	Repeat	Size (bp)	Primer sequence (5′–3′)
BAT 25	4q12	(T)25	~128	TCG CCT CCA AGA ATG TAA GT
				TCT GCA TTT TAA CTA TGG CTC
BAT 26	2p	(A)26	~122	TGA CTA CTT TTG ACT TCA GCC
				AAC CAT TCA ACA TTT TTA ACC C
BAT 40	1p13.1	(T)40	~129	ATT AAC TTC CTA CAC CAC AAC
				GTA GAG CAA GAC CAC CTT G
D5S346	5q21	(CA)26	111–127	ACT CAC TCT AGT GAT AAA TCG
				AGC AGA TAA GAC AGT ATT ACT AGT T
D17S250	17q11	(CA)24	151–169	GGA AGA ATC AAA TAG ACA AT
				GCT GGC CAT ATA TAT ATT TAA ACC
D10S197	10q	(CA)12	161–173	ACC ACT GCA CTT CAG GTG AC
				GTG ATA CTG TCC TCA GGT CTC C
D18S69	18q21	(CA)14	174–189	CTC TTT CTC TGA CTC TGA CC
				GAC TTT CTA AGT TCT TGC CAG
D2S123	2p16	(CA)15	197–227	AAA CAG GAT GCC TGC CTT TA
				GGA CTT TCC ACC TAT GGG AC
MYCL1	1p32	(GAAA)14	169–205	TGG CGA GAC TCC ATC AAA G
				CTT TTT AAG CTG CAA CAA TTT C

[a]Forward primers appear first and reverse primers appear last for each locus.

1. Enrich peripheral blood samples for mononuclear cells by standard density gradient centrifugation.
2. Prepare cytospins and stain with MGG by standard methods, and examine by light microscopy to confirm the absence or low incidence of PCs (*see* **Note 1**).

3.1.2. Source of Tumor DNA

Syndecans are a family of cell-surface proteoglycans of which syndecan-1 is the predominant member. Syndecan-1, also known as CD138, is expressed on normal and malignant PCs and is recognized by the monoclonal antibody B-B4 *(9)*. Thus, superparamagnetic microbeads conjugated to B-B4 allow magnetic cell sorting of PCs.

1. Spin down mononuclear cell suspension and then resuspend in 90 μL of MACS buffer/5×10^6 total cells. For fewer cells, use the same volume.
2. Add 10 μL of CD138 MACS MicroBeads for each 5×10^6 total cells, mix well, and incubate for 15 min at 6–12°C. A shelf in a refrigerator door is appropriate. Again, for fewer cells, still use 10 μL of beads.
3. Wash the cells by adding 10–20 times the labeling volume of buffer, centrifuge at 400*g* for 10 min, completely remove the supernatant, and resuspend the cell pellet in 1 mL of MACS buffer.

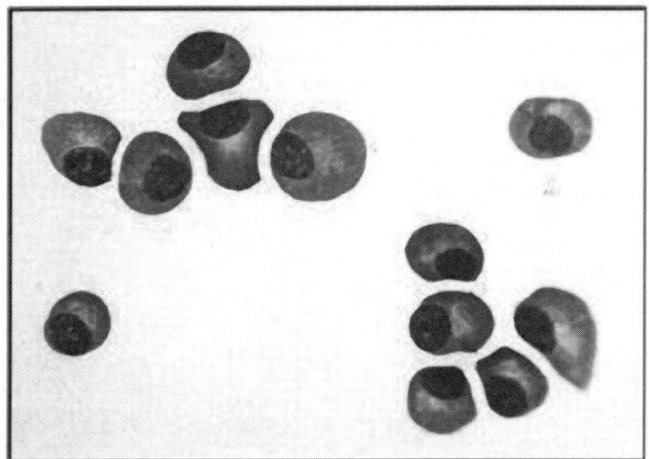

Fig. 1. MGG-stained cytospin preparation of PCs purified from a diagnostic bone marrow aspirate of a patient with myeloma using CD138 magnetic microbeads.

4. Place an LS-separation column with an adapter in a MidiMACS separation magnet. Add 3 mL of MACS buffer to the top of the column for equilibration. Discard the effluent.
5. Pipet the magnetically labeled cell suspension onto the top of the column and allow to run through. Wash with 3 mL of buffer four times. The effluent can be retained as the negative fraction but may have a significant number of PCs.
6. Remove the column from the magnet, pipet 5 mL of MACS buffer, and flush the CD138$^+$ retained cells using the plunger supplied with the column.
7. Spin down the CD138$^+$ cells, count, and prepare cytospin for MGG staining. Assess the purity of the PC preparation morphologically using a light microscope. **Figure 1** shows MACS purified PCs with their characteristic eccentric nucleus and perinuclear halo. Store the remaining cells as pellets at –80°C.

3.2. DNA Extraction From Cell Pellets

1. Extract DNA from paired patient peripheral blood mononuclear cells and CD138$^+$ purified cells using a DNA Minikit (Qiagen) according to the manufacturer's instructions.
2. Estimate the yield and purity by spectrophotometric absorbance at 260 and 280 nm (*see* **Note 2**).

3.3. Microsatellite Analysis

3.3.1. Polymerase Chain Reaction

Since its inception as a technique for the production of large quantities of DNA from few copies of template DNA *(10)*, PCR is now an important molecular biological tool. The PCR reaction uses short synthetic primers to amplify a specific DNA sequence through multiple rounds of denaturation, annealing, and elongation.

3.3.1.1. PCR Setup

1. To avoid inaccuracies associated with pipetting small volumes, combine all reaction components except sample DNA in a PCR master mix as shown in **Table 2.** Prepare sufficient mix for at least one extra volume. Add *Taq* polymerase last, and mix well by inversion or gentle vortexing.
2. Aliquot 24 µL into each reaction tube or well. Add a minimum of 5 ng of sample DNA. A well with no DNA added serves as a reagent blank. Matched constitutive and tumor DNA pairs should be amplified and analyzed in the same run.
3. Place into a thermal cycler and run the program as shown in **Table 3** (*see* **Notes 3** and **4**).

3.3.2. Capillary Gel Electrophoresis

The CEQ 8000 is a fully automated genetic analysis system (Beckman Coulter). The system automatically fills an eight-well capillary array with a linear polyacrylamide gel, denatures, loads fluorescently labeled PCR product, applies the voltage program, and analyzes the data. The separated amplicons are detected by ultraviolet absorbance and laser-induced fluorescence. Automatic calculation of fragment sizes can be achieved by the use of a dye 1-labeled internal size calibration standard added to each PCR product.

3.3.2.1. Sample Loading

1. Add 0.5–1 µL of labeled PCR product to 40 µL of sample loading solution and 0.5–1 µL of size standard-400 (Beckman Coulter) labeled with WellRed dye 1-PA.
2. Transfer the samples onto a 96-well plate and cover with one drop of mineral oil.
3. Load the plate onto a CEQ 8000 Genetic Analysis System and run on the frag-3 program, which is appropriate for the size range of amplicons generated with these primers. The Frag-3 parameters are as follows:
   a. Capillary: temperature (50°C), wait for temperature (yes).
   b. Denature: temperature (90°C), duration (120 s).
   c. Inject: voltage (2 kV), duration (30 s).
   d. Separation: voltage (6 kV), duration 35 min.
4. Analyze the data with fragment analysis software.

Positive MSI is characterized by the appearance of a novel-sized allele in the tumor DNA sample that is absent in the matched constitutive sample. Loss of an allele in the tumor sample compared to constitutive is regarded as complete loss of heterozygosity (LOH). Examples of MSI and LOH in samples from patients with myeloma are shown in **Fig. 2** (*see* **Notes 5–7**).

Table 2
PCR Setup for Microsatellite Analyses

Reagent	Initial concentration	Final concentration/ amount	Volume for single 25-μL reaction	Master mix for 50 tubes
10X buffer	10X	1X	2.5 μL	127.5 μL
MgCl$_2$	25 μM	3 mM	3 μL	153 μL
dNTP	12.5 μM	125 μM	0.25 μL	12.75 μL
Forward primer	20 μM	0.2 μM	0.3	15.3 μL
Reverse primer	20 μM	0.2 μM	0.3	15.3 μL
Water			17.525	893.775 μL
Amplitaq Gold	5 U/μL	0.625	0.125	6.375 μL
DNA	Minimum of 5 ng/μL	5 ng	1 μL	Add 24-μL aliquots to each reaction tube/well

Table 3
Thermal Cycling Program for Microsatellite PCR

Initial incubation step	Melt	Anneal	Extend	Final extension	Final step
Hold at 95°C for 10 min	30 cycles at 95°C for 45 sec	30 cycles at 57°C for 45 sec	30 cycles at 72°C for 1 min	Hold at 72°C for 7 min	Hold at 4°C for infinity

4. Notes

1. For assessment of MSI at more advanced stages of MM or of PC leukemia when PCs may spill over into the peripheral circulation, consider positive selection of T-cells using CD3 MACS beads or depletion of CD138-expressing cells using the MACS method (see MACS information sheet). Alternatively, obtain buccal mucosa samples as a source of constitutive DNA.

2. In our experience, the mean PC yield from a standard bone marrow aspirate from a patient with myeloma at presentation (~2 mL) is about 7×10^5 cells, with a purity invariably >90%. The DNA yields from these preparations range from 25 to 1500 ng.

3. Failed amplification is most commonly owing to an excess of DNA causing substrate inhibition.

4. Theoretically, treatment of the PCR products with T4 DNA polymerase with its 3′ exonuclease activity should remove additional bases added by *Taq* polymerase during the PCR and, thus, should reduce the number of product species and simplify analyses, particularly of mononucleotide repeats (*11*). However, we have not found this additional procedure to be beneficial in our laboratory.

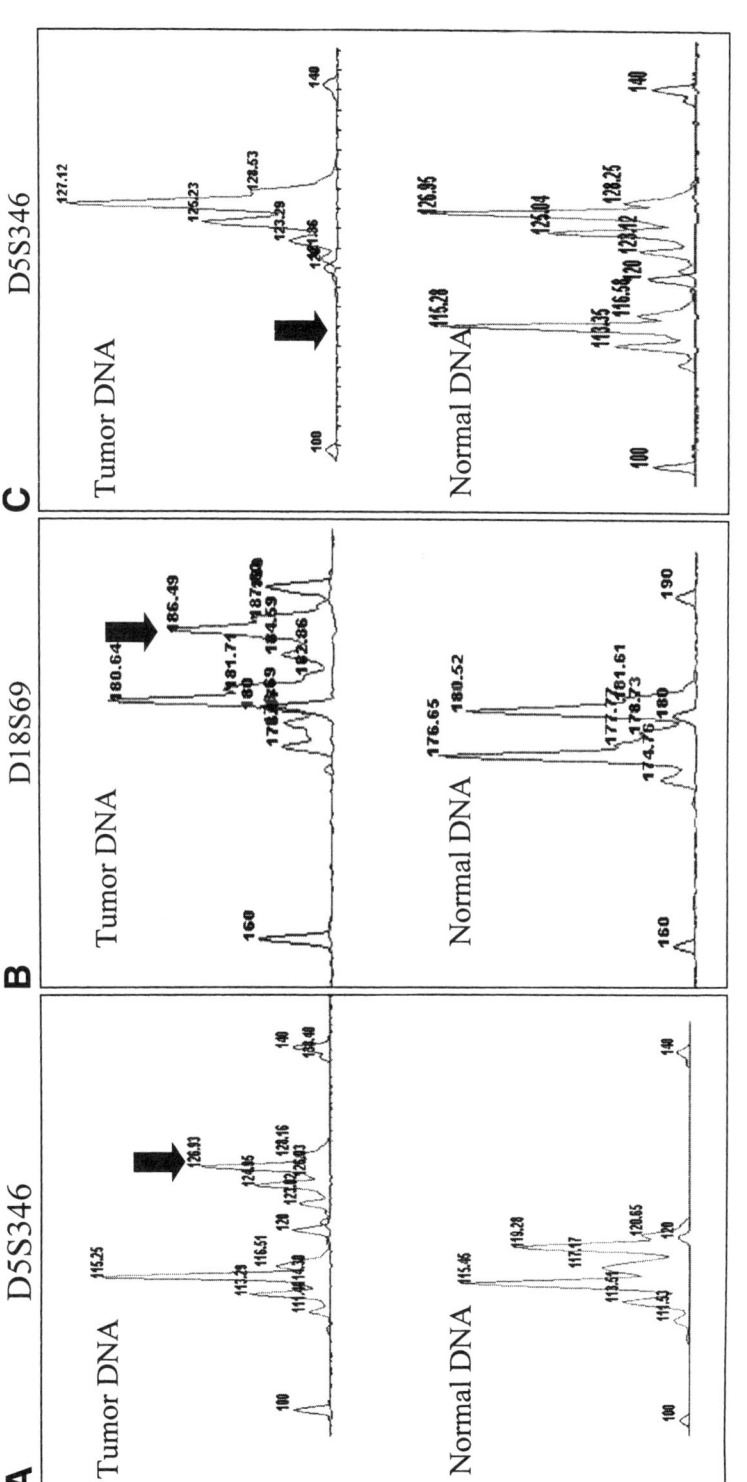

Fig. 2. Electrophoretograms of paired constitutive and tumor DNA from patients with myeloma showing gain of extra allele in tumor compared to constitutive at D5S346 and D18S69 loci (**A**,**B**) indicative of MSI and showing complete loss of allele in tumor compared to constitutive DNA at D5S346 locus (**C**),indicative of LOH.

5. Samples showing MSI should always be confirmed by repeating both the PCR and capillary electrophoresis steps. Disparate results may occur owing to *Taq* polymerase errors in early cycle numbers or migration errors during electrophoresis. In our experience, the reproducibility of this technique is excellent, but disparities have occurred, although they are rare.

6. Maehara et al. *(8)* describe well the identification of MSI and the theoretical patterns that can be generated and highlight the problem of more subtle changes in electrophoretic profiles owing to low levels of MSI-positive cells. In our hands, interpretation of microsatellite analyses of myeloma samples and classification of MSI were relatively straightforward, probably owing to the almost pure tumor cell preparations used.

7. Although the diagnostic criteria for MSI are well defined for the study of hereditary nonpolyposis colorectal cancer (HNPCC), there are few guidelines for other tumors *(12,13)*. Recently, it was proposed that evidence for instability at one or more loci in a set of more than five selected microsatellites is a criterion for positive MSI in other tumors *(8)*. Thus, our approach to the assessment of MMR function in myeloma is to screen 9 of the 10 loci recommended for HNPCC and consider instability at one or more of these loci a significant finding.

Acknowledgment

We gratefully acknowledge the Leukaemia Research Fund for supporting this work.

References

1. Tindall, K. R., Glaab, W. E., Umar, A., et al. (1998) Complementation of mismatch repair gene defects by chromosome transfer. *Mutat. Res.* **402**, 15–22.
2. Peltomaki, P. (2003) Role of DNA mismatch repair defects in the pathogenesis of human cancer. *J. Clin. Oncol.* **15**, 1174–1179.
3. Matheson, E. C. and Hall, A. G. (2003) Assessment of mismatch repair function in leukaemic cell lines and blasts from children with acute lymphoblastic leukaemia. *Carcinogenesis* **24**, 31–38.
4. Aaltonen, L. A., Peltomaki, P., Leach, F. S., et al. (1993) Clues to the pathogenesis of familial colorectal cancer. *Science* **260**, 812–816.
5. Peltomaki, P., Lothe, R. A., Aaltonen, L. A., et al. (1993) Microsatellite instability is associated with tumors that characterize the hereditary non-polyposis colorectal carcinoma syndrome. *Cancer Res.* **53**, 5853–5855.
6. Leach, F. S., Nicolaides, N. C., Papadopoulos, N., et al. (1993) Mutations of a mutS homolog in hereditary nonpolyposis colorectal cancer. *Cell* **75**, 1215–1225.
7. Fishel, R., Lescoe, M. K., Rao, M. R., et al. (1993) The human mutator gene homolog MSH2 and its association with hereditary nonpolyposis colon cancer. *Cell* **75**, 1027–1038.
8. Maehara, Y., Oda, S., and Sugimachi, K. (2001) The instability within: problems in current analyses of microsatellite instability. *Mutat. Res.* **461**, 249–263.

9. Wijdenes, J., Vooijs, W. C, Clement, C., et al. (1996) A plasmocyte selective monoclonal antibody (B-B4) recognizes syndecan-1. *Br. J. Haematol.* **94,** 318–323.

10. Mullis, K. B. and Faloona, F. A. (1987) Specific synthesis of DNA in vitro via a polymerase-catalyzed chain reaction. *Methods Enzymol.* **155,** 335–350.

11. Ginot, F., Bordelais, I., Nguyen, S., and Gyapay, G. (1996) Correction of some genotyping errors in automated fluorescent microsatellite analysis by enzymatic removal of one base overhangs. *Nucleic Acids Res.* **1,** 540–541.

12. Boland, C. R., Thibodeau, S. N., Hamilton, S. R., et al. (1998) A National Cancer Institute Workshop on Microsatellite Instability for cancer detection and familial predisposition: development of international criteria for the determination of microsatellite instability in colorectal cancer. *Cancer Res.* **58,** 5248–5257.

13. Bocker, T., Diermann, J., Friedl, W., et al. (1997) Microsatellite instability analysis: a multicenter study for reliability and quality control. *Cancer Res.* **57,** 4739–4743.

22

Methylation-Specific Polymerase Chain Reaction

Oliver Galm and James G. Herman

Summary

Methylation-specific polymerase chain reaction (MSP) is a method that can rapidly assess the methylation status of virtually any group of CpG sites within a CpG island, independent of the use of methylation-sensitive restriction enzymes. This assay entails the initial modification of DNA by sodium bisulfite, converting all unmethylated cytosines to uracils but leaving the methylated cytosines unchanged, followed by subsequent amplification with primers specific for methylated vs unmethylated DNA. The great sensitivity of this technique allows qualitative methylation analysis from DNA obtained not only from fresh frozen tissues, peripheral blood, bone marrow, or body fluids but also from paraffin-embedded samples. It is a rapid and cost-effective method that does not require radioactive reagents and can be used for the analysis of a large number of clinical samples.

Key Words

DNA methylation; epigenetics; gene silencing; transcriptional repression; tumor suppressor gene; bisulfite treatment; methylation-specific polymerase chain reaction; tumor marker.

1. Introduction

1.1. Background

Multiple myeloma (MM) is a B-cell neoplasm that is characterized by the accumulation of malignant plasma cells (PCs) in the bone marrow. Previous molecular studies have largely focused on the analysis of genetic aberrations in MM. Important changes include chromosomal translocations involving the immunoglobulin heavy chain locus on chromosome 14q32 and various partner genes such as cyclin D1, cyclin D3, fibroblast growth factor receptor 3, and c-maf, as well as mutations of N-ras and K-ras. The accumulation of genetic events is thought to be crucial for the malignant transformation of PCs (1–3). In recent years, there has been increasing evidence that, in addition to those genetic aberrations, epigenetic processes play a major role in carcinogenesis.

From: *Methods in Molecular Medicine, Vol. 113: Multiple Myeloma: Methods and Protocols*
Edited by: R. D. Brown and P. J. Ho © Humana Press Inc., Totowa, NJ

The term *epigenetics* refers to the inheritance of information based on gene expression, which—in contrast to genetic information—is not transmitted on the basis of gene sequence. A major epigenetic modification in humans is DNA methylation at cytosines located 5′ to guanosines. CpG dinucleotides have been depleted from the eukaryotic genome owing to the conversion of methylcytosine to uracil. Most remaining CpGs are methylated. However, there are CpG-rich regions termed *CpG islands*, which are often located near the promoter regions of approx 50% of human genes and normally are unmethylated *(4,5)*. This lack of methylation allows expression of the gene if the appropriate transcription factors are present and the chromatin structure allows access to them. DNA methylation plays an important role in genomic imprinting and X-chromosome inactivation and is essential for normal mammalian development *(6–8)*. **Figure 1** shows the structure of a typical CpG island. Aberrant regional hypermethylation of CpG islands within promoter regions of tumor suppressor genes is associated with transcriptional inactivation and represents an important mechanism of gene silencing in the pathogenesis of neoplasia. This process may act as an alternative to genetic alterations such as mutations or deletions to disrupt tumor suppressor gene function *(4,5)*. A large number of different pathways have been shown to be affected by aberrant hypermethylation in carcinogenesis. These comprise cell-cycle control (p16[INK4a], p15[INK4b], p14[ARF], Rb), DNA damage repair (hMLH1, O[6]MGMT, GSTπ, BRCA1), regulation of apoptosis (death-associated protein [DAP]-kinase), cell invasion (E-cadherin, adenomatosis polyposis coli, tissue inhibitor of metalloproteinase-3), as well as growth factor and cytokine response (estrogen receptor, retinoic acid receptor-β, suppressor of cytokine signaling [SOCS]-1). There is emerging evidence that the methylation profile of individual cancer types might have important prognostic implications for clinical monitoring, risk assessment, and even therapeutic considerations *(9–13)*. Furthermore, in clinical trials, the demethylating drugs 5-aza-2′-deoxycytidine and 5-azacytidine have been shown to be effective in patients with acute leukemia, myelodysplastic syndrome, and chronic myelogenous leukemia *(14–17)*.

Recent reports have identified hypermethylation of p16[INK4a], p15[INK4b], DAP-kinase, and SOCS-1 in MM cell lines and patient samples *(18–21)*, demonstrating that epigenetic events represent an additional mechanism of gene inactivation in the pathogenesis of MM.

1.2. Methods for Methylation Analysis

Various methods have been developed to analyze the methylation status of DNA regions. In earlier studies, methylation patterns at individual CpG sites were assessed by digestion of genomic DNA with methylation-sensitive restriction enzymes followed by Southern blotting *(22)*. However, this approach requires large amounts of high molecular weight DNA, and information about

Normal cell

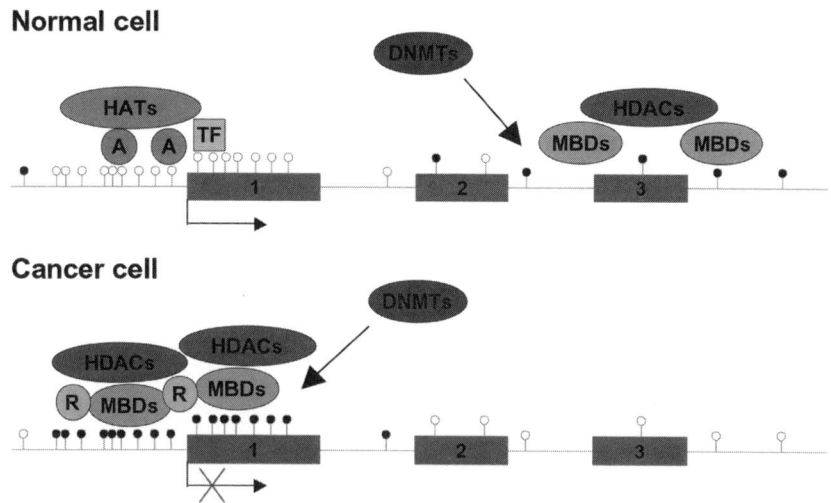

Cancer cell

Fig. 1. A typical CpG island near the transcription start of a tumor suppressor gene is schematically shown in a normal and a cancer cell. The CpG island is constituted by a CpG-rich region that in normal cells is mostly unmethylated (open circles), while the downstream areas within the body of the gene and more 3′ show a lower frequency of CpG dinucleotides. Those downstream CpGs are usually methylated (solid circles). This methylation pattern allows the gene to be actively transcribed. In a cancer cell, the CpG island is hypermethylated and transcriptionally silenced, whereas the downstream areas are hypomethylated. Numbered boxes represent exons 1–3. Each "lollipop" indicates a CpG dinucleotide; open circles represent unmethylated cytosines, and solid circles represent methylated cytosines. HATs, histone acetyltransferases; A, transcriptional activators; TF, transcription factors; DNMTs, DNA methyltransferases; MBD, methyl-binding proteins; HDACs, histone deacetylases; R, transcriptional repressors.

DNA methylation is restricted to methylation-sensitive enzyme recognition sites.

Most newer techniques utilize initial sodium bisulfite treatment of genomic DNA to distinguish methylated from unmethylated cytosines prior to further analysis. This chemical modification, which converts all unmethylated cytosines into uracils, has become the basis for a variety of techniques to analyze DNA methylation *(23,24)*. Subsequent amplification of bisulfite-converted DNA by polymerase chain reaction (PCR) replaces the uracil residues with thymidines and the 5-methylcytosines with cytosines. Several methods rely on amplifying the bisulfite-converted DNA by primers that anneal at locations that lack CpG dinucleotides in the original genomic sequence. Thus, the primers will amplify the sequence in between independent of its original methylation status. This results in a mixture of different PCR products, which all have the same length but are potentially different in their sequence owing to sites of potential DNA methylation at CpG dinucleotides. These PCR products can then be analyzed by different approaches such as bisulfite sequencing, bisulfite restriction analysis *(25,26)*, methylation-sensitive single nucleotide primer extension *(27)*, or enzymatic regional methylation assay *(28)*. All these techniques yield detailed quantitative information about methylation patterns of a particular DNA region and are widely used in basic and translational research regarding DNA methylation. However, these approaches are rather labor- and cost-intensive, may entail the use of radioactive materials or restriction enzymes, and may require larger amounts of high-quality DNA.

Methylation-specific polymerase chain reaction (MSP) *(29)* has been predominantly used for qualitative gene promoter region methylation analysis of multiple tumor suppressor genes in various human malignancies *(9,21,30–32)*. The MSP approach also includes initial bisulfite treatment of genomic DNA, but the subsequent PCR amplification is performed with two different primer pairs that are specific for either the methylated or the unmethylated sequence.

In this chapter, we describe the MSP technique in more detail, because it is a rapid and simple method for the analysis of CpG island hypermethylation.

1.3. Methylation-Specific Polymerase Chain Reaction

The MSP assay is the most widely used technique for studying the methylation of CpG islands in human cancer. **Figure 2** provides a general outline of the MSP technique. After bisulfite treatment of genomic DNA, the subsequent PCR amplification is performed in two separate reactions with two different primer pairs that are specific for either the methylated or the unmethylated sequence. Primers for MSP analysis are designed to discriminate between methylated and unmethylated alleles after bisulfite treatment and to anneal only to DNA that has been bisulfite converted. **Figure 3** illustrates for a sequence example how the DNA sequence is altered by bisulfite treatment dependent on the methylation status and how the two different MSP primer pairs (U primers are specific only for the unmethylated sequence and M primers only for the methylated sequence) anneal to their respective DNA template. MSP primer design is a critical step, because the amplification of bisulfite-modified DNA is more difficult than of native genomic DNA. Bisulfite treatment leads to partial degradation of DNA and results in DNA strands that are no longer complementary. It is necessary to select one strand in the region of interest (ROI) for the primer design and take into account any unequal distribution of bases between the two DNA strands (one strand is C poor and T rich, and the other one is G poor and A rich). Furthermore, the MSP primers must be designed to be specific for bisulfite-converted DNA in order to avoid unwanted annealing

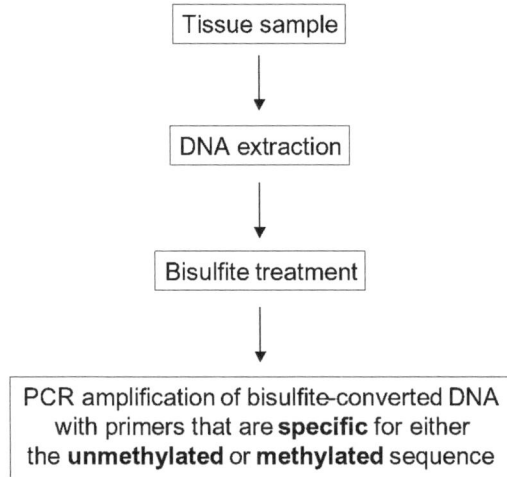

Fig. 2. General outline for MSP procedure. After DNA extraction and bisulfite treatment of genomic DNA, PCR amplification is performed in two separate reactions with two different primer pairs that are specific for either the methylated or the unmethylated sequence.

to unmodified DNA that might be potentially present. To achieve both good sensitivity and specificity, it is often optimal to overlie three CpG dinucleotides within each MSP primer. In the design of M primers, cytosines that are conserved because of their methylation are placed near the 3′ end to increase the specificity of primer annealing. Furthermore, it is advisable to design primers of at least 21–24 bp in length to achieve proper gene specificity. Depending on the DNA source and quality, the total amplicon length should not exceed 200 bp (*see* **Note 1**). When these criteria are taken into account, MSP primers can be designed for the analysis of virtually any DNA sequence.

2. Materials

2.1. Reagents

1. Ammonium acetate, ammonium sulfate, hydroquinone, sodium bisulfite, Tris base, β-mercaptoethanol, deoxynucleotides (dNTPs) (Sigma, St. Louis, MO).
2. *Taq* polymerase (RedTaq, 1 U/μL) (Sigma).
3. Sephadex G-50 minicolumns (BioMax).
4. Wizard DNA cleanup system (Promega A7280; Promega, Madison, WI).
5. *Sss*I methylase (4000 U/mL, includes 32 mM S-adenosylmethionine [SAM] and 10X NE-Buffer 2) (New England Biolabs).
6. 10X PCR buffer stock solution: (166 mM ammonium sulfate; 670 mM Tris, pH 8.8; 67 mM MgCl$_2$; 100 mM β-mercaptoethanol (*see* **Table 1**). Store aliquots at –20°C.

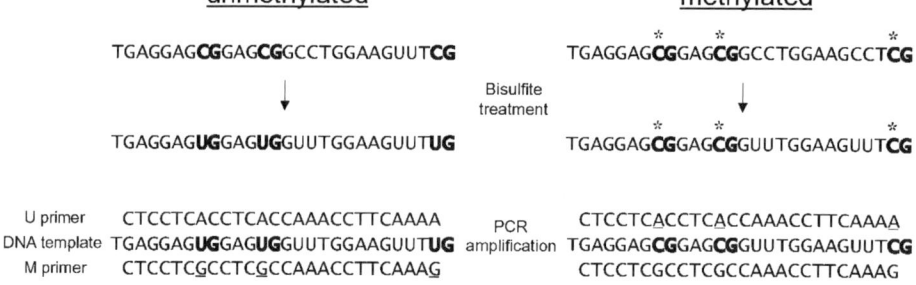

Fig. 3. (**Top**): Effect of bisulfite treatment on a representative DNA sequence dependent on the original methylation status. All cytosines that are not located 5′ to guanosine will be deaminated to uracil. Those cytosines within a CpG dinucleotide that are unmethylated (left) will also be converted into uracils, whereas those cytosines within a CpG dinucleotide that are methylated (right) remain unchanged (bold letters indicate CpG dinucleotides, and asterisks indicate methyl groups). (**Bottom**): Annealing of U and M primers depending on the sequence differences after bisulfite modification. The U primer is specific for the unmethylated sequence (left), whereas the M primer is specific for the methylated sequence (right). Any MSP primer will anneal only to bisulfite-converted DNA, because cytosines not located 5′ to guanosines and thus converted into uracils are also covered by the primer sequence. Thus, the unwanted amplification of possibly unconverted DNA is avoided. Primer mismatches (U vs M primers) are underlined.

7. Final PCR buffer: 16.6 mM ammonium sulfate; 67 mM Tris, pH 8.8; 6.7 mM MgCl$_2$; 10 mM β-mercaptoethanol.

2.2. Equipment

1. Water bath and/or heat block.
2. DNA vacuum drier (e.g., Speed Vac).
3. Vacuum manifold (e.g., Promega A7231).
4. Microcentrifuge.
5. PCR hood.
6. Thermocycler.

3. Methods

3.1. Isolation of Genomic DNA

Genomic DNA can be extracted from cultured cells, primary tissues, or paraffin-embedded sections using standard techniques. The quality of the DNA retrieved from any isolation procedure is crucial for further processing (*see* **Note 1**).

Table 1
10X PCR Buffer Stock Solution

Reagent	Volume (mL)
1 M Ammonium sulfate	16.6
2 M Tris, pH 8.8	33.5
1 M MgCl$_2$	6.7
14.4 M β-Mercaptoethanol	0.7
Distilled H$_2$O	42.5

3.2. Generation of In Vitro-Methylated DNA

As a positive control for the M reaction, it is possible to use DNA from tumor cell lines that have been shown to be hypermethylated at the gene ROI (*see* **Note 2**). In vitro-methylated DNA (IVD) provides the advantage that almost every CpG dinucleotide is methylated, which makes it a universal methylation-positive control for any given DNA sequence. IVD is generated by incubation of normal human DNA (e.g., DNA from peripheral blood cells) with *Sss*I methylase and SAM as a methyl group donor. After a final purification step, IVD is subjected to bisulfite treatment like any other DNA sample to be analyzed.

1. Dilute 50 μg of DNA with 150 μL of distilled H$_2$O (this amount can be scaled for actual needs).
2. Add 2.5 μL of 32 mM SAM, 25 μL of 10X NE-Buffer 2, 6.25 μL (25 U) of *Sss*I methylase and 66.25 μL distilled H$_2$O; mix gently by pipetting.
3. Incubate at 37°C for 4 h, and then add 5 μL of 32 mM SAM and 3 μL (12 U) of *Sss*I methylase; mix gently by pipetting.
4. Incubate at 37°C for another 4 h.
5. For DNA cleanup, it is most convenient to use G-50 spin minicolumns. Prespin the minicolumns at room temperature in a microcentrifuge at 1000g for 3 min.
6. Transfer the minicolumns to a 1.5-mL microcentrifuge tube supplied with the kit, and carefully load up to a 50-μL DNA aliquot to the center of the gel bed surface (i.e., 5 × 50 μL).
7. Centrifuge at 1000g for 3 min at room temperature. After pooling, the purified DNA can then be quantified by spectrophotometry and subjected to bisulfite treatment.

3.3. Bisulfite Treatment of Genomic DNA

1. Add 1 μg of DNA to 50 μL of distilled H$_2$O (*see* **Note 1**).
2. Add 5.5 μL of 2 M NaOH and incubate at 37°C for 10 min in order to denature the DNA.

3. Prepare a fresh solution of 10 mM hydroquinone by adding 55 mg of hydroquinone to 50 mL of distilled H$_2$O, and invert gently until fully dissolved.
4. Prepare a fresh solution of 3 M sodium bisulfite by adding 1.88 g of sodium bisulfite to 5 mL of distilled H$_2$O, invert gently until fully dissolved, and adjust the pH to 5.0 with concentrated NaOH (5 mL of 3 M sodium bisulfite solution is sufficient for nine DNA samples).
5. Add 30 μL of 10 mM hydroquinone and 520 μL of 3 M sodium bisulfite solution to each DNA sample and mix well by pipetting.
6. Layer with mineral oil (10 drops) and incubate at 50°C for 16 h in the dark (*see* **Note 3**).
7. After removing the oil, add 1 mL of DNA Promega wizard cleanup solution to each sample, and transfer the mixture to the miniprep column provided in the kit; it is convenient to use a vacuum manifold for up to 20 samples.
8. Wash with 2 mL of 80% isopropanol.
9. Place the miniprep column in a microcentrifuge tube.
10. Add 50 μL of heated distilled H$_2$O (50°C) to the column.
11. Spin the tube with the column in a microcentrifuge for 1 min at maximum speed.
12. Remove the column, add 5.5 μL of 3 M NaOH, and incubate at room temperature for 5 min; then proceed to ethanol precipitation.
13. Add 1 μL of glycogen (serves as a carrier), 17 μL of 10 M ammonium acetate, and 150 μL of ice-cold 100% ethanol.
14. Precipitate for 3 h at –20°C or for 1 h at –70°C.
15. Spin at maximum speed in a cooling centrifuge for 25–30 min.
16. Pour off the ethanol and add 500 μL of ice-cold 70% ethanol.
17. Spin at maximum speed in a cooling centrifuge for 15 min.
18. Pour off the ethanol and dry the pellet using a vacuum drier; alternatively, pellets can also be air-dried.
19. Carefully resuspend the pellet with 21 μL of distilled H$_2$O and make two aliquots.
20. Store bisulfite-treated samples in a –20°C freezer. If stored properly, bisulfite-treated samples can be used for more than 12 mo (*see* **Note 4**).

3.4. Methylation-Specific Polymerase Chain Reaction

All MSP reactions (U and M reactions) may be performed in a total reaction volume of 25 μL. The standard 1X PCR buffer for MSP contains 16.6 mM ammonium sulfate; 67 mM Tris, pH 8.8; 6.7 mM MgCl$_2$; and 10 mM β-mercaptoethanol (*see* **Subheading 2.1., item 7** and **Note 5**). To prepare a 100-mL stock solution of 10X PCR buffer (i.e., 166 mM ammonium sulfate; 670 mM Tris, pH 8.8; 67 mM MgCl$_2$; 100 mM β-mercaptoethanol), the ingredients listed in **Table 1** are mixed. Aliquots of this 10X buffer should be stored in a –20°C freezer.

Table 2 gives an overview of the components of the MSP master mixes (*see* **Note 5**). Since there are two U primers and two M primers per gene there are always two separate master mixes that differ in the primer pairs used. **Table 3**

Table 2
MSP Master Mixes

Reagent	Volume per sample (µL)	Volume per 10 samples (µL)
10 X PCR buffer	2.5	25
dNTP mix	1.25	12.5
Sense primer (U or M)	0.5	5
Antisense primer (U or M)	0.5	5
Distilled H$_2$O	14.25	142.5

Table 3
MSP Primers for p16^{INK4a}

Primer	Primer sequence (5′ → 3′)	Amplicon length (bp)
U sense	TTATTAGAGGGTGGGGTGGATTGT	151
U antisense	CAACCCCAAACCACAACCATAA	
M sense	TTATTAGAGGGTGGGGCGGATCGC	150
M antisense	GACCCCGAACCGCGACCGTAA	

provides examples of MSP primer sequences for the p16^{INK4a} tumor suppressor gene *(29)*.

For every MSP reaction, 1 µL (~50 ng) of bisulfite-converted DNA is added to 19 µL of the corresponding master mix (U or M). Reactions are hot-started at 95°C for 5 min and held at 80°C before the addition of 5 µL of diluted *Taq* polymerase (0.625 µL of RedTaq + 4.375 µL of distilled H$_2$O per reaction). Standard temperature conditions for PCR are as follows: 35 cycles of 95°C for 30 s, 60°C for 30 s, and 72°C for 30 s, followed by 1 cycle of 72°C for 5 min. The annealing temperature may vary depending on the choice of MSP primers but is usually in the range of 58–60°C. MSP products (10 µL) are then loaded onto either nondenaturing 6% polyacrylamide or 2.5% agarose gels, stained with ethidium bromide, and finally visualized under ultraviolet (UV) illumination. It is very important to include the appropriate controls for every MSP reaction (*see* **Note 2**).

3.5. Interpretation of Results

Figure 4 shows a representative MSP gel for analysis of the O^{6}MGMT gene in human tumor cell lines. As described previously, there are two PCR reactions per sample (one for the unmethylated and one for the methylated

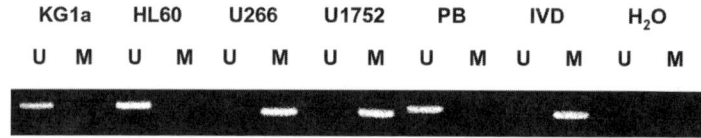

Fig. 4. Representative MSP analysis of methylation status of O⁶MGMT gene in human tumor cell lines. Normal peripheral blood cells (PB), IVD, and distilled H_2O served as controls. Lane U, amplified product with primers recognizing unmethylated O⁶MGMT sequence; lane M, amplified product with primers recognizing methylated O⁶MGMT sequence. MSP products were separated on a 2.5% agarose gel containing ethidium bromide and visualized under UV illumination.

sequence). A fully unmethylated sample will result in a positive signal only in the U reaction, whereas a fully methylated sample will yield only a positive signal in the M reaction. However, it is possible that there are positive signals in both reactions for one DNA sample. This may be owing to the heterogeneity of cells in the samples, because there are often "contaminating" nonmalignant cells in a tumor specimen. On the other hand, even in a pure cell population there may be heterogeneous methylation patterns ("partial methylation") in a given CpG island, which may also result in a mixed MSP result.

4. Notes

1. The quality and quantity of the genomic DNA used for bisulfite treatment are essential for the efficiency of the subsequent PCR amplification. During the process of bisulfite conversion, genomic DNA is separated into single strands and is subject to significant degradation. The type of DNA source is critical for the DNA quality. Fresh frozen tissue, mononuclear cells from bone marrow and peripheral blood, as well as cell lines yield a better DNA quality than paraffin-embedded tissue. The input amount of DNA for bisulfite treatment should be close to 1 μg. Using more DNA carries the risk of incomplete bisulfite conversion, and lesser DNA amounts might result in decreased PCR efficiency.

2. It is essential for every MSP reaction to include three controls: one for the unmethylated sequence, one for the methylated sequence, and one as a negative (i.e., H_2O) control. Normal cells (e.g., peripheral blood mononuclear cells) should give a positive signal only in the U reaction. As a positive control for the M reaction, it is possible to use IVD, which is methylated at almost every CpG dinucleotide, or tumor cell lines that have been shown to be hypermethylated at the gene ROI. It is important to note that in the U control there should be a positive signal only in the U reaction and not in the M reaction (this would indicate a lack of specificity in the M reaction), whereas the M control may also give a positive signal in the U reaction besides a strong positive signal in the M reaction (owing to possible incomplete methylation of IVD or heterogeneous methylation patterns

in cell lines). Whenever there is a positive M signal in the U control, the results of the MSP reaction cannot be interpreted.

3. Bisulfite and hydroquinone solutions are light sensitive and thus should be protected from light, especially during the 16-h incubation period. Hydroquinone serves to prevent the oxidation of sodium bisulfite.

4. Bisulfite-converted DNA is very sensitive to degradation unless stored at –20°C. Repeated thawing and freezing should be avoided, because this will increase the degradation process and result in the inability to amplify template. Therefore, bisulfite-treated DNA samples should be aliquoted and not subjected to thawing and freezing more than five times.

5. As with any PCR reaction, initial optimization of the ingredients of the master mix and thermocycling conditions is important. We have found that most genes can be optimally amplified using the described PCR buffer with 1.25 mM of each dNTP, 400 nM of each primer, and 0.625 U of *Taq* polymerase per reaction using a "hot-start" thermocycling program. The annealing temperature may vary depending on the choice of MSP primers but is usually in the range of 58–60°C. This can most easily be optimized through the use of a gradient block thermocycler. The cycle number should not exceed 35 cycles, owing to the risk of unspecific products and the potential for mispriming/false annealing.

Acknowledgments

This work was supported by National Institute of Health grant CA-84986. Conflict of interest statement: "JGH is a paid consultant to OncoMethylome Sciences. The terms of this arrangement are being managed by the Johns Hopkins University in accordance with its conflict of interest policies."

References

1. Hallek, M., Bergsagel, P. L., and Anderson, K. C. (1998) Multiple myeloma: increasing evidence for a multistep transformation process. *Blood* **91,** 3–21.

2. Kuehl, W. M. and Bergsagel, P. L. (2002) Multiple myeloma: evolving genetic events and host interactions. *Nat. Rev. Cancer* **2,** 175–187.

3. Seidl, S., Kaufmann, H., and Drach, J. (2003) New insights into the pathophysiology of multiple myeloma. *Lancet Oncol.* **4,** 557–564.

4. Baylin, S. B. and Herman, J. G. (2000) DNA hypermethylation in tumorigenesis: epigenetics joins genetics. *Trends Genet.* **16,** 168–174.

5. Jones, P. A. and Baylin, S. B. (2002) The fundamental role of epigenetic events in cancer. *Nat. Rev. Genet.* **3,** 415–428.

6. Constancia, M., Pickard, B., Kelsey, G., and Reik, W. (1998) Imprinting mechanisms. *Genome Res.* **8,** 881–900.

7. Robertson, K. D. and Jones, P. A. (2000) DNA methylation: past, present and future directions. *Carcinogenesis* **21,** 461–467.

8. Jaenisch, R. and Bird, A. (2003) Epigenetic regulation of gene expression: how the genome integrates intrinsic and environmental signals. *Nat. Genet.* **33(Suppl.),** 245–254.

9. Esteller, M., Corn, P. G., Baylin, S. B., and Herman, J. G. (2001) A gene hyper-methylation profile of human cancer. *Cancer Res.* **61,** 3225–3229.

10. Nguyen, T. T., Mohrbacher, A. F., Tsai, Y. C., et al. (2000) Quantitative measure of c-abl and p15 methylation in chronic myelogenous leukemia: biological implications. **Blood** *95,* 2990–2992.

11. Wong, I. H., Ng, M. H., Huang, D. P., and Lee, J. C. (2000) Aberrant p15 promoter methylation in adult and childhood acute leukemias of nearly all morphologic subtypes: potential prognostic implications. *Blood* **95,** 1942–1949.

12. Chim, C. S., Liang, R., Tam, C. Y., and Kwong, Y. L. (2001) Methylation of p15 and p16 genes in acute promyelocytic leukemia: potential diagnostic and prognostic significance. *J. Clin. Oncol.* **19,** 2033–2040.

13. Laird, P. W. (2003) Early detection: the power and the promise of DNA methylation markers. *Nat. Rev. Cancer* **3,** 253–266.

14. Willemze, R., Suciu, S., Archimbaud, E., et al. (1997) A randomized phase II study on the effects of 5-Aza-2'-deoxycytidine combined with either amsacrine or idarubicin in patients with relapsed acute leukemia: an EORTC Leukemia Cooperative Group phase II study (06893). *Leukemia* **11(Suppl. 1),** S24–S27.

15. Wijermans, P., Lubbert, M., Verhoef, G., Bosly, A., Ravoet, C., Andre, M., and Ferrant, A. (2000) Low-dose 5-aza-2'-deoxycytidine, a DNA hypomethylating agent, for the treatment of high-risk myelodysplastic syndrome: a multicenter phase II study in elderly patients. *J. Clin. Oncol.* **18,** 956–962.

16. Silverman, L. R., Demakos, E. P., Peterson, B. L., et al. (2002) Randomized controlled trial of azacitidine in patients with the myelodysplastic syndrome: a study of the cancer and leukemia group B. *J. Clin. Oncol.* **20,** 2429–2440.

17. Kantarjian, H. M., O'Brien, S., Cortes, J., et al. (2003) Results of decitabine (5-aza-2'deoxycytidine) therapy in 130 patients with chronic myelogenous leukemia. *Cancer* **98,** 522–528.

18. Ng, M. H., Chung, Y. F., Lo, K. W., Wickham, N. W., Lee, J. C., and Huang, D. P. (1997) Frequent hypermethylation of p16 and p15 genes in multiple myeloma. *Blood* **89,** 2500–2506.

19. Gonzalez, M., Mateos, M. V., Garcia-Sanz, R., et al. (2000) De novo methylation of tumor suppressor gene p16/INK4a is a frequent finding in multiple myeloma patients at diagnosis. *Leukemia* **14,** 183–187.

20. Ng, M. H., To, K. W., Lo, K. W., et al. (2001) Frequent death-associated protein kinase promoter hypermethylation in multiple myeloma. *Clin. Cancer Res.* **7,** 1724–1729.

21. Galm, O., Yoshikawa, H., Esteller, M., Osieka, R., and Herman, J. G. (2003) SOCS-1, a negative regulator of cytokine signaling, is frequently silenced by methylation in multiple myeloma. *Blood* **101,** 2784–2788.

22. Feinberg, A. P. and Vogelstein, B. (1983) Hypomethylation distinguishes genes of some human cancers from their normal counterparts. *Nature* **301,** 89–92.

23. Frommer, M., McDonald, L. E., Millar, D. S., et al. (1992) A genomic sequencing protocol that yields a positive display of 5-methylcytosine residues in individual DNA strands. *Proc. Natl. Acad. Sci. USA* **89,** 1827–1831.

24. Clark, S. J., Harrison, J., Paul, C. L., and Frommer, M. (1994) High sensitivity mapping of methylated cytosines. *Nucleic Acids Res.* **22,** 2990–2997.
25. Sadri, R. and Hornsby, P. J. (1996) Rapid analysis of DNA methylation using new restriction enzyme sites created by bisulfite modification. *Nucleic Acids Res.* **24,** 5058–5059.
26. Xiong, Z. and Laird, P. W. (1997) COBRA: a sensitive and quantitative DNA methylation assay. *Nucleic Acids Res.* **25,** 2532–2534.
27. Gonzalgo, M. L. and Jones, P. A. (1997) Rapid quantitation of methylation differences at specific sites using methylation-sensitive single nucleotide primer extension (Ms-SNuPE). *Nucleic Acids Res.* **25,** 2529–2531.
28. Galm, O., Rountree, M. R., Bachman, K. E., Jair, K. W., Baylin, S. B., and Herman, J. G. (2002) Enzymatic regional methylation assay: a novel method to quantify regional CpG methylation density. *Genome Res.* **12,** 153–157.
29. Herman, J. G., Graff, J. R., Myohanen, S., Nelkin, B. D., and Baylin, S. B. (1996) Methylation-specific PCR: a novel PCR assay for methylation status of CpG islands. *Proc. Natl. Acad. Sci. USA* **93,** 9821–9826.
30. Bachman, K. E., Herman, J. G., Corn, P. G., et al. (1999) Methylation-associated silencing of the tissue inhibitor of metalloproteinase-3 gene suggest a suppressor role in kidney, brain, and other human cancers. *Cancer Res.* **59,** 798–802.
31. Corn, P. G., Smith, B. D., Ruckdeschel, E. S., Douglas, D., Baylin, S. B., and Herman, J. G. (2000) E-cadherin expression is silenced by 5′ CpG island methylation in acute leukemia. *Clin. Cancer Res.* **6,** 4243–4248.
32. Esteller, M., Garcia-Foncillas, J., Andion, E., et al. (2000) Inactivation of the DNA-repair gene MGMT and the clinical response of gliomas to alkylating agents. *N. Engl. J. Med.* **343,** 1350–1354.

23

Making Sense of DNA Microarray Data

Wei-min Liu, Sunhee K. Ro, and Walter H. Koch

1. Introduction

The fast advance of genomic science and nucleic acid detection technology provides medical researchers new tools for detecting genetic and expressional variations of individuals and their relations to pathology, etiology, and diagnostics. DNA microarrays, also called DNA chips, contain many different single-stranded DNA segments immobilized on specified locations of glass or other solid surfaces (*1,2*). In a DNA microarray experiment, the free DNA or RNA segments in solution hybridize with the immobilized DNA segments with known sequences at known locations owing to base pairing. The immobilized DNA segments are called the probes, and the nucleic acids whose identity or abundance are to be detected are called the targets. Because targets are usually labeled with fluorescent tags, the hybridized targets can be readily detected with laser scanners or charge-coupled device cameras. The locations and intensities of the fluorescent signals on a microarray reveal the sequence and/or abundance of specific targets.

DNA microarray technology makes it possible to analyze many thousands of genes or markers in a single experiment. Therefore, DNA microarrays are high-throughput devices for parallel analysis of DNA or RNA samples and can significantly save time and materials. The results obtained from DNA microarrays are highly concordant with traditional analytical methods such as Northern blots (*3–5*), DNA sequencing-based technology, serial analysis of gene expression (*6*), and reverse transcriptase polymerase chain reaction (*7*).

There are two different types of DNA microarrays: oligonucleotide microarrays and cDNA microarrays. The probes of an oligonucleotide microarray are usually 18–70 bases long. They may be synthesized directly on the microarray

From: *Methods in Molecular Medicine, Vol. 113: Multiple Myeloma: Methods and Protocols*
Edited by: R. D. Brown and P. J. Ho © Humana Press Inc., Totowa, NJ

surface or presynthesized and immobilized by various methods. The probes of a cDNA microarray are usually several hundred or even several thousand bases long. cDNA microarrays are usually spotted with robotic tools and, therefore, are often called spotted DNA microarrays.

A connected area on a DNA microarray where probe molecules of the same sequence are immobilized is called a feature. On cDNA microarrays, a feature is a spot, usually with a diameter of 50–350 μm and with additional space between adjacent spots. On photosynthesized oligonucleotide microarrays, a feature is usually a rectangular cell with side length of 8–50 μm, directly adjacent to its neighboring cells. Hence, in situ synthesized oligonucleotide microarrays provide a higher density of probes than cDNA microarrays. Because oligonucleotide microarrays use shorter probes, they are less likely to form secondary and tertiary structures and can provide better specificity for detection of target sequences. Therefore, oligonucleotide microarrays can not only be used to discover gene expression profiles, but also to detect point mutations including single nucleotide polymorphisms (SNPs), as well as deletions and insertions. DNA microarrays have been used to detect genetic variations important for disease or for response to therapeutics, and to monitor viral drug resistance mutations arising during treatment.

The manufacturing cost of cDNA microarrays with a small number of features can be lower than that of oligonucleotide microarrays. However, the processes of making, purifying, cataloging, and tracking thousands of probes for cDNA microarrays are more complicated.

Fodor et al. (2) applied photolithography, a technique originally used to make computer chips, to make oligonucleotide microarrays. The method uses ultraviolet light passing through masks to control the exposure of a protective layer and, hence, the locations of multiple steps of synthesis of oligonucleotides on a glass wafer. It remains the leading technique for producing oligonucleotide microarrays on a large scale. Currently, Affymetrix uses photolithography to routinely produce oligonucleotide microarrays with 11-μm feature size and probes of up to 25 bases in length. Warrington et al. (8) described the designs and applications of Affymetrix oligonucleotide microarrays before the year 2000.

Singh-Gasson et al. (9) propose the use of a digital micromirror array instead of the expensive photolithographic masks to direct light for synthesis of oligonucleotides on a microarray. Digital micromirrors were originally used in computer display projection systems. NimbleGen uses this technology to make oligonucleotide microarrays with approx 200,000 twenty-four-base probe features. This method can develop and manufacture custom DNA microarrays quickly.

Ink-jet printing is another technology commonly employed for manufacturing microarrays (10–12). The microarrays made by Agilent using ink-jet printing contain 60-base oligonucleotide probes. The feature size is approx 80 μm in diameter, and the distance between features is usually 145–150 μm. Therefore, the feature density is lower than microarrays made with photochemical synthesis, and significantly larger surface areas are required to represent the entire human genome for gene expression analyses.

In the following sections, we discuss the applications of oligonucleotide DNA microarrays in medical research and their potential use in the diagnosis of multiple myeloma (MM).

2. Gene Expression Profiling

2.1. Gene Expression Levels and Calls

An important application of DNA microarrays is to find similarities and differences of gene expression profiles between two or more groups such as cancer tissues vs normal tissues, or treated vs untreated individuals.

To interrogate the expression level of a gene, the Affymetrix oligonucleotide microarray uses a probe set consisting of multiple probe pairs to detect particular segments of a gene. A probe pair includes a perfect match probe feature and a single-base mismatched probe feature. The perfect match cell contains probes of sequence complementary to the target, whereas the Affymetrix mismatch cell contains probes different from the perfect match sequence only at the middle nucleotide, which is usually the same as the corresponding target nucleotide. Affymetrix adopted this probe design strategy because a major challenge to microarray technology is cross-hybridization; that is, probes hybridize not only with targets of exactly matching sequences, but also with nucleotide segments of similar sequences under nonstringent conditions. Although careful selection of probe sequences can significantly reduce the signal noise from cross-hybridization and unwanted secondary structures of probes *(13)*, comparison of perfect match/mismatch probe pairs allows certain cross-hybridization noise to be subtracted.

The Affymetrix software package Microarray Suite 5 (MAS5) uses a robust positive estimate of the differences between perfect match intensities and mismatch intensities as the signal detected by a probe set in an expression microarray. There are also other summaries such as the detection call (whether a gene is present or absent), the comparative call (whether the expression levels of a gene in two different microarray experiments change), and the logarithmic ratio of expression levels (a metric related to the fold change of a gene in two experiments). The signals and log ratios are based on the one-step Tukey's biweight estimation *(14)*, and the detection calls and comparative calls are based on the signed rank test *(15,16)*.

There are other methods to estimate the signals. Li and Wong *(17,18)* proposed a multiplicative statistical model for multiple expression microarrays.

Their approach is to find the common profile of probe effects of a gene on multiple arrays and calculate a model-based expression index, which is essentially a scaled projection of the expression profile at the probe level onto the common profile. The Li-Wong model provides both the expression indices and probe effects. However, it requires multiple experiments, and the expression indices are dependent on which experiments are used to estimate the probe effects. If one uses one more or less experiment, the expression indices values may change. Although the changes may be small, they may make the verification and validation process more difficult.

For multiple array comparisons, Irizarry et al. *(19,20)*, Bolstad et al. *(21)*, and Wu et al. *(22)* proposed the robust multiarray analysis (RMA), also known as the robust multichip average *(21)*. In RMA, only the intensities of perfect match cells are used to estimate the expression levels because subtraction of the mismatch intensities from the perfect match intensities may result in larger variances in data. Bolstad et al. *(21)* compared various normalization methods and recommended the percentile normalization method. Irizarry and coworkers developed the open source software package Bioconductor for RMA in the programming language R (http://www.bioconductor.org). Irizarry et al. *(19)* claimed that RMA outperforms the logarithmic ratio of MAS5 using the receiver operating characteristic curves of spiked-in targets with known concentrations. It is worth noting that they also showed that the comparative calls of MAS5 based on the *p* values of signed rank tests outperform RMA for an Affymetrix Hg_U95A data set publicly available on the Affymetrix Web site and perform similarly to RMA for a GeneLogic data set, whose concentration range is narrower than the Affymetrix data set, according to the descriptions of these two data sets.

2.2. Multiple Hypothesis Tests of Expression Data

A basic problem that researchers wish to solve with gene expression microarray analyses is finding the genes that are expressed significantly differently in two or more different groups of experiments. One approach to solve this problem is to use *t*-tests for two groups and analysis of variance for multiple groups, or nonparametric tests such as the Mann-Whitney tests and Kruskal-Wallis tests. For example, Jin et al. *(7)* use the Mann-Whitney tests to study the effects of early angiotensin-converting enzyme inhibition on cardiac gene expression after acute myocardial infarction.

For expression microarray data, the number of genes is usually much larger than the number of experiments. This causes difficulty when using the classic type I error rate (false positive rate). For example, multiple hypothesis tests for 20,000 genes with a significance level of 0.05 may yield 1000 false positive genes from random data. The statistical theory and computational methods developed by Westfall and Young *(23)* can be used to solve this problem. They refine the concepts of weak, exact, and strong controls of familywise errors to address the different combinations of null hypothesis and apply the resampling technique to adjust *p* values to take care of the dependency of hypothesis. The false discovery rate proposed by Benjamini and Hochberg *(24)* and the positive false discovery rate developed by Storey *(25)* are also useful. Dudoit et al. *(26)* compared these methods with the significance analysis of microarrays (SAM) proposed by Tusher et al. *(27)*, as well as the neighborhood analysis method proposed by Golub et al. *(28)*. They claimed that these multiple testing methods are statistically better than SAM and neighborhood analysis methods. Ge et al. *(29)* summarize the applications of the results of multiple-hypothesis testing to expression microarray data and propose a fast computational algorithm.

2.3. Clustering and Classification

Classification is the procedure that optimally allocates observations into classes. Clustering is the technique that groups observations based on the similarities or distances between observations. In a classification problem, the number of classes is fixed, whereas in a clustering problem, the number of groups is usually not fixed. Classification is often a supervised learning procedure and requires training data with known class labels, whereas clustering is usually an unsupervised learning procedure. Because classification and clustering methods can put similarly expressed genes in a group and put differentially expressed genes in different groups, they are frequently used in gene-profiling studies.

Because the number of genes is usually much more than the number of experiments for expression microarray data, to obtain reliable results for classification and regression problems, the number of independent variables (genes, or their expression levels) needs to be reduced. There are essentially three different approaches for this purpose: (1) grouping the similarly expressed genes together, (2) using a small number of linear combinations of many genes, and (3) reducing the number of genes for analysis. All clustering techniques such as the hierarchical clustering algorithms and k-means or k-medoids algorithms can group similarly expressed genes. The principal component analysis (PCA) and partial least squares methods use linear combinations of expression levels of different genes. Alter et al. *(30)* suggested the singular value decomposition *(31)* format of PCA for analysis of expression microarray data. They also coined the terms *eigengenes* for linear combinations of expression levels of genes in every experiment and *eigenexperiments* for the linear combinations of expression levels of every gene in various experiments. Most works in gene expression profile analysis use certain rules to eliminate the genes that have low expression levels or do not vary significantly. Guyon et al. *(32)* proposed the recursive feature elimination based on the support vector machine (SVM) for the cancer classification problem. They present the method in the binary classification format, but it can also be generalized to multicategory classification problems.

Tamayo et al. *(33)* used the self-organization map (SOM) to cluster genes in their study of hematopoietic differentiation. They also compared their method with the hierarchical clustering methods. The SOM *(34,35)* is a robust and scalable clustering method that maps a small number of nodes in a low dimensional space to the high dimensional space of observations. The nodes should have a simple topology and distance measure, such as $(p \times q)$ rectangular grid points on the two-dimensional plane. The number of nodes, pq, should be smaller than the number of observations. The algorithm iteratively adjusts the map function so that observations in the original data space can be represented by these nodes and the original neighbor relations can be preserved as much as possible.

2.4. Gene Expression-Based Classification of Hematopoietic Cancers

Golub et al. *(28)* used the gene expression pattern obtained using Affymetrix Hu6800 microarrays for the classification of acute myeloid leukemia (AML) and acute lymphoblastic leukemia (ALL). Such classification can be used to guide therapy choice. They named their classification method the "neighborhood analysis." The method is based on their correlation measures between the class label vector and the expression profile, in this case of bone marrow mononuclear cells from 11 patients with AML and 27 patients with ALL. For a particular gene, their correlation measure is motivated by the signal-to-noise ratio and is similar to the t-statistic. It is defined as

$$P(g, c) = (m1(g) - m2(g)) / (s1(g) + s2(g)),$$

in which g denotes a particular gene or its expression vector; c is the class label vector; $m1(g)$ and $m2(g)$ are, respectively, the sample means of expression levels of gene g in class 1 and class 2 (AML and ALL); and $s1(g)$ and $s2(g)$ are the corresponding standard deviations. They call the genes with large absolute values of $P(g, c)$ the informative genes. Their discriminant is the sum of $P(g, c)(x_g - b_g)$ over all informative genes. Here x_g is the expression level of gene g in the to-be-classified sample: $b_g = (m1(g) + m2(g))/2$ is the average of the two sample means. A positive sum indicates class 1 and a negative sum indicates class 2.

Armstrong et al. *(36)* used the Affymetrix Hg_U95A and Hg_U95Av2 expression microarrays to show that mixed-lineage leukemia (MLL) translocations form a type of leukemia different from ALL and AML (it had previously been included together with other ALLs in the literature). They first used the unsupervised PCA with 8700 genes to show that 20 ALL, 17 MLL, and 20 AML samples are well separated. Further analysis with 500 genes that best distinguish ALL and AML still confirmed that MLL forms a separate cluster in the space of the first three principal components.

Yeoh et al. *(37)* used the Affymetrix Hg_U95Av2 microarrays to classify six known ALL subtypes and a newly found subtype using bone marrow samples from 327 pediatric patients. The six known subtypes are T-cell lineage ALL (T-ALL), E2A-PBX1 (t[1;19]), BCR-ABL (t[9;22]), TEL-AML1 (t[12;21]), MLL rearrangement on chromosome 11 band q23, and hyperdiploid with over 50 chromosomes. These investigators applied various gene selection and classification methods. Their gene selection methods include the χ^2, *t*-statistic, Wilkins metric (a weighted average of three measures about the discriminant ability of a gene between two classes), correlation-based feature selection, SOM, and discriminant analysis with variance. The clustering and classification methods that they employ include the two-dimensional hierarchical clustering, k-nearest neighbor, SVM, artificial neural network, prediction by collective likelihood of emerging patterns, and weighted votes. Here the different methods all lead to similar results.

Similarly, Kohlmann et al. *(38)* used the Affymetrix Hg_U133A microarrays to classify adult leukemia samples with SVM based on the genes suggested in **refs. 36** and *37*) from the pediatric samples.

2.5. Prognosis of Time to Recurrence of Cancer

Microarray expression data are also being used to help predict the time to recurrence of cancer after treatment. In their studies of breast cancer samples, West et al. *(39)*, Nevins et al. *(40)*, and Huang et al. *(41,42)* used the k-means clustering method to group similarly expressed genes. They represent a group of such genes with the first principal component and call it a metagene. They then use metagenes and clinical metrics, such as the number of involved lymphnodes and the multiple decision trees based on the Bayesian factors *(43)*, to predict the time to recurrence of breast cancer after the surgery. If validated in broader populations, such analysis can help guide clinical decisions about cancer patient treatment.

Nguyen and Rocke *(44)* proposed to apply the partial least squares and proportional hazard regression to solve the problem of time to recurrence of cancer with microarray data. In fact, the partial least squares method can also be used to solve the classification problem *(45,46)*. The critical point of this method is to find linear combinations of expression levels that maximize their squared covariance with recurrent time or class labels subject to certain constraints for orthogonality.

3. Applications to MM

MM is a malignancy of a terminally differentiated antibody secreting plasma cells (PCs). Its clinical outcome can vary tremendously, with survival ranging from 2 mo to more than 10 yr. Microarray analysis can help in the diagnosis, prognosis, and development of new treatments for this morphologically homogeneous but clinically heterogeneous disease *(47)*.

Shaughnessy and Barlogie provided a detailed review of the applications of gene expression profiling to research on MM *(48)*. They applied the gene expression profiles to MM classification and survival analysis. These analyses revealed that the coexpressed and upregulated cell-cycle genes are linked to abnormal cytogenetics. A linear discrimination model was used to predict the deletion status of chromosome 13 of MM. The genes related to MM-associated translocations t(11;14)(q13;q32), t(4;14)(p16;q32), and t(6;14)(p21;q32) were also identified.

Chauhan et al. *(49)* found that 2-methoxyestradiol (2ME2), an estrogen derivative, induces apoptosis in MM cells in vitro and in vivo. Because 2ME2 also induces apoptosis in MM cells resistant to conventional therapies such as dexamethasone, 2ME2 may be used to improve the treatment of MM.

Davies et al. *(50)* applied microarrays to study the pathways involved in the multistep transformation process of normal PCs to monoclonal gammopathy of uncertain significance and MM. They identified several differentially expressed genes including oncogenes, tumor suppressor genes, cell-signaling genes, DNA-binding and transcription factor genes, as well as genes involved in developmental regulation.

Tian et al. *(51)* studied a microarray data set of 45 control subjects, 36 patients with MM whose focal lesions of bone could not be detected by magnetic resonance imaging (MRI), and 137 patients with MRI-detected lesions. They found 57 genes showing significant different expression patterns, and 4 of these 57 genes were overexpressed in PCs of patients with focal lesions. One of the genes identified was *dickkopf 1*, whose DKK1 protein product is an inhibitor of osteoblast differentiation and is associated with the lytic bone lesions in patients with MM.

4. Discussion

Currently, most research applications of DNA microarrays focus on gene expression profiling of mRNA. DNA microarrays can also detect inherited or somatically acquired variations in DNA. SNPs may either directly change gene expressions or relate to more complicated disease-associated genetic variations. Lindblad-Toh et al. *(52)* applied an early genotyping array, HuSNP, with approx 1000 SNPs to study the relation between loss of heterozygosity and lung carcinoma. Recently, Affymetrix produced the Mapping 10k array for genotyping of >10,000 SNPs *(53,54)*. The details of the algorithms of the genotyping microarrays for whole-genome analysis have been presented *(55)*. It will be interesting to see whether this type of high-throughput genotyping microarray for whole-genome analysis can help discover genetic markers of MM or other cancer and markers associated with the efficacy of various treatments.

Acknowledgment

We thank P. Mickey Williams for helpful discussions.

References

1. Khrapko, K. R., Lysov, Y. P., Khorlyn, A. A., Shick, V. V., Florentiev, V. L., and Mirzabekov, A. D. (1989) An oligonucleotide hybridization approach to DNA sequencing. *FEBS Lett.* **256,** 118–122.
2. Fodor, S. P., Read, J. L., Pirrung, M. C., Stryer, L., Lu, A. T., and Solas, D. (1991) Light-directed, spatially addressable parallel chemical synthesis. *Science* **251,** 767–773.
3. Jelinski, S. A. and Samson, L. D. (1999) Global response of *Saccharomyces cerevisiae* to an alkylating agent. *Proc. Natl. Sci. USA* **96,** 1486–1491.
4. Harkin, D. P., Bean, J. M., Miklos, D., et al. (1999) Introduction of GADD45 and JNK/SAPK-dependent apoptosis following inducible expression of BRCA1. *Cell* **97,** 575–586.
5. Lee, S. B., Huang, K., Palmer, R., et al. (1999) The Wilms tumor suppressor WT1 encodes a transcriptional activator of amphiregulin. *Cell* **98,** 663–673.
6. Ishii, M., Hashimoto, S., Tsutsumi, S., Wada, Y., Matsushima, K., and Kodama, T. (2000) Direct comparison of GeneChip and SAGE on the quantitative accuracy in transcript profiling analysis. *Genomics* **68,** 136–143.
7. Jin, H., Yang, R., Awad, T. A., et al. (2001) Effects of early angiotensin-converting enzyme inhibition on cardiac gene expression after acute myocardial infarction. *Circulation* **103,** 736–742.
8. Warrington, J. A., Dee, S., and Trulson, M. (2000) Large-scale genomic analysis using Affymetrix GeneChip(R) probe arrays, in *Microarray Biochip Technology* (Schena, M. ed.), Natick, MA, pp. 119–148.
9. Singh-Gasson, S., Green, R. D., Yue, Y., et al. (1999). Maskless fabrication of light-directed oligonucleotide microarrays using a digital micromirror array. *Nat. Biotechnol.* **17,** 974–978.
10. Blanchard, A. P., Kaiser, R. J., and Hood, L. E. (1996). High-density oligonucleotide arrays. *Biosens. Bioelectron.* **6/7,** 687–690.
11. Okamoto, T., Suzuki, T., and Yamamoto, N. (2000). Microarray fabrication with covalent attachment of DNA using bubble jet technology. *Nat. Biotechnol.* **18,** 384–385.
12. Hughes, T. R., Mao, M. Jones, A. R., et al. (2001) Expression profiling using microarrays fabricated by an ink-jet oligonucleotide synthesizer. *Nat. Biotechnol.* **19,** 342–347.
13. Mei, R., Hubbell, E., Bekiranov, S., et al. (2003) Probe selection for high-density oligonucleotide arrays. *Proc. Natl. Acad. Sci. USA* **100,** 11,237–11,242.
14. Hubbell, E., Liu, W.-M., and Mei, R. (2002) Robust estimators for expression analysis. *Bioinformatics* **18,** 1585–1592.

15. Liu, W.-M., Mei, R., Bartell, D. M., Di, X., Webster, T. A., and Ryder, T. (2001) Rank-based algorithms for analysis of microarrays. *Proc. SPIE* **4266,** 56–67.
16. Liu, W.-M., Mei, R., Di, X., et al. (2002) Analysis of high-density expression microarrays with signed-rank call algorithms. *Bioinformatics* **18,** 1593–1599.
17. Li, C. and Wong, W. H. (2001) Model-based analysis of oligonucleotide arrays: expression index computation and outlier detection. *Proc. Natl. Acad. Sci. USA* **98,** 31–36.
18. Li, C. and Wong, W. H. (2001) Model-based analysis of oligonucleotide arrays: model validation, design issues and standard error applications. *Genome Biol.* **2,** 0032.1–0032.11.
19. Irizarry, R. A., Bolstad, B. M., Collin, F., Cope, L. M., Hobbs, B., and Speed, T. P. (2003). Summaries of Affymetrix GeneChip probe level data. *Nucleic Acids Res.* **31,** 1–8.
20. Irizarry, R. A., Hobbs, B., Collin, F., et al. (2003) Exploration, normalization, and summaries of high density oligonucleotide array probe level data. *Biostatistics* **4,** 249–264.
21. Bolstad, B. M., Irizarry, R. A., Astrand, M., and Speed, T. P. (2003). A comparison of normalization methods for high density oligonucleotide array data based on variance and bias. *Bioinformatics* **19,** 185–193.
22. Wu, Z., Irizarry, R. A., Gentleman, R., Martinez-Murillo, F., and Spencer, F. (2004) A model based background adjustment for oligonucleotide expression arrays. *J. Amer. Stat. Assoc.* **99,** 909–917.
23. Westfall, P. H. and Young, S. S. (1993) *Resampling-Based Multiple Testing: Examples and Methods for p-Value Adjustment*, Wiley, New York.
24. Benjamini, Y. and Hochberg, Y. (1995) Controlling the false discovery rate: a practical and powerful approach to multiple testing. *J. Roy. Stat. Soc.* **B57,** 289–300.
25. Storey, J. D. (2002) A direct approach to false discovery rates. *J. Roy. Stat. Soc.* **B64,** 479–498.
26. Dudoit, S., Shaffer, J. P., and Boldrick, J. C. (2003) Multiple hypothesis testing in microarray experiments. *Stat. Sci.* **18,** 71–103.
27. Tusher, V. G., Tibshirani, R., and Chu, G. (2001). Significance analysis of microarrays applied to the ionizing radiation response. *Proc. Natl. Acad. Sci. USA* **98,** 5116–5121.
28. Golub, T. R., Slonim, D. K., Tamayo, P., et al. (1999) Molecular classification of cancer: class discovery and class prediction by gene expression monitoring. *Science* **286,** 531–537.
29. Ge, Y., Dudoit, S., and Speed, T. P. (2003) Resampling-based multiple testing for microarray data analysis. *Sociedad Estadistica Investigacion Operativa Test* **12,** 1–77.
30. Alter, O., Brown, P. O., and Botstein, D. (2000) Singular value decomposition for genome-wide expression data processing and modeling. *Proc. Natl. Acad. Sci. USA* **97,** 10,101–10,106.
31. Golub, G. H. and van Loan, C. F. (1996) *Matrix Computations*, 3rd ed., Johns Hopkins University Press, Baltimore.

32. Guyon, I., Weston, J., Barnhill, S., and Vapnik, V. (2002). Gene selection for cancer classification using support vector machines. *Machine Learning* **46,** 389–422.

33. Tamayo, P., Slonim, D., Mesirov, J., et al. (1999) Interpreting patterns of gene expression with self-organizing maps: methods and application to hematopoietic differentiation. *Proc. Natl. Acad. Sci. USA* **96,** 2907–2912.

34. Kohonen, T. (1982) Self-organizing formation of topologically correct feature maps. *Biol. Cybern.* **43,** 59–69.

35. Kohonen, T. (1989) *Self-Organization and Associative Memory,* 3rd ed., Springer-Verlag, Berlin.

36. Armstrong, S. A., Staunton, J. E., Silverman, L. B., et al. (2002) MLL translocations specify a distinct gene expression profile that distinguishes a unique leukemia. *Nat. Genet.* **30,** 41–47.

37. Yeoh, E.-J., Ross, M. E., Shurtleff, S. A., et al. (2002) Classification, subtype discovery, and prediction of outcome in pediatric acute lymphoblastic leukemia by gene expression profiling. *Cancer Cell* **1,** 133–143.

38. Kohlmann, A., Schoch, C., Schnittger, S., et al. (2004) Pediatric acute lymphoblastic leukemia (ALL) gene expression signatures classify an independent cohort of adult ALL patients. *Leukemia* **18,** 63–71.

39. West, M., Blanchette, C., Dressman, H., et al. (2001) Predicting the clinical status of human breast cancer by using gene expression profiles. *Proc. Natl. Acad. Sci. USA* **98,** 11,462–11,467.

40. Nevins, J. R., Huang, E. S., Dressman, H., Pittman, J., Huang, A. T., and West, M. (2003). Towards integrated clinico-genomic models for personalized medicine: combining gene expression signatures and clinical factors in breast cancer outcomes prediction. *Human Mol. Genet.* **12,** R153–R157.

41. Huang, E., Chen, S. H., Dressman, H., et al. (2003) Gene expression predictions of breast cancer outcomes. *Lancet* **361,** 1590–1596.

42. Huang, E., Ishida, S., Pittman, J., et al. (2003) Gene expression phenotypic models that predict the activity of oncogenic pathways. *Nat. Genet.* **34,** 226–230.

43. Kass, R. and Raftery, A. (1995) *J. Am. Stat. Assoc.* **90,** 773–795.

44. Nguyen, D. V. and Rocke, D. M. (2002) Partial least squares proportional hazard regression for application to DNA microarray survival data. *Bioinformatics* **18,** 1625–1632.

45. Nguyen, D. V. and Rocke, D. M. (2002) Tumor classification by partial least squares using microarray gene expression data. *Bioinformatics* **18,** 39–50.

46. Nguyen, D. V. and Rocke, D. M. (2002) Multi-class cancer classification via partial least squares with gene expression profiles. *Bioinformatics* **18,** 1216–1226.

47. Claudio, J. O., Masih-Khan, E., and Stewart, A. K. (2004) Insights from the gene expression profiling of multiple myeloma. *Curr. Hematol. Rep.* **3,** 67–73.

48. Anderson, K. C., Shaughnessy, J. D., Jr., Barlogie, B., Harousseau, J.-L., and Roodman, G. D. (2002) Multiple myeloma. *Hematology—ASH Education Program Book* 214–240.

49. Chauhan, D., Li, G., Auclair, D., et al. (2003) Identification of genes regulated by 2-methoxyestradiol (2ME2) in multiple myeloma cells using oligonucleotide arrays. *Blood* **101,** 3606–3614.
50. Davies, F. E., Dring, A. M., Li, C., et al. (2003) Insights into the multistep transformation of MGUS to myeloma using microarray expression analysis. *Blood* **102,** 4504–4511.
51. Tian, E., Zhan, F., Walker, R., et al. (2003) The role of the Wnt-signaling antagonist DKK1 in the development of osteolytic lesions in multiple myeloma. *N. Engl. J. Med.* **349,** 2483–2494.
52. Lindblad-Toh, K., Tanenbaum, D. M., Daly, M., et al. (2000) Loss of heterozygosity analysis of small-cell lung carcinomas using single nucleotide polymorphism arrays. *Nat. Biotechnol.* **18,** 1001–1005.
53. Kennedy, G. C., Matsuzaki, H., Dong, S., et al. (2003) Large scale genotyping of complex DNA. *Nat. Biotechnol.* **21,** 1233–1237.
54. Matsuzaki, H., Loi, H., Dong, S., et al. (2004) Parallel genotyping of over 10,000 SNPs using a one primer assay on a high density oligonucleotide array. *Gen. Res.* **14,** 414–425.
55. Liu, W.-M., Di, X., Yang, G., et al. (2003) Algorithms for large scale genotyping microarrays. *Bioinformatics* **19,** 2397–2403.

Index